YogaExplained

This book is
dedicated to
all learners.

Without students,
where would
teachers be?

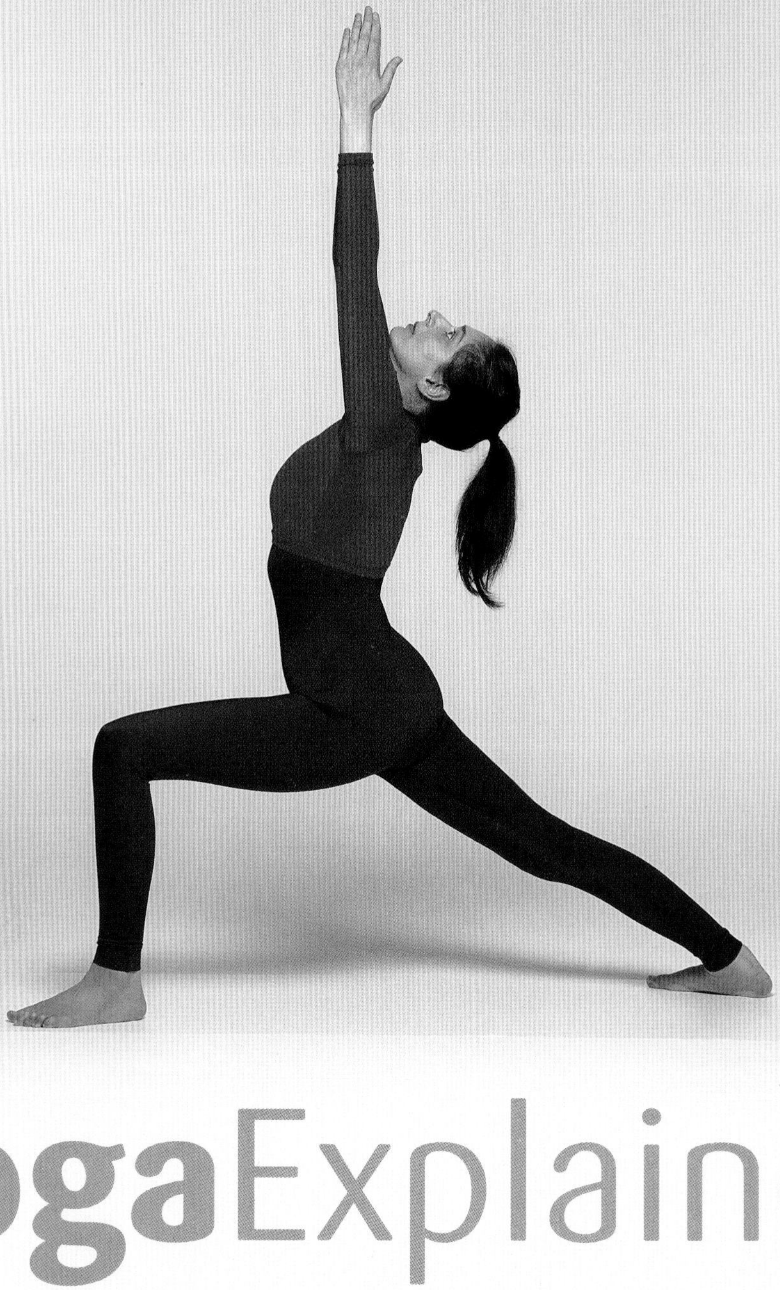

YogaExplained

A NEW STEP-BY-STEP APPROACH TO UNDERSTANDING AND PRACTICING YOGA

MIRA MEHTA

with Krishna S. Arjunwadkar

kyle books

This edition published in 2005 by Kyle Books
An imprint of Kyle Cathie Limited
general.enquiries@kyle-cathie.com
www.kylecathie.com

Distributed by National Book Network
4501 Forbes Blvd., Suite 200
Lanham, MD 20706
Phone: (301) 459 3366 Fax: (301) 429 5746

ISBN 1 90492 017 9

Inside cover and pages 7, 17, 28, 33, 48, 51, 66, 71, 82, 85, 98, 101, 112, 117, 129, 133, 146, 149, 164, 169, 182, 187, 203, 207 and 218: The Bhandarkar Oriental Research Institute, Pune, India.
Page 9: The Ashmolean Museum, Oxford, U.K.

Project editor: Sarah Epton
Copy editor: Ruth Baldwin
Editorial assistant: Vicki Murrell
Americanizer: Delora Jones
Designer: Heidi Baker
Production by Sha Huxtable and Alice Holloway

The Library of Congress Cataloguing-in-Publication Data is available on file.
Color separations by Scanhouse, Malaysia
Printed and bound by C & C Offset

Other books by Mira Mehta:
Yoga: The Iyengar Way (with Silva and Shyam Mehta)
Health Through Yoga
Cascade of Stars

Acknowledgments

The authors wish to thank the following:
Prashant S. Iyengar for his encouragement;
Shyam Mehta for checking the posture programs;
Paul Heyda for discussing problems and solutions;
John Harrison, Paul Heyda, Shyam Mehta, and Damian and Maggie Treanor for suggesting amendments to the text;
Sallie Sullivan for supervising the photo-shoots;
Michael Alcock for finding a publisher;
Kyle Cathie, the publisher;
Sarah Epton, the project editor;
Ruth Baldwin, the copy editor;
Heidi Baker, the designer;
Guy Hearn, the photographer;
Gandolfi, the costume maker;
Fiona Leech for hair and makeup;
Yoga Matters for the loan of props;
Deep Space for the use of their studio;
the Bhandarkar Oriental Research Institute, Pune, India, for permission to reproduce photographs of manuscripts in their collection;
S. L. Khot for photographing the manuscripts;
the Ashmolean Museum, Oxford, for permission to reproduce the photograph of the statuette of **Patañjali** on anonymous loan to them;
Shepheard-Walwyn (Publishers) Ltd. for the twelve poems from Mira Mehta's book *Cascade of Stars*.

Contents

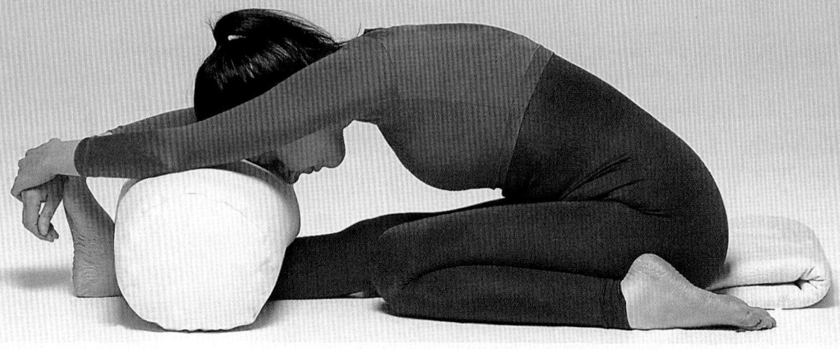

Preface

This book arose almost as an afterthought. I was planning a comprehensive book on Yoga that would integrate theory with practice. It struck me, however, that such a book would need to stand on the shoulders of a basic introduction to the complex ideas and practices embraced by Yoga. This idea took root and swiftly grew into its own independent shape.

I asked my dear friend Professor Krishna Arjunwadkar to collaborate with me for the portions on philosophy, for he has spent a lifetime browsing in the vast fields of Sanskritic knowledge, which represent the ancient Indo-European heritage of language, logic, and philosophy.

There is a celebrated Indian book of fables, analogous to Aesop's fables. Its framing story concerns a teacher who is engaged to educate the sons of a king. His method is to teach through stories, so that the princes imbibe knowledge imperceptibly and pleasurably. This method is also used in ancient Indian philosophical works to impart the wisdom gained by sages through their meditations on the world, life, and intelligence. Emulating this time-tested pedagogical device, Professor Arjunwadkar has, wherever possible, introduced stories and examples, both traditional and modern, to illustrate the concepts of Yoga philosophy.

In a practical subject such as Yoga, personal tuition is of paramount importance to progress, and a book, however informative, can never replace a teacher. I have tried to bridge the gap of anonymity between writer and reader by presenting material as if to students in a class. Drawing on my teaching of numerous foundation courses, I have addressed the common questions and problems encountered by students, for what is troubling to one is usually troubling to many.

Embarking on a new venture can be both exciting and daunting. I have heard many people say that they would like to learn Yoga but feel that it deserves a commitment in time and effort that they are unable to give to it. Therefore, they do not begin at all. My reaction is always, "What a pity!"; for they are missing out on a most rewarding experience. To begin Yoga does not require a huge commitment. Nor is it necessary to consider the plenitude of the subject. In the words of a Sanskrit proverb, encouraging the diffident beginner:

> **How can one gain wealth except piece by piece?**
> **How can one gain learning except moment by moment?**

It is from small beginnings, little by little, that one acquires mastery.

Mira Mehta, January 2004

Introduction

A tree is only as healthy as its roots, and a building only as sound as its foundations. Likewise in Yoga, the quality of the foundation is crucial. This is a subject whose area of study is the human being; it prescribes a training of every aspect of the personality, with the goal of reaching a pinnacle of spiritual experience. That summit cannot be reached—or even envisaged—without proper groundwork.

If Yoga is treated as merely physical exercise, an explanation of principles is not essential, for the utilitarian benefits of the postures and breath training techniques speak for themselves. With this approach, too, an emphasis on perfection is not crucial, since results are seen even from imperfect practice. However, to probe beyond the physical sphere into the inner person requires both a grasp of theory and an accurate application of the tools of the inquiry—namely, the body and the mind. Without exactness the value of practice is diminished, and insight into the subject is hindered. Without a grasp of the subject, the purpose of precision is not understood, and progress is effectively barred.

For these reasons, this book presents an introduction to Yoga practice hand in hand with the basics of its philosophy.

Viṣṇu reclines on the immortal Serpent, Ananta. Patañjali, the author of the *Yoga Sūtras* is said to be an incarnation of Ananta.

Plan of the Book

The plan of this book is modeled on classroom teaching. The material is divided into twelve Units of study, each incorporating three components: a short reflective essay on a philosophical theme; an explanation of an aspect of practice followed by a program of postures; and a philosophy topic, which is expanded by notes giving a wider perspective.

The Units are progressive, together forming a comprehensive foundation course, covering a wide range of basic poses. (Head Balance, though a basic pose, is excluded, as it requires a grounding in all these poses.) No time limit is set for learning; readers may progress at their own pace and repeat a Unit as often as they feel necessary.

Each Unit opens with a reflection on an aspect of life, in the form of a short poem, and then gives the Yoga view. This is based on the most authoritative ancient work on Yoga, the *Yoga Sūtra* (aphorisms) of Patañjali and its commentary by Vyāsa.

In the practical section of each Unit, a principle of practice is first explained. Instructions for a program of postures that exemplify this principle are then given. In addition to the basic method, guidance is offered on how to progress and how to work with difficulties such as stiffness or pain. Each pose is briefly described; touching on various aspects, these descriptions provide a conceptual framework for the poses.

The bulk of the poses introduced in the course are standing ones. This is because movements performed on the feet are the easiest for the body to learn. The feet are the base from which the body stands erect.

Standing poses activate the feet and legs and bring mobility to the hips, spine, shoulders, and arms. This training is essential for all other postures.

However, concentrating on just one set of postures does not form a balanced practice. This is especially true of standing poses, which are fairly strenuous. Therefore, other simple poses are also introduced, which involve different kinds of stretches, spinal rotation, and, most importantly, inverting the body. Inverted poses counteract the effect of gravity on the body and are enormously beneficial to health.

Last but not least, the art of relaxation is explained. Every fourth Unit is devoted to postures and practices that effectively de-stress the body, mind, and senses. With this preparation a simple breathing technique is explained in the final Unit.

The method of postures and breathing techniques followed is that of B. K. S. Iyengar, a contemporary Yogin of world-wide influence, whose classic work *Light on Yoga* is recognized by all schools as authoritative. His lineage of learning can be traced back in the traditional manner to a Yogin living in the Himalayas, in Nepal.

In the theory section of each Unit, a topic of Yoga philosophy is explained. This explanation is supplemented by discursive notes. Key concepts are defined at the beginning, and the thread of the argument is reiterated in simple verse summaries.

The topics place Yoga in both a historical and a universal frame. The sources of Yoga are discussed, together with a summary of the principal works, schools, and authors associated with it.

To set Yoga in a wider context, the origin of Indian philosophical speculation is traced to the question "What is the one thing by which all things can be known?" and to the quest for knowledge of the inner world. The concept of Ultimate Reality is introduced and the relevance of Yoga to the spiritual goal explained. Topics relating to these are discussed: the evolution of the world, fate as the consequence of actions, self-realization, liberation from repeated reincarnation, and the eight divisions of Yoga.

The inner search requires an understanding of how the mind operates. Accordingly, the nature, functions and instigators of the mind are explained. Finally, the concept and process of meditation is discussed: it is a means to mastery and, ultimately, transcendence of the mind.

The exposition of philosophy follows closely the most respected ancient text on Yoga, the *Yoga Sūtra* of Patañjali. Over two thousand years old, this work summarizes the entire subject in under two hundred gnomic sentences. It also draws on the fourth-century commentary on the *Yoga Sūtra* by Vyāsa. For the illustrative stories it draws on works of even greater antiquity, the *Upaniṣads*, which are treasure-houses of ancient Indian thought.

A summary of the main tenets of Yoga, "Yoga Concepts at a Glance," is given at the beginning of the book. It serves both to introduce the topics and as a reference tool.

The essential teaching of the philosophy is lightheartedly recapitulated in the Afterword, in the shape of an allegorical dialogue between a doctor and his patient.

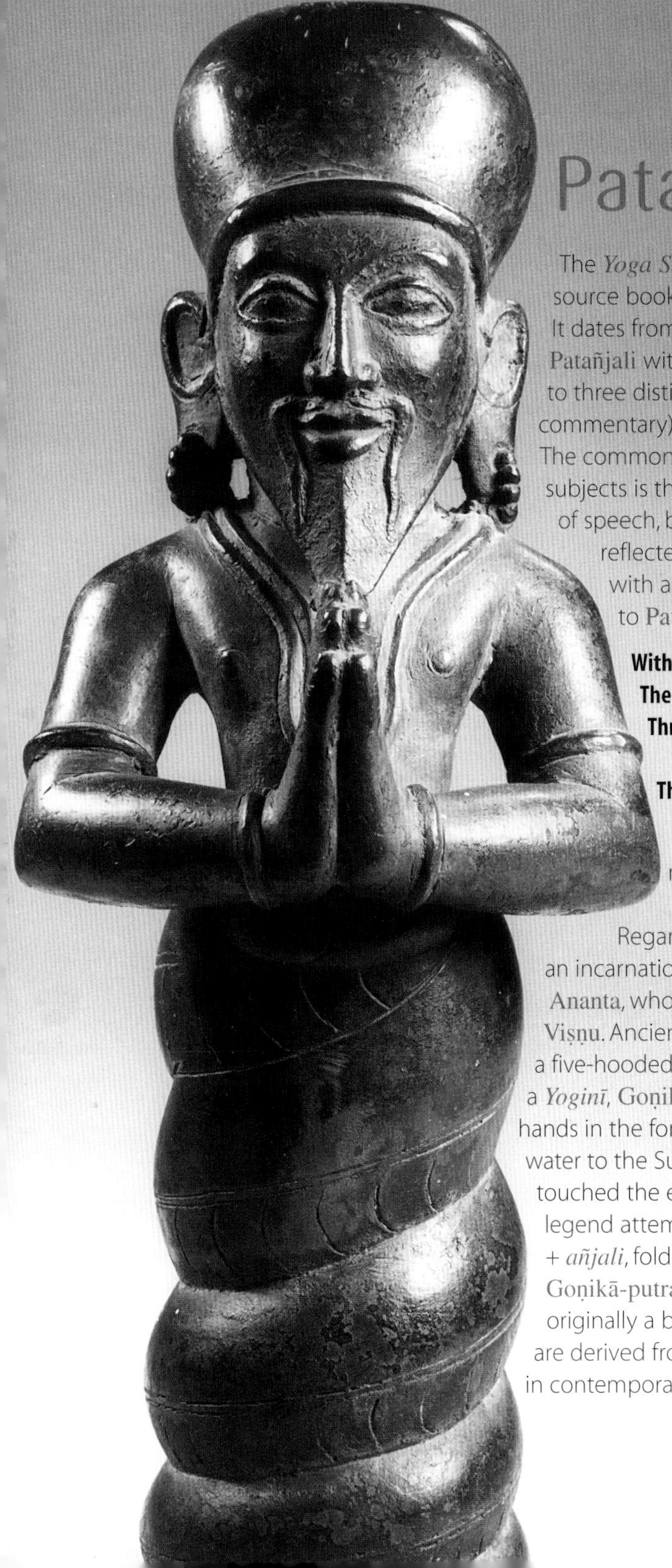

Patañjali

The *Yoga Sūtra* of Patañjali has remained the major source book as well as inspiration for later writers on Yoga. It dates from the second century B.C. Tradition credits Patañjali with the authorship of substantial works relating to three distinct areas of study: grammar (an exhaustive commentary), medicine (a major compendium), and Yoga. The common thread that binds these apparently unrelated subjects is that they are designed to achieve purity—of speech, body, and mind, respectively. This belief is reflected in a traditional verse, thought to originate with an authority on grammar, paying homage to Patañjali:

With folded hands I salute Patañjali
The foremost sage, who removed
Through Yoga impurity of mind, through grammar that of speech,
Through medicine that of body.

Anecdotes about great personalities are numerous in the Sanskrit tradition, but little is known about them beyond such stories. Regarding Patañjali, we are informed that he was an incarnation of the divine serpent Śeṣa, also known as Ananta, whose coiled body provided a bed for the god Viṣṇu. Ancient stone images of Patañjali show him with a five-hooded snake behind his head. He was adopted by a *Yoginī*, Goṇikā, as her son. He descended into her folded hands in the form of a miniature child while she was offering water to the Sun god during her morning rites. As the water touched the earth he grew into an ordinary child. This legend attempts to explain Patañjali's name (*patat*, falling + *añjali*, folded hands), as well as his traditional epithet, Goṇikā-putra (son of Goṇikā). Most probably, it was originally a bird name: the names of many old sages are derived from those of birds. This custom also exists in contemporary Indian society.

Guidelines for practice

Food
Do not do Yoga on a full stomach. Allow two to three hours to pass after a snack and five to six hours after a heavy meal. Wait for half an hour after practice before taking food.

Water
Do not drink during practice. All drinks, including water, need to be digested, and digestion is not compatible with exercise.

Clothes
Wear loose clothing, as tight clothes restrict movement. Have bare feet, as this allows them to stretch and become sensitive.

Bowel Movements
Evacuate the bowels if practicing in the morning. It is difficult to move well when constipated.

Menstruation
Avoid inverted poses, as these inhibit the exit of blood from the body. Also avoid standing poses and other strenuous poses. Do a program of supine poses and restful forward bends (see Unit 8). This supports the physiological changes of the menstrual cycle and helps to alleviate any difficulties experienced with it.

Illness and Operations
If suffering from a serious or chronic medical condition or recovering from recent surgery, seek the advice of an experienced teacher. A beginners' program that includes strenuous standing poses is not likely to be suitable; a program of restful and recuperative postures will be more beneficial.

Pregnancy
Seek the advice of an experienced teacher. A special program of postures geared toward the constantly changing physical condition of the mother-to-be, and including plenty of restful postures, is necessary.

Repetition of Poses
Standing poses, forward bends, and twists are normally repeated twice. Repetition reduces stiffness, making the poses easier to do.

Timings in Poses
Supine and inverted poses are normally held for a length of time. Staying enhances their physiological effect, such as the expansion of the chest and lungs. The capacity to stay in the poses increases with practice.

Contraindications
Inverted poses are contraindicated in certain circumstances; please read the cautions included in the instructions for these poses.

Props
To make it easier to learn the postures, simple props are sometimes used. They give support, a sense of direction, and a more effective experience of the pose. With the help of props, it is possible to stay in a pose with comfort and confidence, thereby deriving the maximum benefit. Most of these props are household items, such as a nonslip mat, blankets, a chair, a stool, a bolster (pillow), a brick, a bench or coffee table, and a wall.

Guide to Sanskrit pronunciation

The spelling of Sanskrit words in this book follows the international convention of transliteration. A guide to pronunciation is as follows:

Vowels

There are long and short vowels. A bar sign over a vowel indicates that it is long.

Pure vowels

a as in about; **ā** as in arm; **i** as in it; **ī** as in eat; **u** as in pull; **ū** as in pool

Diphthongs

e as in eight; **ai** as in eye; **o** as in ore; **au** as in owl

Vocalic r

ṛ as ri or ru (approximate equivalents)

Nasalized vowel

ṁ or **ṃ**: the nasal is modified by the following consonant: **sāṁkhya** as saankhya.

Aspiration

ḥ indicates the breathy repetition of the preceding vowel: **aḥ** as aha; **iḥ** as ihi; **uḥ** as uhu (approximate equivalents).

Consonants

These are grouped according to the place of articulation. Many have both unvoiced and voiced, and unaspirated and aspirated forms. There is a nasal in most groups.

Guttural

k as in kind; **kh** as in backhand; **g** as in give; **gh** as in aghast; **ṅ** as in sink and sing.

Palatal

c as in chin; **ch** as in church hall; **j** as in jam; **jh** as in hedgehog; **ñ** as in inch and engine

Retroflex

ṭ, ṭh, ḍ, ḍh, ṇ: the tongue curls back and hits the upper palate.

Dental

t, th, d, dh, n: the tip of the tongue touches the back of the upper teeth.

th as in outhouse; **dh** as in childhood

Labial

p, ph, b, bh, m

ph as in haphazard; **bh** as in abhor

Semi-vowels

y, r, l, v

Sibilant

ś, ṣ, s

ś: palatal **sh** as in sheet; **ṣ**: retroflex **sh** as in push

Aspirate

h

Summary

A bar sign over a vowel indicates that the vowel is long.

An accent on s makes the pronunciation sh.

A dot under r makes the sound vocalic.

A dot under t, d, or n makes it retroflex.

A dot above n makes it guttural.

A tilde above n makes it palatal.

A dot above or under m modifies it according to the following consonant.

Yoga concepts at a glance

This section outlines the basic concepts used in the explanation of Yoga philosophy in this book. The original Sanskrit terms are given in parentheses after the English entry. The concepts are arranged in four groups:

1. The Framework of Philosophical Inquiry This gives general information on Indian philosophical systems relevant to Yoga.

2. The World and Life This includes fundamental concepts such as the soul, God, and primordial matter.

3. Mind and its Realm This includes concepts relating to the analysis of the mind.

4. Yoga This summarizes the key terms of Yoga.

The Framework of Philosophical Inquiry

School of philosophy (*darśana*—"view"): Indian philosophical schools offer views on the world, the soul, God, and the relationships between them. The nature of these views is defined by which means of knowledge (see below) is given priority by the school concerned.

Sāṃkhya **school** (*sāṃkhya-darśana*—"the view of intellectuals"): a school of philosophy giving priority to inference or rational thinking. Concentrating on metaphysical inquiry, it analyzes Ultimate Reality into two distinct, contrasting categories, Matter (see right) and Spirit or soul (see right). The teachings of this school are accepted by Yoga.

Yoga school (*yoga-darśana*—"the view on the means of spiritual experience"): This school studies the mind and how to transcend it. It analyzes the modes of the mind, shows how it causes worldly sufferings, and specifies an eightfold plan to control and nullify it. The authoritative work on Yoga is the *Yoga Sūtra* of Patañjali, dating from the second century B.C.

Means of knowledge (*pramāṇa*—"means of measuring, that is, knowing"): All schools of Indian philosophy state the means of knowledge on which they base their arguments. Those accepted by Yoga are:

1. Perception (*pratyakṣa*—"open to the sense organs"): knowledge received directly through the sense organs. Examples: we hear a sound, feel heat or cold, and so on.
2. Inference (*anumāna*—"subsequent means of measuring"): knowledge of the unknown by means of the known. Example: from visible smoke, we infer the existence of an invisible fire.

3. Authority (*āgama*—"what has come down through a tradition"): the knowledge of old masters obtained by them through established means or intuition and transmitted to later generations. Examples: Indian scriptures, the classic works on Yoga, and so on.

The World and Life

Soul, Spirit, or Self (*puruṣa, ātman*): the conscious, eternal principle in all living bodies. It is also viewed as an all-pervading principle when shorn of its worldly associations. Though single as a principle, Spirit consists of an infinite number of individual souls, which become entangled with the material world.

God (*īśvara*): the supreme Soul who is untouched by the limitations of normal souls. Knowing everything, He is the ultimate and supreme teacher. The syllable *Om* is His symbol.

Primordial Matter or Matter (*prakṛti*—"the original"): the insentient, ultimate, eternal principle. It has three qualities: light (*sattva*), activity (*rajas*), and inertia (*tamas*). All worldly phenomena are permeated by and can be analyzed according to these qualities. As a result of the presence of the conscious soul (see above), Primordial Matter is activated and evolves into the phenomenal world, including the body complex that imprisons the soul in life (see right).

Evolution of the world There are 24 products of Primordial Matter (see above) that evolve from it in order, beginning with the principles of intelligence and individualization. From these evolve living creatures with capacities to act and react and the insentient elements—space, air, fire, water, and earth.

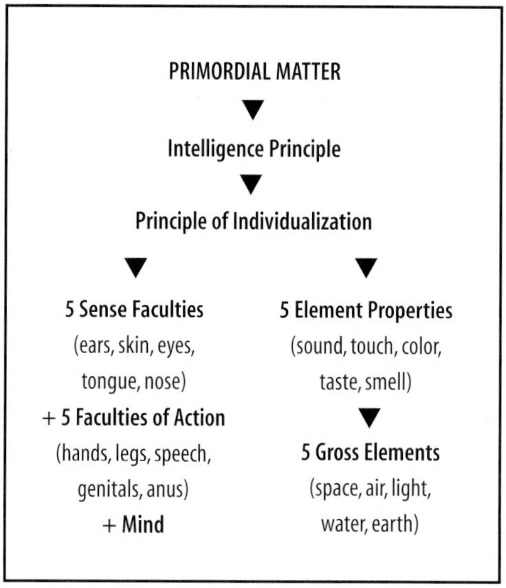

Life (*saṃsāra*—"course, passage"): In the Yoga context life is a chain of actions (see below) and transmigration, involving the soul in suffering. Permanent release from suffering is liberation (see page 15), attainable only through discriminating knowledge (see page 15).

Reincarnation (*punar-janma*): an aspect of the soul's worldly existence consisting of a series of births and deaths with life in between. Birth and death belong to the physical body. The soul with its subtle body (see page 14) continually passes through a series of such physical bodies in the process of transmigration. This ends only on liberation (see page 15).

Actions (*karmas*): The soul performs actions with the aid of the body-mind complex. It is considered that no action is finished until it has borne consequences. This has led to the theory of an invisible power of action that survives the short-lived physical or mental action. The term *karma* is used in both these connotations.

Subtle body (*sūkṣma-śarīra*): The soul possesses a subtle, invisible body in addition to the perishable, physical body. The subtle body has faculties corresponding to those of the physical body, but it is not subject to the same limitations—for example, it can move anywhere and through anything. It stays with the soul unless the soul attains liberation (see right), upon which it merges into its source, Primordial Matter (see page 13).

The Mind and its Realm

Mind (*manas, citta*): (a) the instrument by which the soul has worldly experiences and is prompted to act. It receives knowledge from the sense organs, which it interprets as welcome or not, thereby involving the soul in pleasure or pain. (b) At the same time, the mind is a huge storehouse of imprints (see below) of experiences which cause memory.

Imprints and instincts (*saṃskāras* and *vāsanās*): These are the mental records of experiences. Instincts are deep-rooted, carried through many incarnations and aroused by birth in a particular species. Other imprints of experience do not depend on such conditions, as is shown by dreams, which are classed as memories caused by the imprints of day-to-day life.

Modes of the mind (*vṛttis*): The mind has five modes of operation:

1. Valid knowledge (*pramāṇa*): This is based chiefly on perception, inference and authority (see "Means of knowledge," page 12).
2. Mistaken knowledge (*viparyaya*): the knowledge of an object as what it is not (for instance, mistaking a rope for a snake).
3. Conceptualization (*vikalpa*): Knowledge arising through the processes of language.
4. Deep sleep (*nidrā*): the mode in which the operations of the senses and mind are suspended.
5. Memory (*smṛti*): the mode caused by the imprints of experiences. It also includes the dream state.

Sufferings (*kleśas*): These are five basic causes of worldly suffering, deep-rooted in the mind. They are: ignorance (*avidyā*), sense of self (*asmitā*), attachment (*rāga*), aversion (*dveṣa*), and clinging to life (*abhiniveśa*). Ignorance is said to be the root cause from which the subsequent sufferings emerge.

Ignorance (*avidyā*): the perverse view that treats as eternal, pure, pleasurable, and spiritual what is actually their opposite—transitory, impure, painful, and non-spiritual. It results from not knowing the distinction between the soul (associated with the former qualities) and the mind (associated with the latter qualities). Ignorance is the root cause of the soul's worldly sufferings (see above).

Yoga

Yoga: This term is used in two senses:

1. The school that specializes in the analysis of the mind and shows the way to isolate the soul from the mind
2. Deep absorption (see below), forming the ultimate goal of this discipline

Knowledge (*khyāti, jñāna*): In Indian philosophy, knowledge does not imply mere intellectual information, but actual experience, also termed realization.

Discriminating knowledge (*viveka-khyāti*): the knowledge (*khyāti*) that the soul is distinct (*viveka*) from the mind. This begins with intellectual knowledge and matures into experience leading to liberation (see below). It requires persistent practice of Yoga. When the goal is achieved, discriminating knowledge, being basically intellectual, ceases to exist.

Liberation or isolation (*mokṣa*—"freedom"; *kaivalya*—"aloneness"): a state of the soul in which it remains in its natural condition of pure consciousness, unaffected by worldly sufferings. As this state involves disentangling the soul from the mind, it is known in Yoga as "isolation." It is achieved through discriminating knowledge (see above).

Aids of Yoga (*yogāṅgas*—"limbs of Yoga"): the means that progressively lead to Yoga (see above), signifying in this context deep absorption (see right) of the mind in the soul. There are eight aids:

1. Moral disciplines (*yamas*): These are non-injury (*ahiṃsā*), truth (*satya*), abstention from theft (*asteya*), celibacy (*brahmacarya*), and nonacquisitiveness (*aparigraha*).
2. Observances (*niyamas*): These are purity or cleanliness (*śauca*), contentment (*saṃtoṣa*), penance (*tapas*), study of sacred texts (*svādhyāya*), and surrender of all actions to God (*īśvara-praṇidhāna*).
3. Posture (*āsana*): This implies a stable and comfortable sitting posture for meditation. The term also refers to the variety of postures used to establish a healthy physical and mental base for spiritual practices.
4. Breath training (*prāṇāyāma*): a system of practices based on the operations of inhaling, exhaling, and holding the breath.
5. Withdrawal of sense organs (*pratyāhāra*): the withdrawal of the sense organs from their stimuli, the preparatory step toward focusing the mind on an inner object.
6. Concentration (*dhāraṇā*): the fixing of the mind on an external object or an inner part of the body, such as the heart.
7. Meditation (*dhyāna*): the steady, continued awareness of an object uninterrupted by other objects.
8. Absorption (*samādhi*—"right placement"): the total absorption of the mind, initially in an external object, and subsequently into its source, Primordial Matter (see above), leaving the soul in its pure state of consciousness. This is the ultimate in Yoga practice.

Unit 1

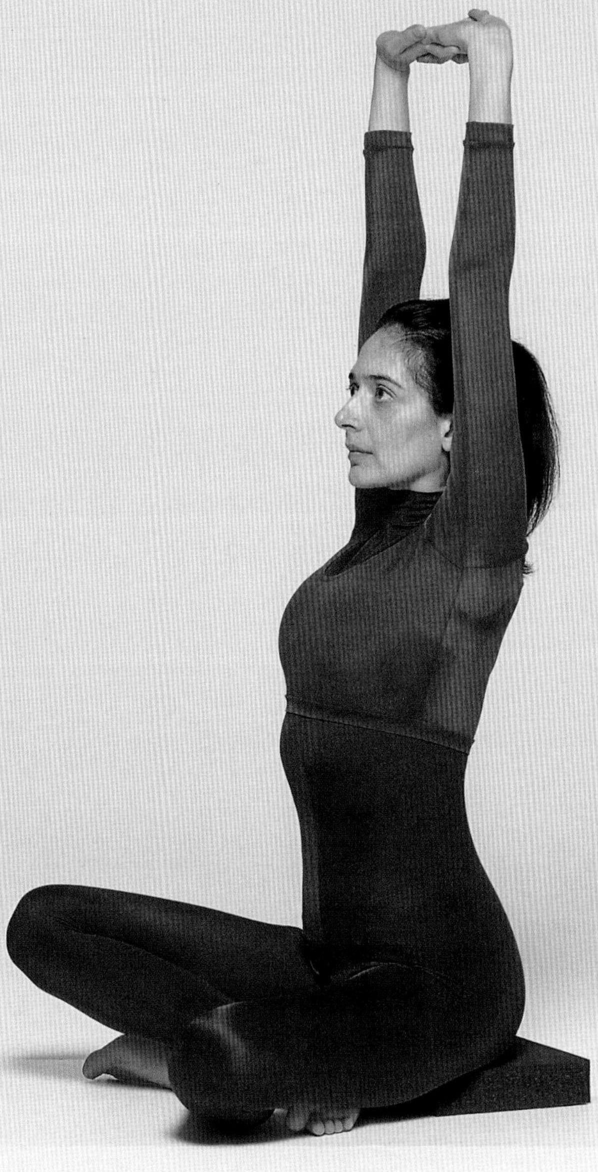

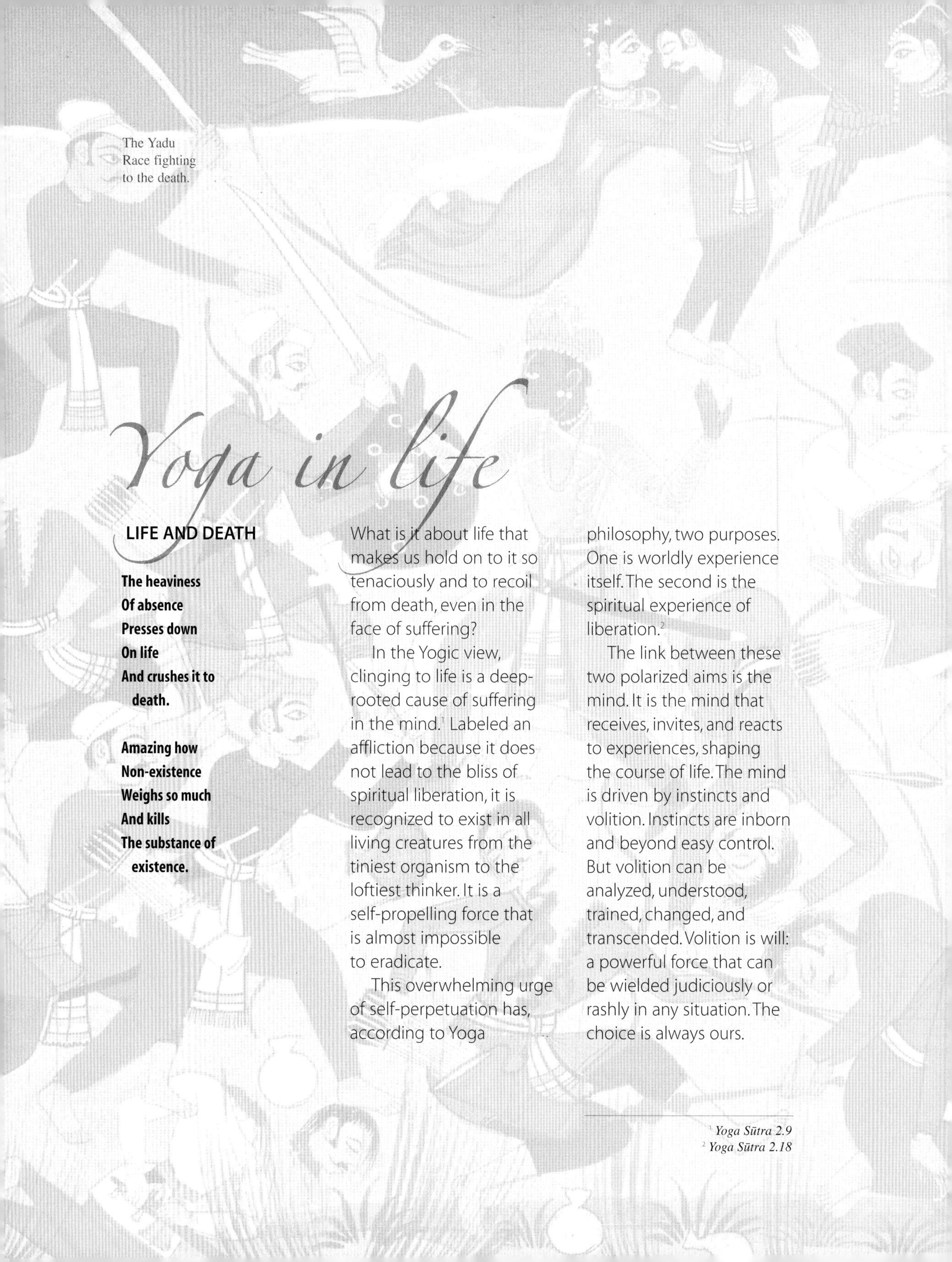

The Yadu
Race fighting
to the death.

Yoga in life

LIFE AND DEATH

The heaviness
Of absence
Presses down
On life
And crushes it to death.

Amazing how
Non-existence
Weighs so much
And kills
The substance of existence.

What is it about life that makes us hold on to it so tenaciously and to recoil from death, even in the face of suffering?

In the Yogic view, clinging to life is a deep-rooted cause of suffering in the mind.[1] Labeled an affliction because it does not lead to the bliss of spiritual liberation, it is recognized to exist in all living creatures from the tiniest organism to the loftiest thinker. It is a self-propelling force that is almost impossible to eradicate.

This overwhelming urge of self-perpetuation has, according to Yoga philosophy, two purposes. One is worldly experience itself. The second is the spiritual experience of liberation.[2]

The link between these two polarized aims is the mind. It is the mind that receives, invites, and reacts to experiences, shaping the course of life. The mind is driven by instincts and volition. Instincts are inborn and beyond easy control. But volition can be analyzed, understood, trained, changed, and transcended. Volition is will: a powerful force that can be wielded judiciously or rashly in any situation. The choice is always ours.

---

[1] *Yoga Sūtra 2.9*
[2] *Yoga Sūtra 2.18*

Shapes and directions

The first step in beginning Yoga postures or poses (*āsanas*) is to become familiar with their shapes. This involves learning their geometrical configuration, their alignment, and the direction of the stretches required to form them.

This inner sense of direction is acquired gradually through repeated practice. While the mind may be quick to understand what is required, the body is often slow, needing the crutch of habit to become adept at new movements. The joy is great, however, when mind and body synchronize in their understanding.

The first thing to be learned is how to stand straight. In the ideal upright stance, the body does not lean forward or back. Kept within a plane, the skeletal structure, soft tissue, and organs are properly aligned. The parts designed to bear weight do so and do not offload their burden onto other parts. For example, when high-heeled shoes are worn, undue weight is thrown onto the front of the foot, and the body leans to the front. This affects the musculature and alignment of the feet and legs, and, by a knock-on effect, of the entire body. The resultant loss of spinal strength may be gauged by comparison with the deportment of people who still live relatively natural lifestyles: with unshod feet and superbly erect back and neck, they can carry heavy loads on their heads.

Thus, the proper upright stance is the foundation of posture, in both its general sense and in the sense of Yogic posture. On the basis of this understanding, various standing poses form the first and fundamental group of postures to be learned.

In this Unit two standing poses are introduced as well as Mountain or Palm Tree Pose (*Tāḍāsana*). All standing poses take this as their starting and finishing point.

In addition to standing straight, it is important to sit straight. The most natural way of sitting for humans is to be cross-legged on the floor. However, the use of chairs has made the floor a distant prospect for many people, with the consequent loss of their birthright of hip flexibility and lower back strength. In Yoga practice, therefore, sitting postures start with this simple yet basic pose.

Limberness, however, is merely a consequence of the goal of Yoga, which is to harness physical, mental, and emotional energies toward higher aims. Recognizing the drain of energy that occurs from the strains of everyday life, Yoga includes many restorative poses. Pre-eminent among these are inverted poses; they revitalize the body and mind and induce calm.

After the body has stretched and relaxed and the mind is quiet, the preoccupations of the day recede in importance. The inward journey can begin. This is done in Corpse Pose (*Śavāsana*). Here attention is turned to the instruments of knowledge, the mind and senses, as entities in themselves, not just as the means of engaging with the world.

ताडासन *Tāḍāsana*

Mountain or Palm Tree Pose

Drawn up to its full height, the body stands straight like a mountain or a palmyra palm.

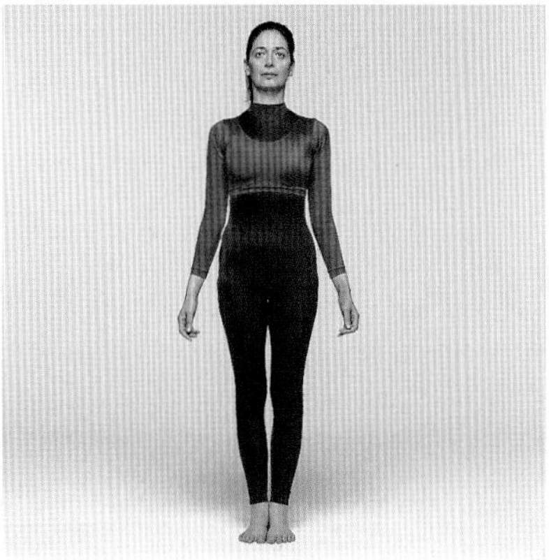

Stand with the feet together. Join the big toes, inner heels, and inner ankles. Tighten the kneecaps and pull up the thigh muscles. Extend the trunk away from the legs.

Take the shoulders back and down, and press the shoulder blades in. Stretch the arms and hands downward and then relax them. Let the palms face the thighs.

Extend the neck upward and keep the head straight. Relax the eyes and face, and look ahead. Breathe evenly.

Stay in this pose for 20 to 30 seconds.

To Progress

Bring the weight of the body a little back onto the heels. Learn to stand with equilibrium, balancing the weight evenly on both sides.

त्रिकोणासन *Trikoṇāsana*

Triangle Pose

The limbs and trunk form a design of triangles in a vertical plane.

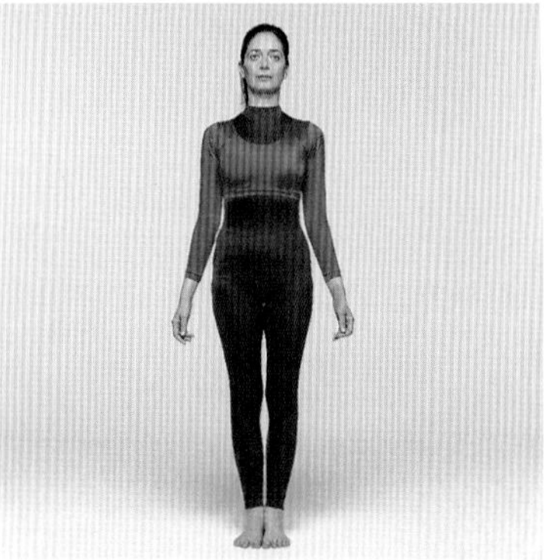

Stand in *Tāḍāsana* (see page 19).

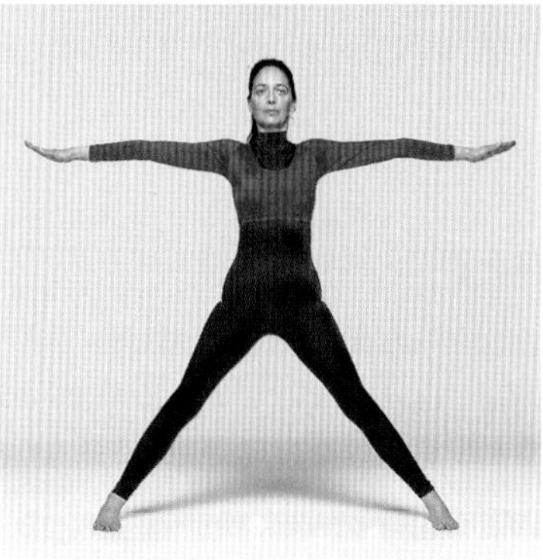

Take a deep inhalation and jump the feet 3½–4 feet apart, simultaneously extending the arms sideways to shoulder level with the palms facing down. Align the feet and make them parallel.

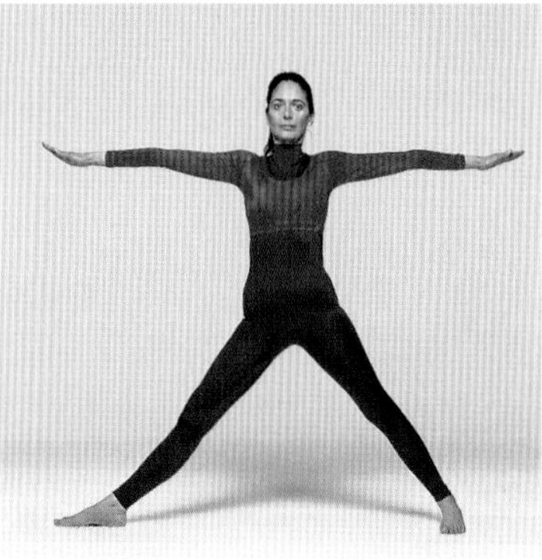

Turn the left foot 15 degrees in and the right foot 90 degrees out. Align the center of the right heel with the center of the left arch. Revolve each leg outward. Tighten the kneecaps, and pull up the thigh muscles.

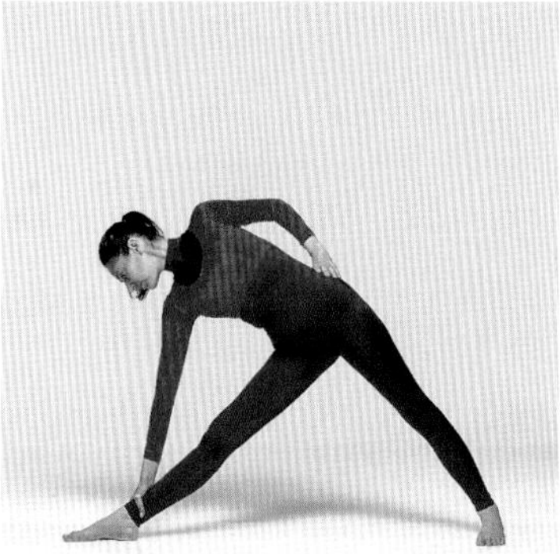

Exhale and take the trunk sideways down to the right; hold the right ankle or shin with the right hand. Rest the left hand on the hip and revolve the trunk strongly upward.

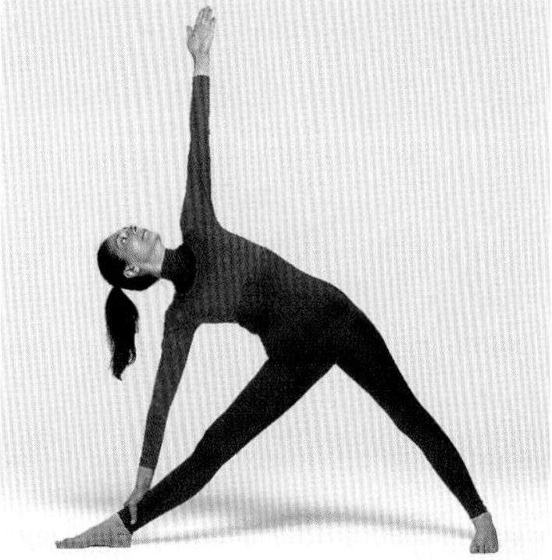

Stretch the left arm up and turn the palm to face forward. Turn the neck and head, and look up at the hand. Breathe evenly.

Stay in the pose for 20 to 30 seconds. Inhale and come up. Turn the feet to the front and rest the arms. Then repeat on the other side.

Inhale and come up. Exhale and jump the feet together, simultaneously bringing the arms down.

To Progress

Press the outer edge of the back foot down. Continue stretching the legs and revolving them away from each other. Lengthen the trunk and maintain the strength of its upward turn.

Help (All Standing Poses)

- **For back and knee problems, step the legs apart; do not jump.**
- **The distance between the feet varies according to body height and length of the legs: it is wider for a tall person than for a short person.**

पार्श्वकोणासन *Pārśvakoṇāsana*

Side Angle Pose

On the base of a quadrilateral formed by the legs and ground, the laterally held trunk revolves upward, aided by the arms.

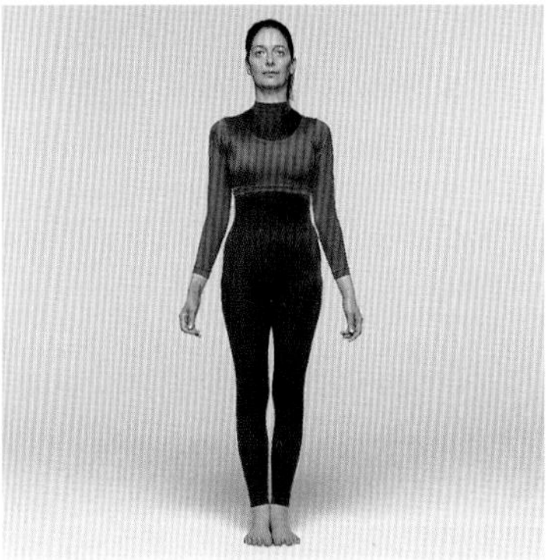

Stand in *Tāḍāsana* (see page 19).

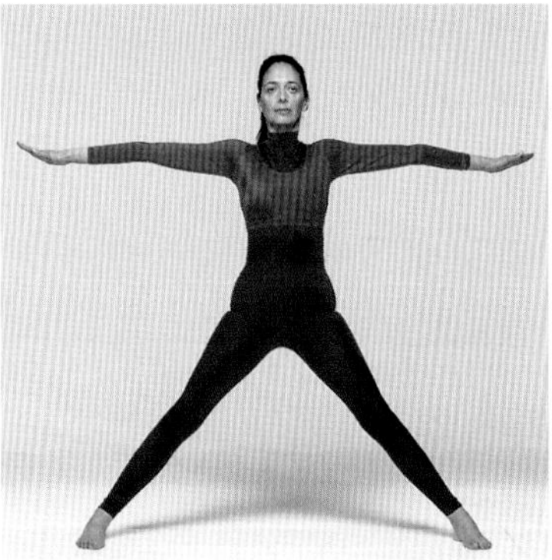

Take a deep inhalation and jump 4–4½ feet apart, simultaneously extending the arms sideways to shoulder level with the palms facing down. Align the feet and make them parallel.

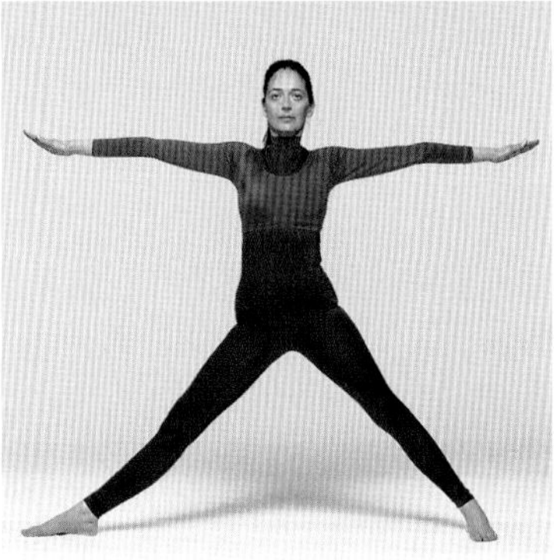

Turn the left foot 15 degrees in and the right foot 90 degrees out. Align the center of the right heel with the center of the left arch. Revolve each leg outward. Tighten the kneecaps, and pull up the thigh muscles.

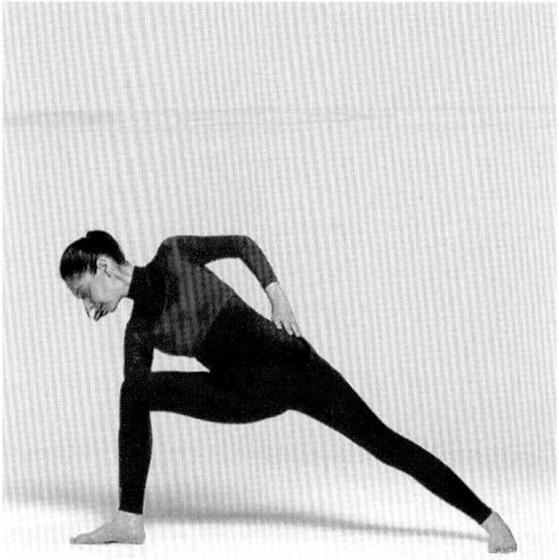

Exhale and bend the right leg to form a right angle, with the shin vertical and the thigh horizontal. Simultaneously take the trunk sideways down toward the thigh, and place the right hand (fingertips) on the floor beside the foot. Rest the left hand on the hip. Revolve the trunk upward.

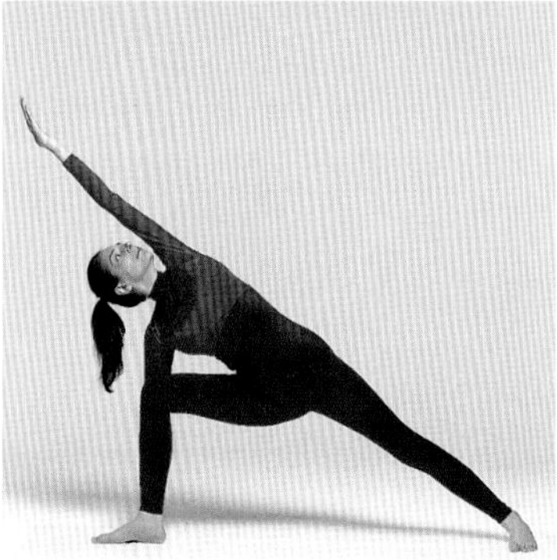

Take the left arm over the head, palm facing down. Turn the neck and head, and look up at the arm. Breathe evenly and without strain.

Stay in the pose for 20 to 30 seconds. Inhale and come up. Turn the feet to the front and rest the arms. Then repeat on the other side.

Inhale and come up. Exhale and jump the feet together, simultaneously bringing the arms down.

To Progress

Press the outer edge of the back foot down. Create a continuous stretch along the back leg, the side of the trunk, and the top arm and hand.

सुखासन *Sukhāsana*

Comfortable Pose

In this natural sitting position, the back is trained to hold itself erect.

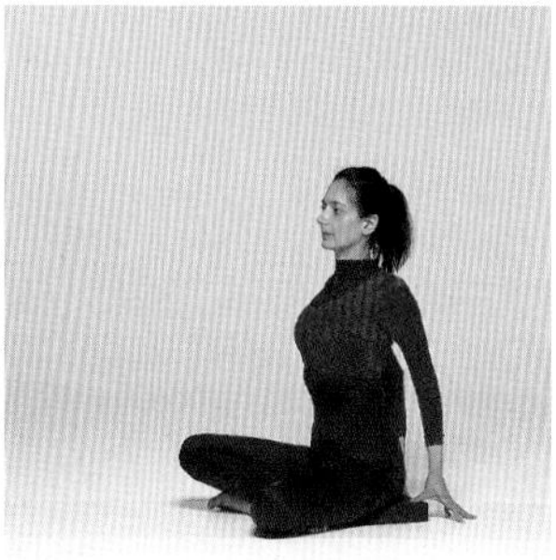

Sit on the floor with the legs crossed simply. If the lower back feels collapsed, sit on a support, such as one or two folded blankets. The support is the correct height when the lower back feels light. Place the fingertips on the floor beside the hips, and stretch the trunk up. Take the shoulders back and the shoulder blades in. Keep the head straight. Breathe evenly.

Stay in the pose for 30 to 60 seconds. Cross the legs the other way and repeat.

To Progress

Keep the body erect. If the back lifts well, place the hands on the knees.

पर्वतासन *Parvatāsana*

Mountain Pose

Like the foot of a mountain, the legs form a broad and stable base from which the trunk and arms stretch up loftily.

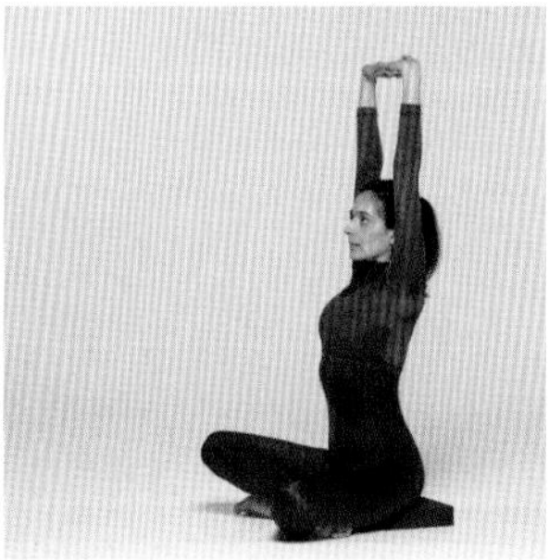

Sit in *Sukhāsana* (see above). Interlock the fingers. Turn the palms outward and stretch the arms up. Tighten the elbows. Keep the face and neck relaxed.

Stay in the pose for 20 to 30 seconds. Bring the arms down, change the interlock of the fingers by crossing them the other way, and repeat.

To Progress

Stretch the sides of the trunk upward with the help of the arms.

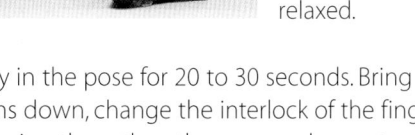

ऊर्ध्व-प्रसारित-पादासन

Ūrdhva-Prasārita-Pādāsana

Upward Leg Extension

The body takes a perpendicular shape by resting itself against the floor and wall.

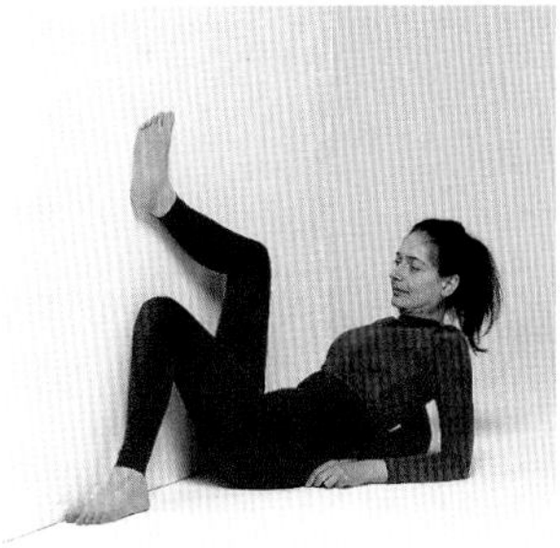

Sit on the floor sideways to the wall with one buttock against it. Lean back onto the elbows, and raise the legs one by one onto the wall, at the same time swiveling the body around.

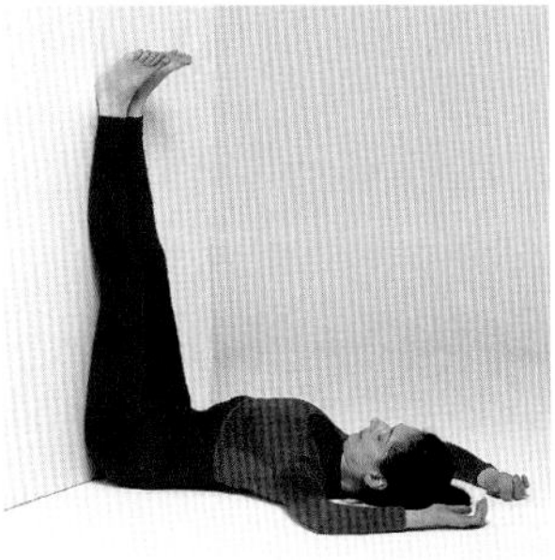

Lie down and straighten the legs up. Keep the buttocks against the wall. Take the arms over the head and relax.

Stay in the pose for up to 5 minutes. To come down, bend the knees and turn to the side.

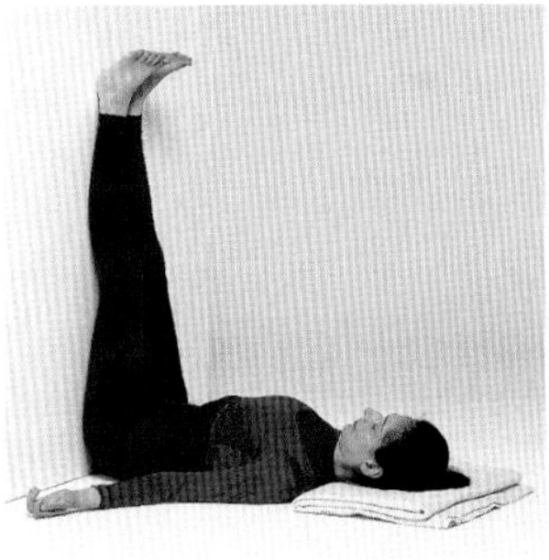

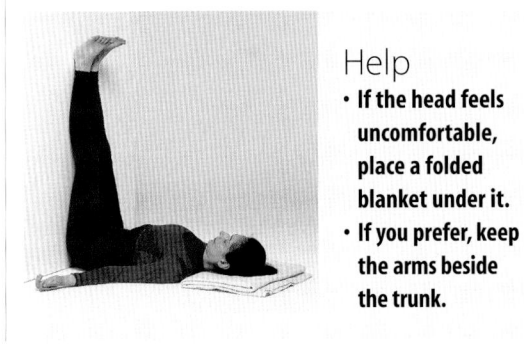

Help

- **If the head feels uncomfortable, place a folded blanket under it.**
- **If you prefer, keep the arms beside the trunk.**

To Progress

Press the outer hips down. Tighten the kneecaps and stretch the legs. Stretch the arms. Maintain the active stretch for 20 to 30 seconds, then relax.

शवासन *Śavāsana*

Corpse Pose

Horizontal and motionless, the body lies as if dead; this simulation is an art in itself.

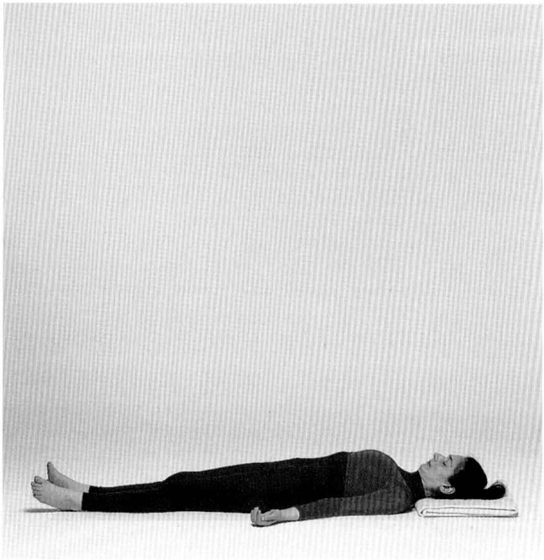

Sit on the floor with the legs stretched out in front. Bend the knees and lie back, making sure the body is in a straight line. Place a folded blanket under the head and neck. Stretch the legs, and then let them drop to the sides. Press the shoulders down and move the shoulder blades in. Turn the upper arms so that the biceps face the ceiling. Stretch the arms and let them drop to the sides. Relax the hands, allowing the fingers to curl.

Close the eyes and relax the face.

Stay in the pose for 5 to 10 minutes. Turn to the side in order to get up.

To Progress

Continuously relax the face and the sense organs: eyes, ears, nose, tongue, and skin. Relax the throat. Whenever tension creeps into the body, let go.

The quest of philosophy

KEY CONCEPTS

Soul The inner, sentient principle in all live bodies, viewed also as an all-pervading principle when shorn of its worldly associations. It is said to have three aspects: existence, consciousness, and bliss.

Immortality When used in the philosophical context, this word means liberation (see pages 163–7), different from the limited immortality of gods in heaven.

Renunciation Giving up routine life and ties for the achievement of a higher, spiritual goal called liberation.

Cognition and Consciousness The two words are used to distinguish between the particular and the general aspects of the process of knowledge. Cognition is consciousness marked by the triple attribute—the knower, the means of knowledge, and the object; consciousness is the general awareness, shorn of specificity, that underlies all cognitions.

Philosophy, briefly, is an attempt to discover the foundation of the outer and the inner worlds. Two stories from ancient works in the Indian philosophical tradition, related below, illustrate how this search begins.

The Probe into the Outer World

Śvetaketu was a lazy boy, more interested in playing than in studies. He reached the age of twelve without schooling.

His father, Āruṇi, was worried. One day he said, "Śvetaketu, no one in our family line has so far been illiterate, deserving to be treated as a dunce. Do you wish to be one? It is high time you attended school, as other boys do."

The admonition worked. Śvetaketu went to stay in a teacher's house, as was the custom in times past. He began his studies in earnest, learning all the traditional texts. At the age of twenty-four he returned home, proud of his learning; however, he had become haughty and full of airs and graces.

His father observed his attitude. It was understandable: inflation of the ego due to achievement. He was concerned about his son's future. He asked him, "Śvetaketu, during your stay with your teacher, did you ever ask him about the knowledge that makes everything in the world known?"

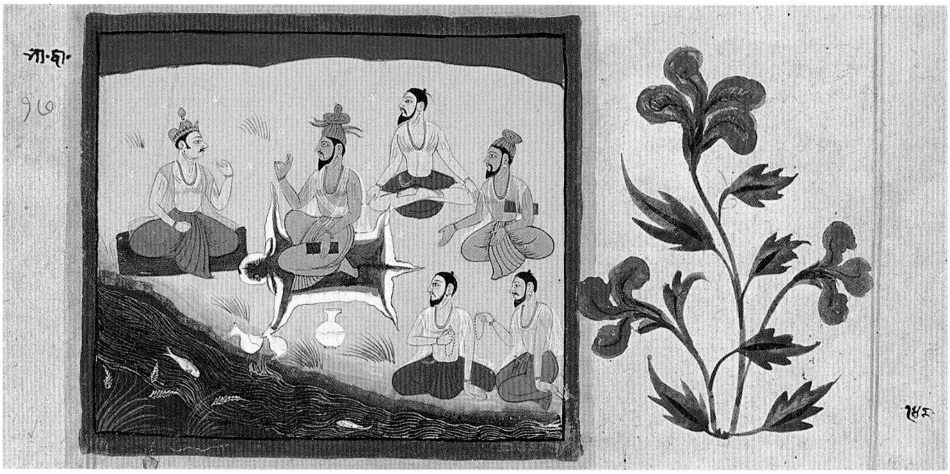

The sage Śuka instructs his disciples on the Body and Spirit.

Śvetaketu was puzzled. No such knowledge had figured in his course of study. He asked, "Father, what you say is a riddle to me. What kind of knowledge could this possibly be?"

"Look, my dear son, it is like this. When you know a clod of earth in essence, you therefore also know everything that is made of it, do you not?"

The son nodded.

"When you know a bead of gold in essence, you know everything made of gold. When you know an iron nail-clipper in essence, you know everything made of iron. The knowledge I am talking about is of this nature."

The son was afraid that he would be asked to go to the teacher again for another twelve years. He thought of a way out that was in keeping with the attitude he had developed. He replied, "I think, Father, my teacher could not have known this. Otherwise would he not have taught it to me? So, will you teach it to me?"

The father smiled, seeing through the son's ruse. However, he said, in the kind tone of a father, "All right, Son, I will."

The first lesson began: "Before the world assumed its present form, it was all only pure, undifferentiated existence, unique and without a second. There are some who think that there was only nonexistence before. But how can existence come out of nonexistence? Hence, it was definitely existence that existed before."

The tuition went on, day after day, point after point, with theory, illustrations, and, occasionally, a practical experiment. (*Chāndogya Upaniṣad*, VI)

The Probe into the Inner World

Yājñavalkya, a scholar-philosopher, wished to renounce the world. One day he announced to Maitreyī, his wife, that he was giving up the householder's life, and he deemed it his duty to make the final settlement of his property between her and his other wife, Kātyāyanī. Of the two, Maitreyī had philosophical leanings, while Kātyāyanī was a woman with normal womanly aspirations. On realizing her husband's intention, Maitreyī asked him: "Tell me, Sir, if, indeed, I were to own the whole earth with all its wealth, should I thereby become immortal—that is, liberated?"

"No," said Yājñavalkya, "you would enjoy a life like that of the well-to-do. As to immortality, there is not even the slightest hope of obtaining it through wealth."

This made the picture absolutely clear to Maitreyī. She said that she would have nothing to do with that which would not bring her immortality, and she wished to learn her husband's knowledge.

Yājñavalkya was delighted. Maitreyī was all the more dear to him because of her philosophical yearnings, he said. He asked her to listen closely to what he was going to explain, and to think deeply over it.

He shocked her as he spoke: "Not, indeed, for the sake of the husband does a woman love him, but for her own sake." He did not spare husbands either: "Not, indeed, for the sake of the wife does a man love her, but for his own sake."

And this truth is not restricted to man and woman; everything in life comes under its sway, as Yājñavalkya exemplifies in a long series of instances. This is a fact that has absolutely no exception. Denial of it is equivalent to self-deception. This truth persuades a thinking mind to focus its attention on the soul, the ultimate source of love. As Yājñavalkya concluded: "One should know the soul, and for that purpose, one should study it, and ponder and meditate on it. When the soul is known, and is made the subject of thinking and meditation, everything becomes known. For nothing exists besides the soul. Not to know this is to sever oneself from the rest of the world."

Yājñavalkya illustrates this point further, to prove conclusively that by knowing a single thing, one can know everything emerging from it. It is not possible for the mind to grasp the individual beats of a drum without first understanding drum and drum beat. This is because multiplicity emerges out of unity, as clouds of smoke issue from fire burning damp fuel. The material body has limited specific consciousness which does not survive its death. But cognition as a universal is eternal. Why is it not "seen," then, if it is there all the time? Because the process of worldly cognition depends on the duality of subject and object. This duality terminates when the pure nature of the soul, the subject, asserts itself. Who else is there to know the soul when the soul is the sole knower?
(*Bṛhadāraṇyaka Upaniṣad*, IV)

Overview

The two stories start from different angles but arrive at a single conclusion: that it is possible to know all phenomena by knowing a single thing, their essence. Further, the essence of the outer world is identified with that of the inner world; and this essence is nothing other than the soul. What is within is also without. This is the keynote of the ancient Indian philosophical tradition.

The second story also reflects the view that liberation is the highest goal of life and no price is too great to pay for it. The sole means to it is the knowledge of the soul, the ultimate source and goal of love.

Following the message reflected in these stories, but in keeping with its fidelity to rational thinking, Yoga views Reality as consisting of two ultimate principles: Matter and Spirit, or soul.

Physics and Metaphysics

The field of inquiry implied in these dialogues is broadly known as metaphysics. Metaphysics, like physics, is a way of thinking supported by evidence that leaves no scope for human will. This character of metaphysics or philosophy is expressed in the *Upaniṣads* when they explain the nature of Ultimate Reality as beyond duties and taboos. Thus, the difference between physics and metaphysics lies not so much in their approach as in their targets. Physics explores the outer world, the object; metaphysics explores the inner world, the subject. If physics is the science of Matter, metaphysics is the science of Spirit, or soul.

Metaphysics and Ethics

Metaphysics, the science of being, is concerned with what is or is not. It explains the soul in its true nature beyond all worldly adjuncts such as pleasure and pain, good and bad, virtue and sin. Metaphysics is, therefore, distinct from ethics, which is concerned with what one should or should not do. Metaphysics is based on universal means of knowledge, such as perception and inference, that do not change with cultural traditions. Ethics is based on collective human will, which shapes the diverse minds and traditions of societies. It is the element of will in ethics, absent in metaphysics, that makes a world of difference between the two.

In Brief

A clod of earth being understood, everything earthen is known.
The underlying essence being understood, the whole world is known.

The essence of the visible world is established in the soul, the seer.
It is the core of all, the most cherished, the experience of all.

Hence, the soul being understood, nothing remains unknown.
It alone should be understood through study, meditation, and deep absorption.

That is called philosophy which explains, of things outer and inner,
The quintessence that is eternal and beyond conventions.

For a wider perspective ...

Education in Ancient India

In ancient India, schooling was conducted by teachers in their own houses. An initiation sacrament at the age of eight marked the beginning of education, when the boy approached the teacher, lived in his house, served him, and received learning according to a method characterized by oral transmission and memorization. This pattern was followed by sons from learned, royal and rich families. There was a rigorous daily routine including religious rites and the study of the Vedic literature of the Veda branch to which he traditionally belonged. This scheme continued for twelve years. At the end of this period, the student offered the teacher whatever he could afford as a token of his gratitude and went home to embark on the second stage of his life—marriage and a householder's duties, which included the regular revision of his studies. Not receiving regular fees, these schools were supported by kings and well-to-do members of society. There are no references to women's education in a similar pattern, although learned women, participating in open, scholarly debates and displaying profound philosophical knowledge, are found in the *Upaniṣads*.

Renunciation

Life in ancient Indian society was conventionally organized into four successive stages:

1. Celibacy (for study)
2. Householder (for religious and social duties)
3. Forest living (a retired life marked by simple living and high thinking, preparatory to the fourth stage)
4. Renunciation (the rigorous life of an ascetic, who rejects worldly comforts and pleasures, devoted to seeking and experiencing Ultimate Reality)

The first two stages were commonly undertaken; the rest were optional and depended on the mind and intellect of the individual concerned. In the stories above, the boy Śvetaketu was in the first stage; the seer Yājñavalkya was on the verge of leaving the second stage and entering the fourth stage directly, omitting the third one.

Unit 2

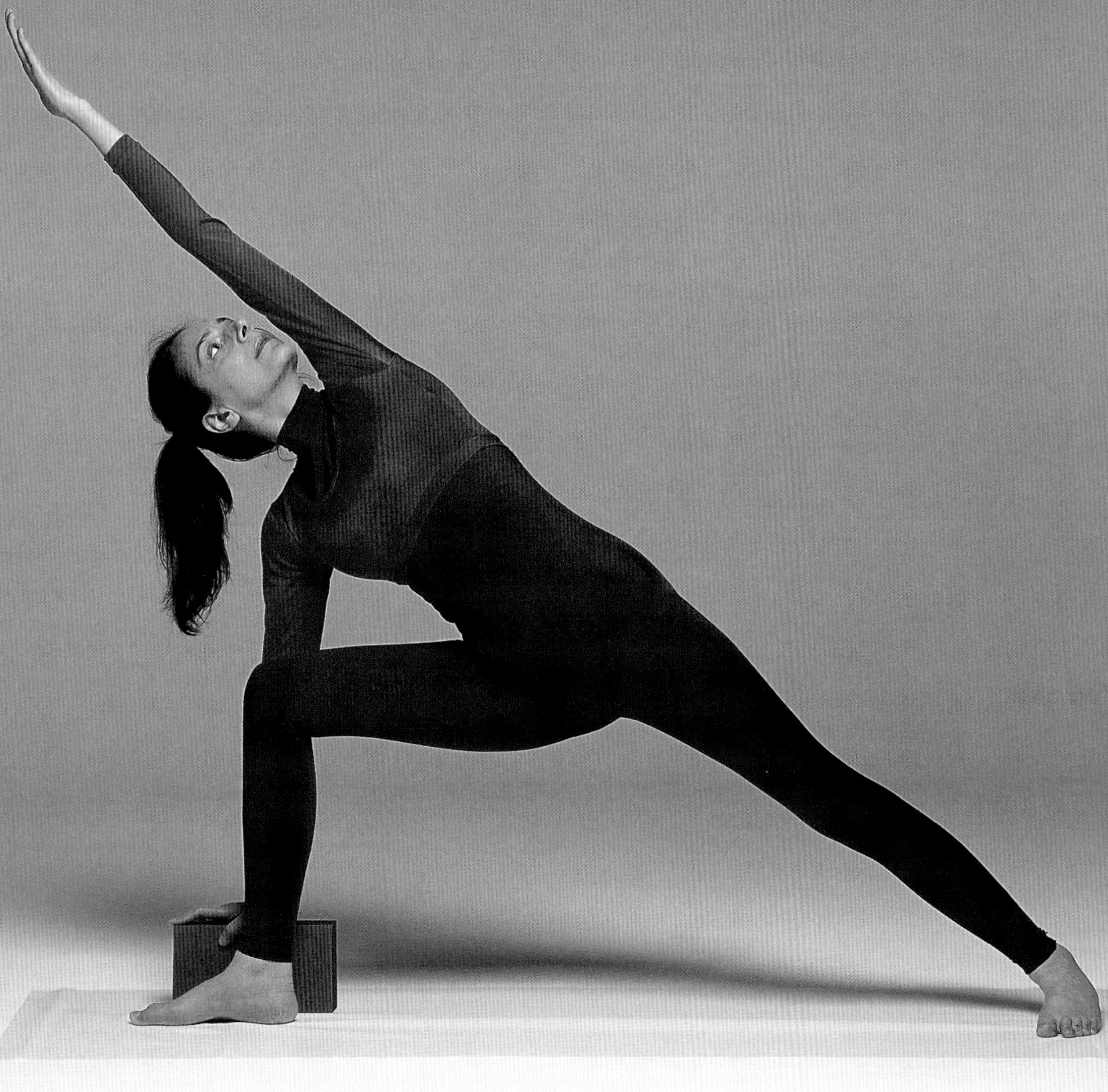

The Yadu men fighting each other at Prabhāsa, from an illustrated manuscript dated A.D. 1648.

Yoga in life

FREEDOM FROM PAIN

A ravaged wilderness where grows
Nothing save a thorny thicket
Piercing one who seeks its flowers:

A challenge to the gardener's skills,
To tame and coax wild nature
Into gentle cultivation.

Suffering is part and parcel of the experience of living. It is defined in the Yoga literature as that which all creatures seek to avoid, and it gives rise to aversion, one of the root causes of suffering that shape the mind.[1]

Fully acknowledging the painful reality of existence, Yoga is optimistic with regard to the removal of future pain. It asserts that a remedy is known for every avoidable cause of pain.[2]

The example is given of a thorn pricking the foot; avoidance of this pain lies in not treading on the thorn or in wearing shoes. The solution begins with knowledge: that a thorn can prick and that a foot can be pricked. Applying this knowledge creates the remedy.

Understanding the factors responsible for hurtful situations and realizing our areas of vulnerability enable us to find the cure. However thorny the path of life may be, means of protection can be identified.

[1] *Yoga Sūtra 2.8*

[2] *Commentary on Yoga Sūtra 2.17*

How to stretch

The incessant pull of gravity on the body acts to contract it: joints are compacted, muscles shortened, and soft tissue compressed. This reduces the circulation to these parts and further encourages degeneration and atrophy. In childhood the upward force of growth maintains space and free energy flow within the body; when growth stops, decline sets in, either slowly or rapidly.

Stretching involves the elongation of muscles and the decompression of joints and soft tissue; for these reasons it has the power to inhibit decline. It can even bring about regeneration. Animals in their natural habitat stretch routinely after waking and are constantly on the move, retaining a beautiful coordination of limbs until old age.

When the body has lost the innate habit of stretching, nature has to be restored through knowledge. The action of stretching is exemplified by elastic. One way to stretch elastic is to hold one end firm while pulling on the other end. Similarly, in order to stretch one part of the body, an adjacent part is held firm. For example, in order to stretch the palms, the fingers need to be extended and the knuckles tightened. In order to stretch the thigh muscle (quadriceps), the knee joint has to be kept tight.

There is a complex interplay between joints and muscles: muscles cannot stretch when the joints are lax, and joints cannot be extended without accompanying muscle extension. As extensions become more effective, muscles become toned and knit more efficiently to the bones that underlie them. Ultimately, when deep muscles are activated in the stretch, bone and muscle can act together. In this way a high level of energy is maintained in all parts of the body.

Standing poses are supreme for learning how to stretch. They strengthen the feet and legs and bring mobility to the knees, hips, and spine. Surprisingly, they also strengthen the arms. This is because they involve keeping the arms in a raised position. The wide span their shapes encompass makes the body lengthen in all directions. Several standing poses are introduced in this Unit.

It is also useful to learn to stretch while lying down. When on the floor, the back gets a sense of direction as well as a support. The horizontal stretch is not opposed by gravity, and therefore the body lengthens more easily.

Standing poses are strenuous, particularly for the legs. Therefore, they need to be balanced by other poses. Kneeling, one of the other basic human resting positions, gives quick relief to the legs. Bending forward is restful for the heart. Combining the two, by kneeling and bending forward with the head supported, removes any strain incurred through the standing poses.

ताडासन *Tāḍāsana*

Mountain or Palm Tree Pose

Coordination of stretches and concentration are needed to maintain balance on both sides of the body in this seemingly simple pose.

Follow the method given in Unit 1 (page 19).

To Progress

Lift the toes, stretch them forward, and place them down again. Lift the heels, stretch them back away from the arches, and place them down again. Stretch the legs up from the ankles. Stretch the calves and backs of the thighs, as well as the fronts of the legs. Draw the hips up, and stretch the sides of the trunk. Try to stretch evenly on both sides.

ऊर्ध्व-हस्तासन *Ūrdhva-Hastāsana*

Mountain Pose with Arms Up

The body reaches up and up with the help of this arm stretch.

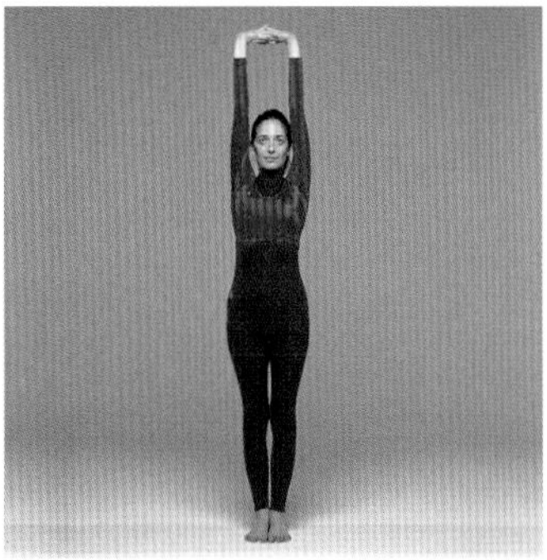

Stand in *Tāḍāsana* (see Unit 1, page 19). Interlock the fingers and turn the palms outward. Inhale and stretch the arms over the head. Tighten the elbows and press the wrists up.

Stay in the pose for 10 to 15 seconds. Exhale and bring the arms down. Change the interlock of the fingers, by crossing them the other way, and repeat.

To Progress

Pull the sides of the trunk up with the help of the arms. Do not collapse the trunk when bringing the arms down.

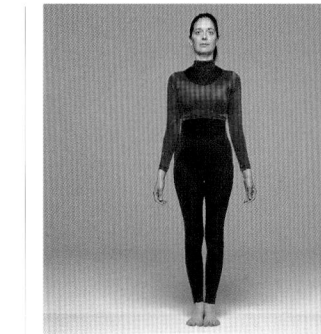

त्रिकोणासन *Trikoṇāsana*

Triangle Pose

Arms, legs, and trunk stretch simultaneously in different directions —vertically, horizontally and diagonally— creating space and energy in the body.

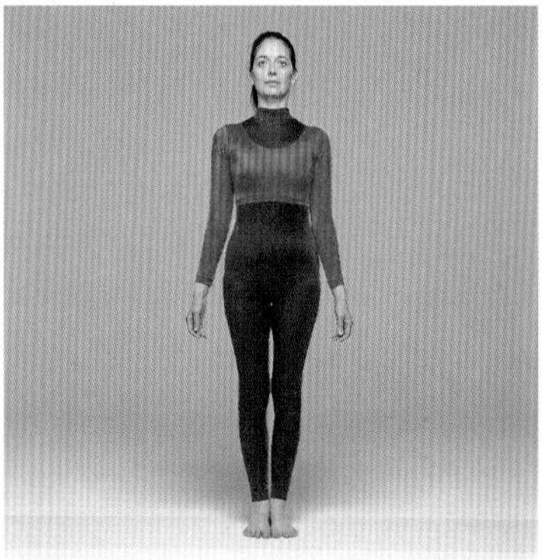

Stand in *Tāḍāsana* (see Unit 1, page 19).

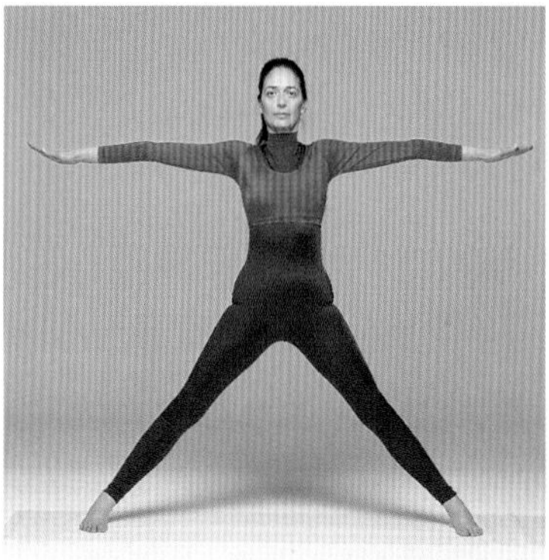

Take a deep inhalation and jump the feet 3½–4 feet apart, simultaneously extending the arms sideways to shoulder level with the palms facing down. Align the feet and make them parallel.

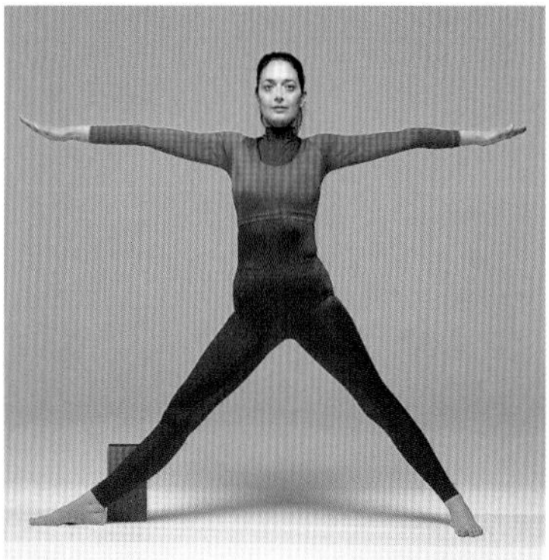

Place a brick upright behind the right foot. Turn the left foot 15 degrees in and the right foot 90 degrees out. Align the center of the right heel with the center of the left arch. Revolve each leg outward. Tighten the kneecaps, and pull up the thigh muscles.

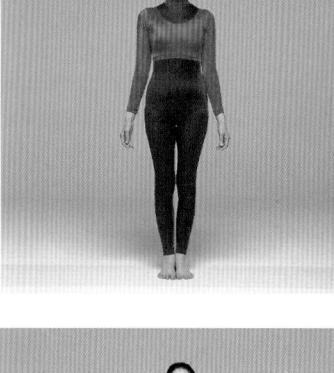

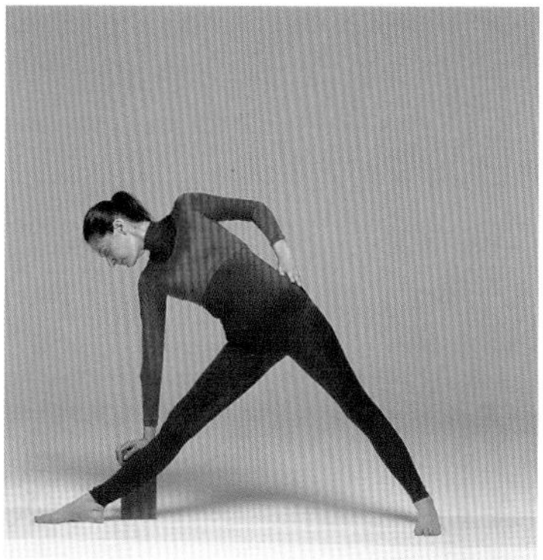

Exhale and take the trunk sideways down to the right; place the right hand on the brick. The brick is used so that the hand does not have so far to reach and the trunk does not collapse. Rest the left hand on the hip and revolve the trunk upward.

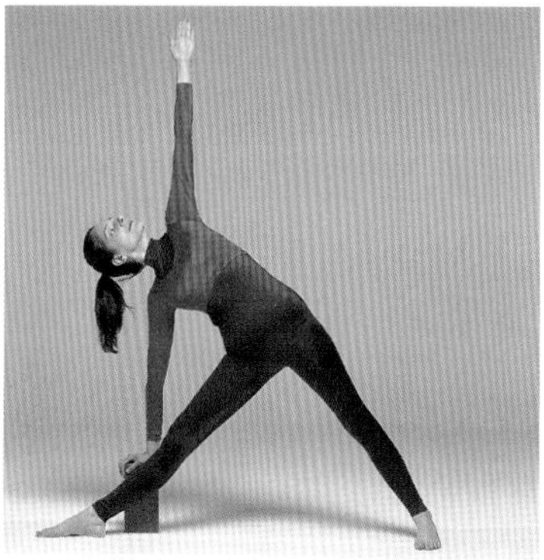

Stretch the left arm up, and turn the palm to face forward. Turn the neck and head, and look up at the hand. Breathe evenly.

Stay in the pose for 20 to 30 seconds. Inhale and come up. Turn the feet to the front and rest the arms. Then repeat on the other side.

Inhale and come up. Exhale and jump the feet together, simultaneously bringing the arms down.

To Progress

Stretch the toes. Keep the knees firm. Lift the left inner ankle and press the outer edge of the left foot down. Stretch the leg up away from the foot. Keep the right ankle firm, and extend the leg away from the foot.

Stretch the trunk in the direction of the head. Keep the elbows firm. Stretch the arms as if from the center of the chest.

Keep the left wrist firm, and stretch the palm and fingers. Keep the fingers together.

पार्श्वकोणासन *Pārśvakoṇāsana*

Side Angle Pose

Buttressed by the front leg and one arm, the diagonal stretch of this pose spans from the back foot, through the trunk, to the top hand.

Stand in *Tāḍāsana* (see Unit 1, page 19).

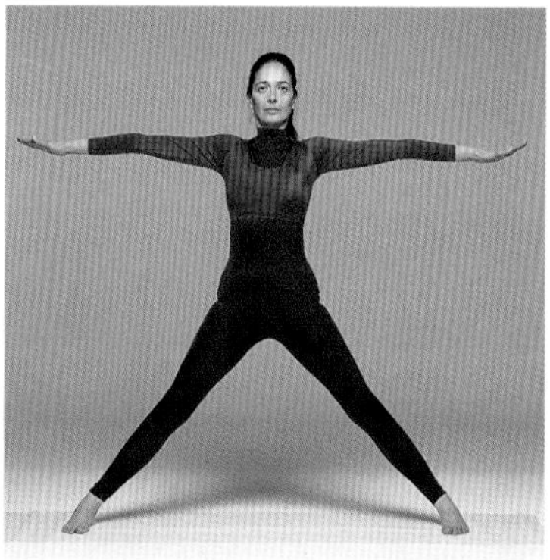

Take a deep inhalation and jump 4–4½ feet apart, simultaneously extending the arms sideways to shoulder level, with the palms facing down. Align the feet and make them parallel.

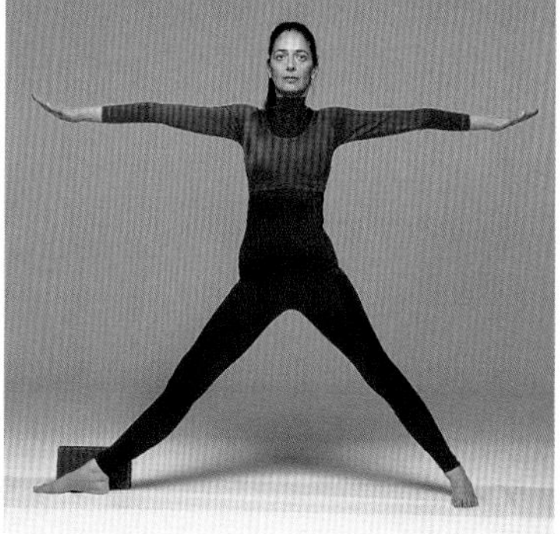

Place a brick horizontally behind the right foot. Turn the left foot 15 degrees in and the right foot 90 degrees out. Align the center of the right heel with the center of the left arch. Revolve each leg outward. Tighten the kneecaps, and pull up the thigh muscles.

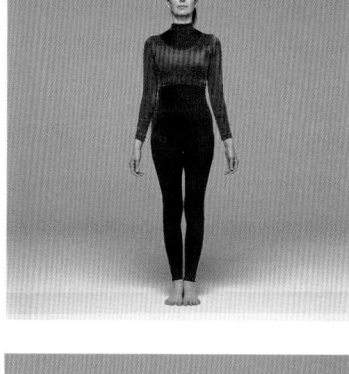

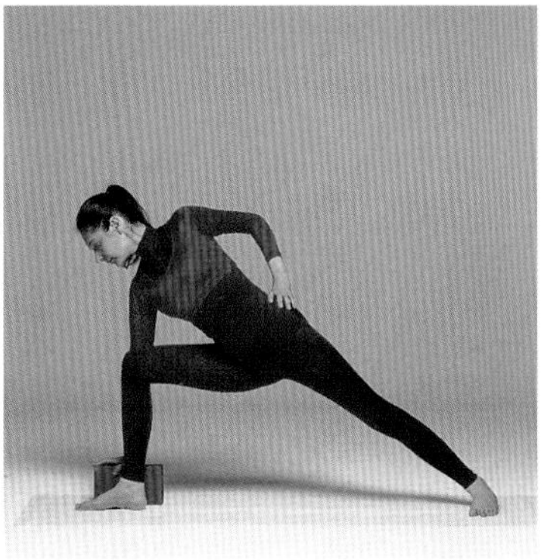

Exhale, and bend the right leg to form a right angle, with the shin vertical and the thigh horizontal. Simultaneously take the trunk sideways down toward the thigh and place the right hand on the brick. The brick support gives the trunk height from the floor so that it does not collapse. Rest the left hand on the hip. Revolve the trunk upward.

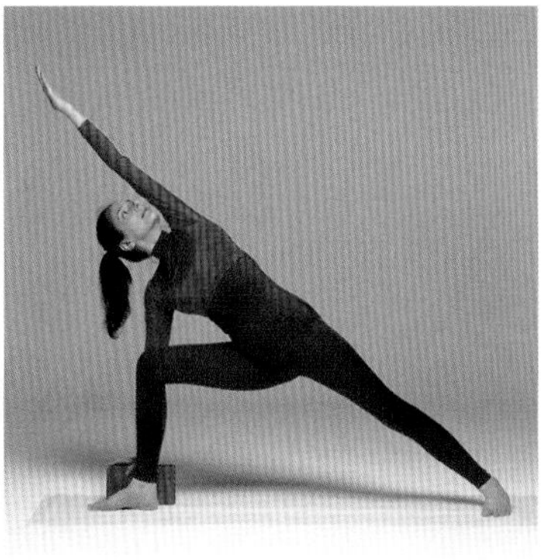

Take the left arm over the head with the palm facing down. Turn the neck and head and look up at the arm. Breathe evenly and without strain.

Stay in the pose for 20 to 30 seconds. Inhale and come up. Turn the feet to the front, and rest the arms. Then repeat on the other side.

Inhale and come up. Exhale and jump the feet together, simultaneously bringing the arms down.

To Progress

Stretch the toes. Lift the left inner ankle, and press the outer edge of the left foot down. Stretch the leg up away from the foot. Keep the knee firm.

Stretch the left side of the trunk from hip to armpit. Lengthen the right side of the trunk and bring it forward.

Open the left armpit, turn the left arm more, so that the palm faces down, and stretch the arm. Keep the elbow, wrist, and knuckles firm. Open the palm and stretch the fingers.

वीरभद्रासन २ *Vīrabhadrāsana 2*

Warrior Pose 2

Horizontal arms extend from a vertical trunk on asymmetrically placed legs: the strength of the straight leg and the back are the invisible supports of this stretch.

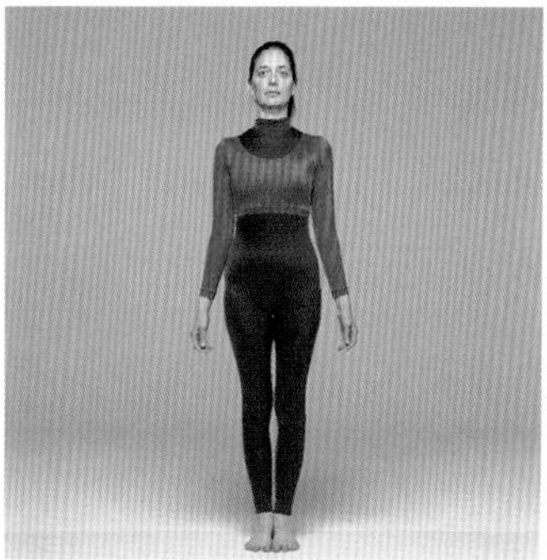

Stand in *Tāḍāsana* (see Unit 1, page 19).

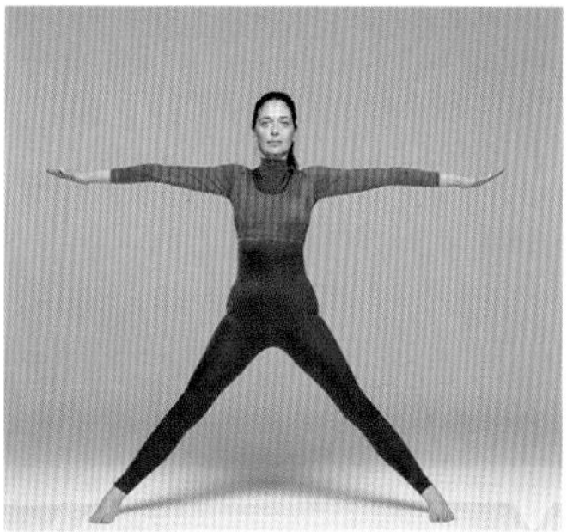

Take a deep inhalation, and jump the feet 4–4½ feet apart, simultaneously extending the arms sideways to shoulder level, with the palms facing down. Align the feet and make them parallel.

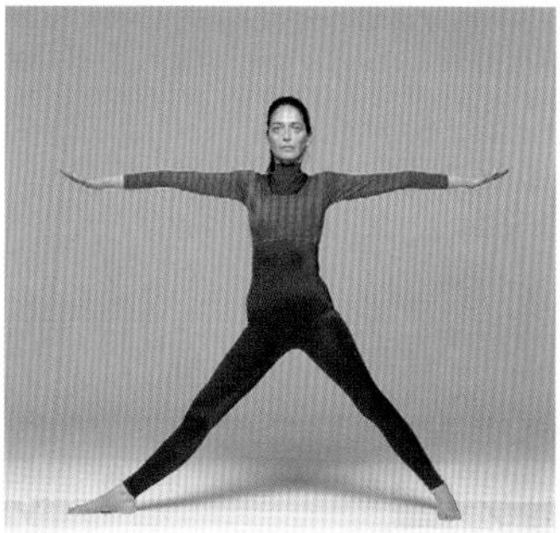

Turn the left foot 15 degrees in and the right foot 90 degrees out. Align the center of the right heel with the center of the left arch. Revolve each leg outward. Tighten the kneecaps, and pull up the thigh muscles.

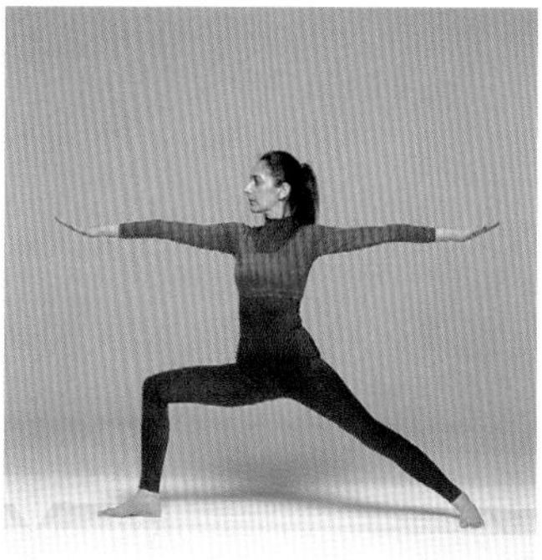

Exhale and bend the right leg to form a right angle, with the shin vertical and the thigh horizontal. Keep the trunk vertical and facing forward, with the arms parallel to the floor.

Turn the neck and head, and look to the right. Breathe evenly and without strain.

Stay in the pose for 20 to 30 seconds. Inhale and come up. Turn the feet to the front and rest the arms. Then repeat on the other side.

Inhale and come up. Exhale and jump the feet together, simultaneously bringing the arms down.

To Progress

Lift the left inner ankle and press the outer edge of the foot down. Stretch the leg away from the foot. Keep the knees firm.

Pull the left arm farther to the left, in order to keep the trunk upright. Stretch the sides of the trunk up but keep the shoulders down.

Keep the elbows firm. Extend the arms as if from the center of the chest. Keep the wrists firm and stretch the hands.

अर्ध-उत्तानासन *Ardha-Uttānāsana*

Half Intense Stretch

Supported by the hands and arms at one end and the hips at the other, the horizontal spine extends beautifully and without strain.

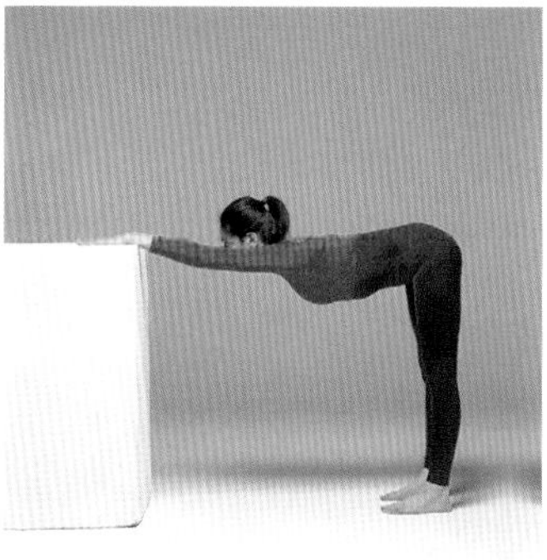

Stand 2–2½ feet away from a ledge of hip-height. Take the feet hip-width apart. Bend forward from the hips and place the hands on the ledge. Keep the knees tight and stretch the legs up. Draw the hips slightly back and move the trunk down without bending the elbows. Breathe evenly.

Stay in the pose for 20 to 30 seconds. Inhale and come up. Bring the feet together.

To Progress

Adjust the position of the feet so that the legs are perpendicular to the floor. Stretch the spine more and more.

अधो-मुख-वीरासन *Adho-Mukha-Vīrāsana*

Hero Pose, Head Down

This kneeling forward bend relaxes legs, back, and head.

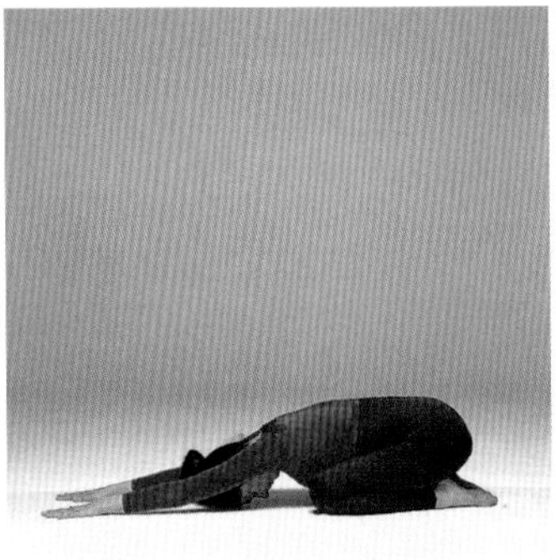

Kneel. Bring the toes together and take the knees apart. Stretch the trunk up and bend forward from the hips, with the sides of the trunk touching the thighs. Take the arms forward, and rest the head on the floor.

Stay in the pose for 20 to 30 seconds, or longer if more rest is required. Inhale and come up. Bring the legs to the front.

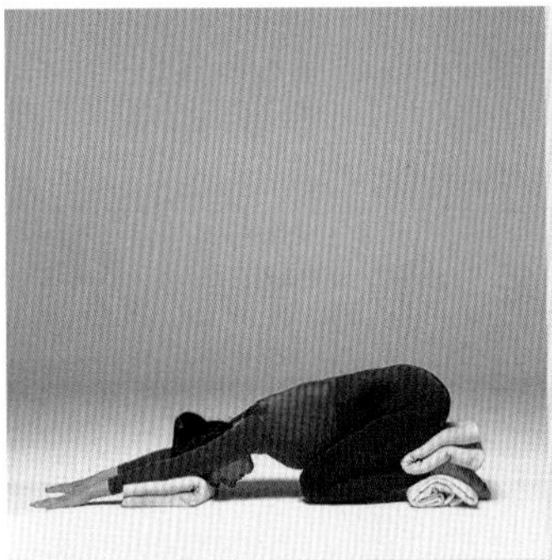

Help

- **If the ankles are stiff, place a rolled blanket under the lower shins.**
- **If the buttocks do not rest on the heels, place a folded blanket on the heels.**
- **If the head does not reach the floor, rest it on a folded blanket.**

To Progress

Press the hips down, and stretch the arms farther forward.

पर्वतासन *Parvatāsana*

Mountain Pose

The stretch of the arms and trunk unite to give a towering height to this sitting pose.

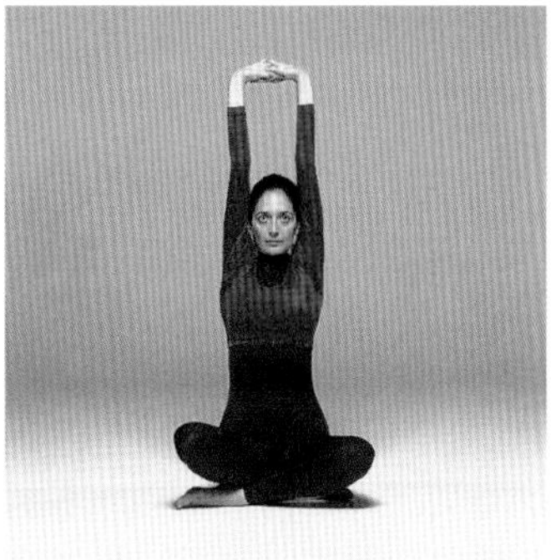

Follow the method given in Unit 1 (page 24).

To Progress

Incorporate the shoulder region in the stretch: move the shoulder blades in, and open the armpits.

शयित-ऊर्ध्व-हस्तासन *Śayita-Ūrdhva-Hastāsana*

Lying-Down Arm Stretch

A two-way stretch dividing at the waist elongates the body.

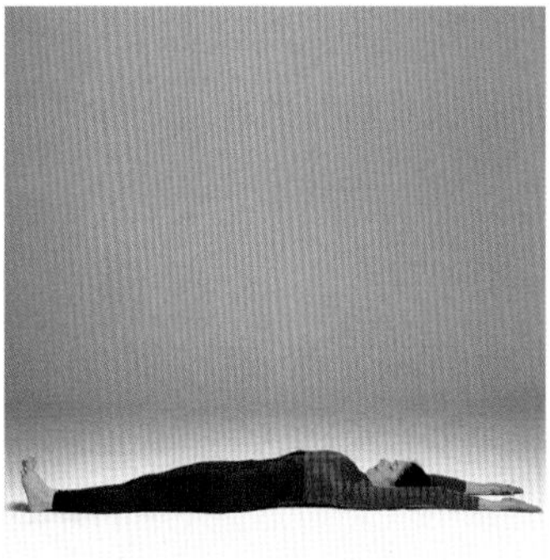

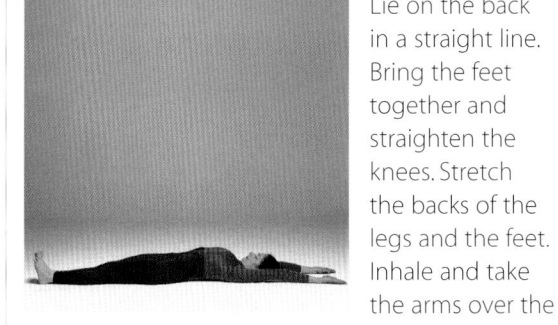

Lie on the back in a straight line. Bring the feet together and straighten the knees. Stretch the backs of the legs and the feet. Inhale and take the arms over the head. Tighten the elbows and stretch the fingers. Stretch from the waist down toward the feet and up toward the hands.

Stay in the pose for 10 to 15 seconds. Bring the arms down and relax the arms and legs.

To Progress

Keep the legs and arms poker-stiff. Lengthen the sides of the trunk.

मत्स्यासन *Matsyāsana*

Fish Pose

The crossed legs anchor the pelvis, enabling a strong stretch of the upper body and arms. A Yogin is said to be able to float in this pose when the legs are fully crossed in the Lotus Pose.

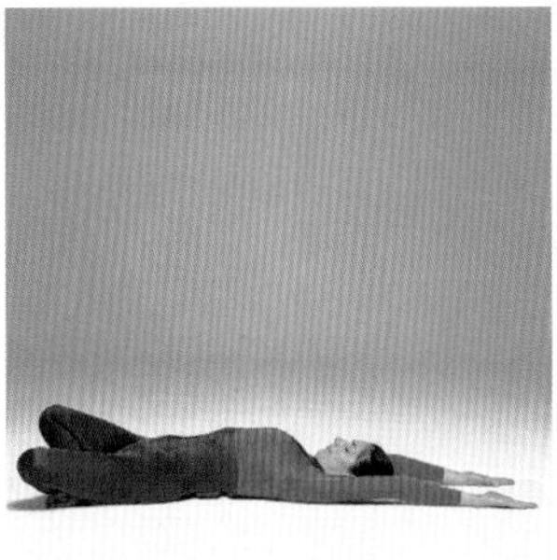

Sit with the legs simply crossed. Lie down and stretch the arms over the head. Tighten the elbows. Adjust the hips so that they are level.

Stay in the pose for 1 to 2 minutes. Come up and repeat with the legs crossed the other way.

To Progress

Use the arms to help stretch the sides of the trunk. Relax the arms intermittently in order to stretch with renewed vigor.

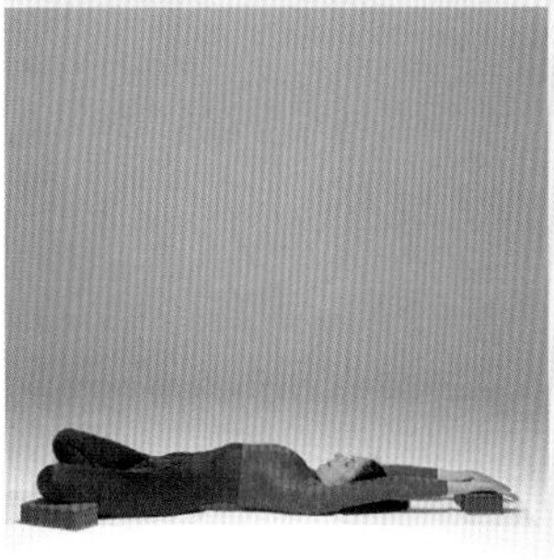

Help

- **If the groins feel strained, place supports under the thighs.**
- **Hold a brick between the palms to give strength to the arm stretch.**
- **If the hands do not touch the floor, place them on a support.**

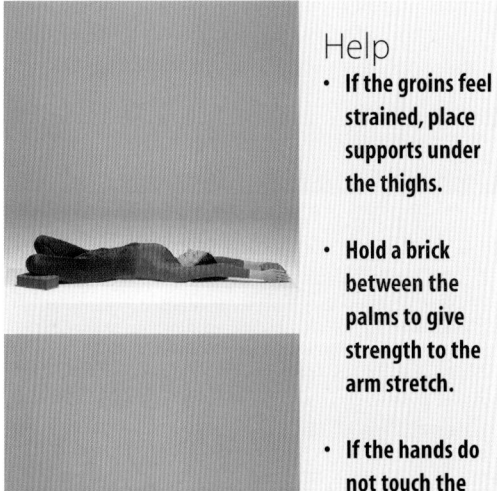

ऊर्ध्व-प्रसारित-पादासन *Ūrdhva-Prasārita-Pādāsana*

Upward Leg Extension

Inverting the legs against the wall brings fast recovery from fatigue.

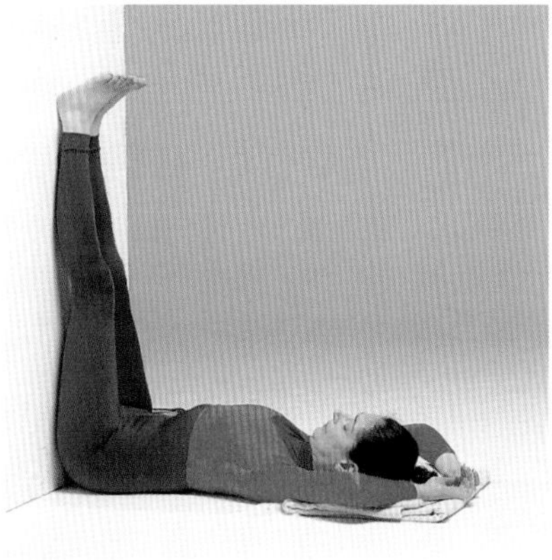

Follow the method given in Unit 1 (page 25).

To Progress

Understand that relaxation is an important adjunct to stretching, allowing the muscles to renew their energy. Learn to stay still.

शवासन *Śavāsana*

Corpse Pose

Lying flat in pseudo-sleep, the body is receptive to imprinting the memory of actions and stretches in the various poses.

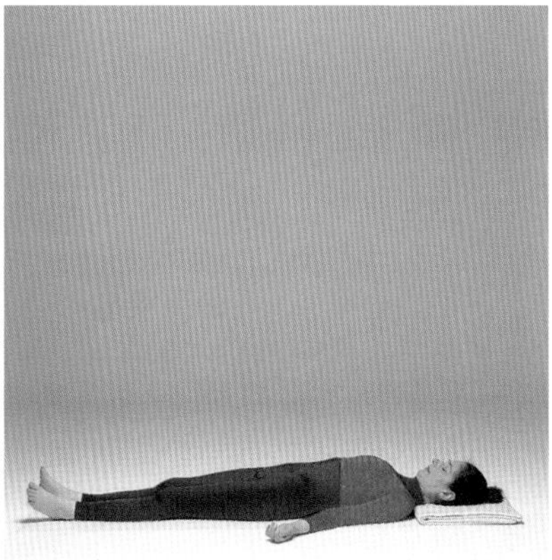

Follow the method given in Unit 1 (page 26).

To Progress

Subdue any urge to move. If there is discomfort somewhere, observe the reason for it, then adjust carefully without disturbing other parts of the body. Keep the eyes still; this maintains the inner focus of the mind.

The soul

KEY CONCEPT

God of Death According to Indian mythology, there is a supernatural world of gods commanding natural phenomena beyond human control. Such a god in charge of dying creatures is Yama, also called Death. He is believed to take charge of the soul after the death of its physical body and subject it to the consequences of its actions. The author of the following story takes a poetic flight in assigning to the god of Death himself the task of throwing light on the post-death destiny of souls.

We have seen how the philosopher investigates the outer and inner worlds to find their essence and also how the concept of the soul, being the ultimate source of love, is at the center of the search into the inner world. We can now go deeper into the nature of the soul. The following story, well known in the Indian philosophical tradition, highlights this topic.

A Dialogue with Death

A precocious boy, Naciketas (whose name means "ignorant"!), was sent to the god of Death by his father. As the story goes, the father was giving malnourished, lame cows as religious gifts. The boy realized that this was against the spirit of gift and repeatedly asked him: "Father, to whom will you give *me* as a gift?"

"To Death," replied the father, irritated by his son's persistence.

Naciketas took his father at his word and went to the abode of the god of Death. He found the god away on business. For three days he waited at the door, fasting and refusing the hospitality offered by the god's family. This worried the god on his return, and, as compensation for his failure in his duty as a householder, he offered three boons to the boy. For the first wish, Naciketas requested reconciliation with his father. His second request was for knowledge about the fire worship that leads to life in heaven.

For the third boon, he asked what happens to the soul after death. The god considered this topic too lofty for a young boy and offered to give him, instead, everything a worldly man would seek—wealth, progeny, land, long life, and so on. The boy was obstinate; he did not budge an inch from his demand. Finally, the god yielded and explained to him the nature of the soul.

In the course of the dialogue Naciketas pinpointed his interest: "Tell me that which is beyond virtue and sin, cause and effect and past and future." In brief, he wanted to know what was beyond the limitations of all that is worldly. The phrase "beyond virtue and sin" implies that philosophy in essence is not concerned with morality and ethics. In reply the god of Death pointed out to Naciketas: "The soul is neither born, nor does it die when the body dies. It is eternal. It is incorporeal, though it is housed in bodies. It is all-pervading. Its knowledge leads the knower to a state beyond grief"—that is, to liberation. (*Kaṭha Upaniṣad*)

The Existence of the Soul

This passage takes us deeper into the subject introduced in the last Unit, namely, metaphysics. It states in brief that the soul is beyond limitations that characterize worldly objects. This raises the question as to what makes the soul or spirit differ from the mind. This problem engaged the minds of *Upaniṣadic* thinkers, who argued that the soul as the viewer of the body-mind complex had to be identified as a separate entity, for no object can view itself. They attempted also to analyze the various states of consciousness—waking, dream and deep sleep—in order to determine the nature of the soul. They arrived at the conclusion that the soul's essential character—consciousness and bliss untouched by worldly pleasure and pain—is revealed in deep sleep.

One popular argument for the independent existence of the soul is based on the case of a woman arousing distinct responses in people with different attitudes. On seeing her, her lover is delighted; a rejected suitor is sad; and a stranger is indifferent. This example shows that responses to the same object vary according to different mind-sets and that the woman exists independently of the minds that view her.

The Mind as Knowable

Patañjali, whose work on Yoga is pre-eminently a treatise on the mind, examines the problem logically, and by analyzing universal experience arrives at a conclusive proof. The mind takes the "shape" of objects it views, both with and without the aid of the sense organs. It is thus an ever-changing entity. We are aware of the mind changing, and this indicates that there is some constant, invariable principle that acts as observer. The mind cannot function both as object and observer, since an object cannot logically be its own observer.

Another argument for the existence of the soul is founded on the way the mind and soul function. The mind operates in association with many guiding factors, such as memory imprints, prejudices, sentiments, and so on. This manner of functioning is found in all cases where the functionary acts not for itself but for another, just as a house, constructed of many components, serves the purpose of its inhabitant. For the mind, this "other" is the soul whose sole function is observation. In fact, the view is that the soul does not function (that is, operate) at all, since its intrinsic nature is awareness. This position leads to the corollary that the observer, the soul, lacking characteristics (color, form, smell, and so on) that are the basis on which the sense organs and mind function, is beyond their ability to know.

The Soul as Knower

What, then, is the proof of the existence of the soul? This question can be answered by a counter question: What is the proof of the existence of the mind, which lacks characteristics—color, form, smell and so on—that can be perceived by the senses? The reply is that we cannot account for the interpretation of data received by our sense organs and the decision for actions based on this unless we assume the existence of the mind.

A similar explanation can be offered for the existence of the soul: cognition of the functions of the mind cannot be explained unless the soul's existence is assumed. The most conclusive proof is, of course, the self-awareness experienced by everyone. There can be no dispute about the fact that perception is superior to inference, as the latter is ultimately founded on the former.

As an *Upaniṣadic* thinker asks, How can one know that which is the foundation of all knowing? Everything in the world is contained in space; in what is space contained? In other words, it is useless to insist on a proof of the existence of the soul that must fit in the accepted framework of knowledge, which is bounded within the limits of the mind.

The god Viṣṇu manifests himself in his cosmic form.

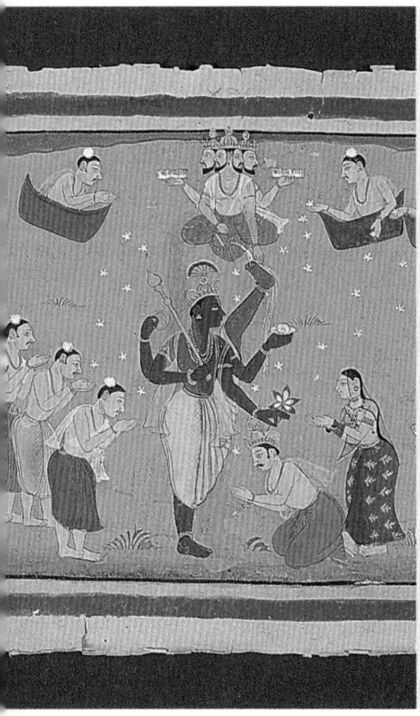

In Brief

What is called philosophy is an inquiry into Ultimate Reality.
That consists of soul and non-soul, as is everyone's objective experience.

The soul is the seer, and the world that which is seen; who can dispute this?
What is the nature of the soul? On this point debaters disagree.

Its nature is consciousness and bliss; worldly existence settles on it through ignorance.
Realization of this leads to liberation, which is the restoration of the soul's intrinsic state.

Morality and immorality, sin and virtue, pleasure and pain, comings and goings.
All this is rooted in ignorance and resembles experience in a dream.

The mind is changeable and observed; the soul, the observer, is ever unchanging;
As the unique viewer of the mind, its existence is demonstrable.

For a wider perspective ...

The World of Gods

According to Indian mythology there is a supernatural world of beings that corresponds to the human world in essential features. It consists of both good and evil elements, represented respectively by gods and demons. In keeping with the fundamental logic of the concept, specific gods are thought to manage natural phenomena beyond human control. Thus, the god **Indra** is in charge of rains, **Varuṇa** in charge of sea waters, **Vāyu** of air, **Agni** of fire, and so on. In this scheme, **Brahmā** (masculine in gender, different from the philosophical concept of *brahman*, neuter in gender, as the impersonal, universal principle) is in charge of creation, or birth, and **Yama** of death. These gods derive their powers from, and are responsible to, the supreme God (with a capital G) variously called **Viṣṇu**, **Śiva**, and so on. Their duties are guided in a general way by the fates (*karmas*) of souls. *Karma* is thus conceived to correspond to law in human society; it is this power that saves the world from turning into chaos. Officiating gods have a have a habitat of their own. What is called heaven is the habitat of the god **Indra**. Virtuous souls go to these superior habitats after death and enjoy pleasures there till their merit is finished. Sinners go to hell (corresponding to human prisons) under the control of **Yama** to experience sufferings matching their sins till their sins are finished.

Aspects of the Soul

The soul is defined as the "immaterial essence of an individual life; the spiritual principle embodied in human beings." The latter definition may not be considered relevant in philosophy, as it restricts the usage of the term to human beings, excluding other forms of life. Even the former definition leaves some aspects of the concept untouched, aspects that Indian philosophy prefers to specify and for which it uses a different term.

Indian philosophy views the "immaterial essence" in two capacities: (a) essence as restricted by aspects of worldly life such as pleasure and pain, love and hate, and so on; (b) essence in its pure form unrelated to life. It limits the term "living soul" (*jīva*) to the first definition and employs the term "self" (*ātman*) for the second. Although such a usage does not make a difference to the essential meaning, Indian philosophy has the practical aim of restoring the essence, the conscious principle, to its pure state, untouched by worldly experiences—a state of unspecified bliss, as exemplified by the experience in deep sleep. This restoration, called liberation, is comparable to that of sound health, free from diseases in normal life. As life is inseparably associated with breathing, ego, and emotions, liberation is conceived to be free from these limitations. Since the subtle distinction between the two meanings does not exist in English, the same term "soul" is used throughout.

Unit 3

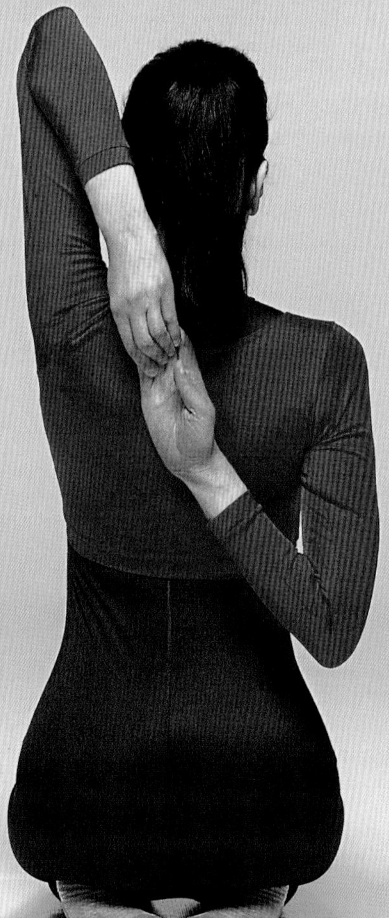

Box pictures showing the diversity of life, from an illustrated *Bhāgavata Purāṇa* manuscript.

Yoga in life

CHANCE AND DESTINY

Windward swept
By chance and circumstance
Into the lee
Of its natural support,
The creeper basks
In the living of the tree
And blooms in its shelter
With embrace.

Life seems to be a haphazard mix of chance and planned encounters, brief and lasting relationships, inconsequent and fateful decisions, and happy and sorrowful times. Surely everyone has tried at some stage to seek a pattern in their own particular chain of events and ties, and to answer the question, *Why*?

Yoga philosophy holds that this current life can be understood only in the context of an unending series of incarnations which each soul undergoes. The unfinished business of past lives must be finished in a future life, in accordance with the law of cause and effect. This is *karma*, the sum of actions that we all carry about with us as invisible baggage and that transmigrates along with the soul.

It is stated that the consequences of actions are seen in three aspects of reincarnation: species type, lifespan, and experiences.[1] Experiences are happy or painful in accordance with previous good or bad actions.[2]

Thus, Yoga philosophy asserts that our destiny is in our own hands. Just as the present is shaped by the past, so the future is shaped by the present which becomes the past. Following this logic, Yoga concludes that suffering in times to come can be avoided.[3]

---

1 *Yoga Sūtra 2.13*
2 *Yoga Sūtra 2.14*
3 *Yoga Sūtra 2.16*

The plane of the body

When the body stands erect, its various parts are held in place within the vertical plane. If any part tilts out of the plane, the body's structural strength and functional efficiency are impaired. For the sake of health, therefore, it is worthwhile to strive for this alignment.

Standing poses are designed with the plane of the body in mind. They form various geometrical shapes with angles, diagonals, and straight lines, but their core direction is the vertical.

It is difficult to achieve this postural ideal in free space because space accommodates any distortion of the body. A sense of line is more easily gained when standing against a wall. The wall concretely parallels the invisible plane of the body and does not allow movements beyond it.

Furthermore, with the physical support of the wall, the effects of standing poses are maximized. For example, a basic instruction in Triangle Pose (*Trikoṇāsana*) is to turn the trunk upward. This rotation is facilitated when the back rests against the wall.

Although the wall is a support, doing the poses against it is, paradoxically, more strenuous than doing them in the middle of the room because of the increased accuracy and range of movement demanded of the body. Exertion is balanced by rest: vigorous standing poses are followed by poses that involve sitting, to rest the legs; bending forward, to rest the head and heart; and inverting the body, to revitalize the whole being.

While the emphasis in standing poses is naturally on the feet and legs, the arms should not be neglected. They have to learn to bend as well as to stretch. Arm positions, as in Cow-Head Pose (*Gomukhāsana*), work not just on the arms but on the whole area of the upper back, neck, and shoulders.

The mobility and lightness developed through these various standing and sitting poses are needed for inverted poses. To maintain an upside-down position requires strength and freedom in the upper back and shoulders. An extremely important posture in this regard, and one that gives a supreme stretch to the whole body, is Dog Pose (*Adho-Mukha-Śvānasāna*). Although introduced here after standing poses, it is often done at the beginning of a practice session. Strong work for the arms, shoulders, and legs, it is at the same time restful because the head and heart are lower than the hips. This means that it can be repeated many times without strain.

The unfamiliar actions involved in the postures need to be assimilated into the body's "memory." This needs time and a period of stillness. Corpse Pose (*Śavāsana*) provides just such a setting. Lying down quietly, without mental or physical distractions, makes body and mind receptive to the imprints of what has been learned.

ताडासन *Tāḍāsana*

Mountain or Palm Tree Pose

Our sense of verticality is challenged by the wall, which tells us that we habitually tilt or zigzag off the true.

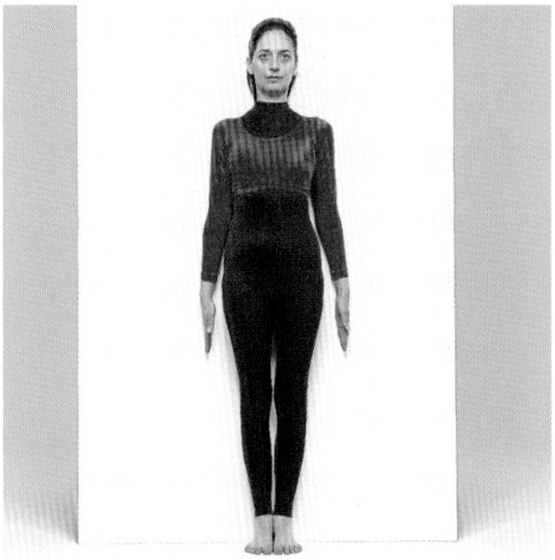

Stand with the heels, buttocks, shoulders, and back of the head against the wall. Pass the hands downward along the lower back, and release it away from the waist. Keep the feet together, joining the big toes, inner heels, and inner ankles. Tighten the kneecaps, join the inner knees, and pull up the thigh muscles. Press the legs toward the wall. Extend the trunk away from the legs.

Draw the abdomen up and, without collapsing the chest, press the waist toward the wall. Take the shoulders back and down, and press the shoulder blades in. Press the thoracic spine in, especially between the shoulder blades. Stretch the arms and hands downward, with the palms facing the thighs. Lift the base of the skull, and extend the neck upward. Keep the head straight. Relax the eyes and face, and look ahead. Breathe evenly.

Stay in the pose for 20 to 30 seconds.

To Progress

Feel the back of the body against the wall, and draw the front of the body toward it.

ऊर्ध्व-हस्तासन *Ūrdhva-Hastāsana*

Upraised Arm Stretch

We should perhaps admire our ape cousins, who keep their arms upraised with ease, thanks to powerfully active hands, flexible shoulder joints, and well extended armpits!

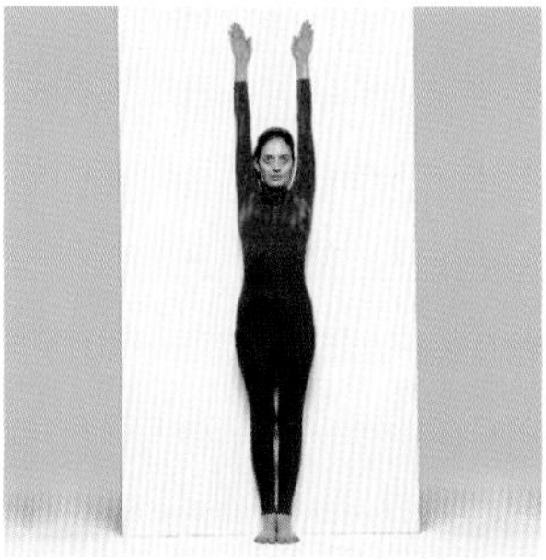

Stand in *Tāḍāsana* against the wall (see page 53). Inhale and raise the arms above the head, palms facing forward. Tighten the elbows and stretch the arms up. Breathe evenly.

Stay in the pose for 20 to 30 seconds. Exhale and bring the arms down.

To Progress

Stretch from shoulder to elbow, elbow to wrist, and wrist to fingertips.

वृक्षासन *Vṛkṣāsana*

Tree Pose

With the wall for support, stretching in the pose can be perfected without concern for balance.

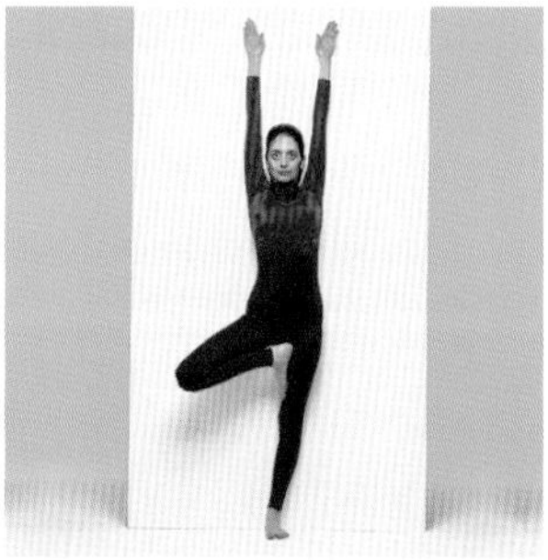

Stand in *Tāḍāsana* against the wall (see page 53). Bend the right leg outward, hold the base of the shin, and place the foot against the top of the inner left thigh. Fit the heel into the groove of the groin. Keep the left leg firm. Inhale, and raise the arms forward and up, resting the backs of the hands against the wall. Tighten the elbows and stretch the arms and hands. Breathe evenly.

Stay in the pose for 20 to 30 seconds. Exhale and bring the arms and leg down. Repeat on the other side.

To Progress

Press the left hip in and the bent knee back toward the wall. Stretch the arms up along the wall, and extend the sides of the trunk.

त्रिकोणासन *Trikoṇāsana*

Triangle Pose

With the wall at the back, the body is coaxed into the perpendicular plane of the pose.

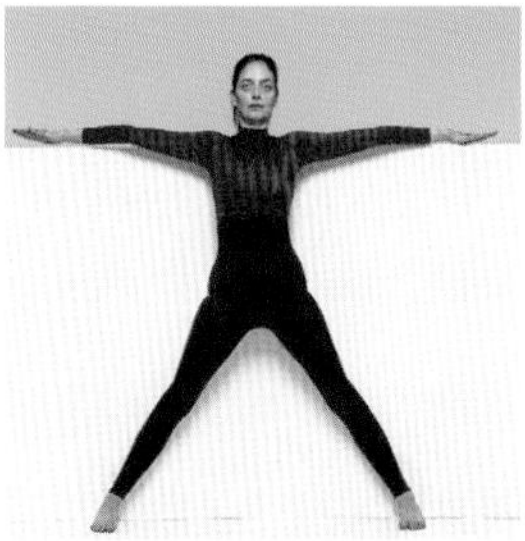

Stand in *Tāḍāsana* (see page 53) against a wall or ledge. Inhale and step the feet 3½–4 feet apart, extending the arms sideways to shoulder level, with the palms facing down. Align the feet and make them parallel.

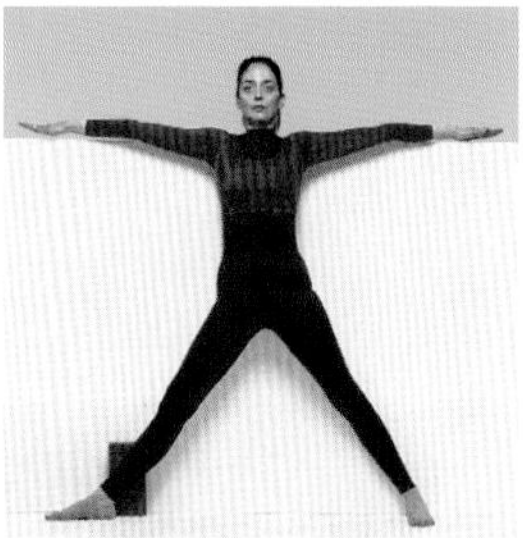

Turn the left foot 15 degrees in and the right foot 90 degrees out. Place a brick upright behind the right foot. Align the center of the right heel with the center of the left arch. (If possible, keep the left heel against the wall.) Revolve each leg outward. Tighten the knee caps and pull up the thigh muscles.

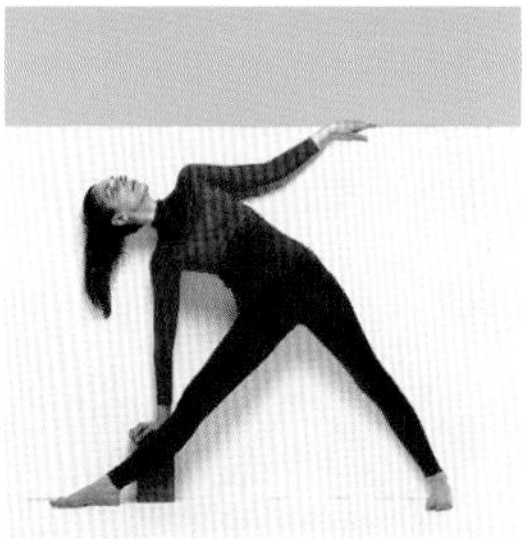

Exhale and take the trunk sideways down to the right; place the right hand on the brick. The brick is used so that the hand does not have so far to reach and the trunk does not collapse. Rest the left hand on the hip or ledge, and revolve the trunk toward the wall. Press the left shoulder back.

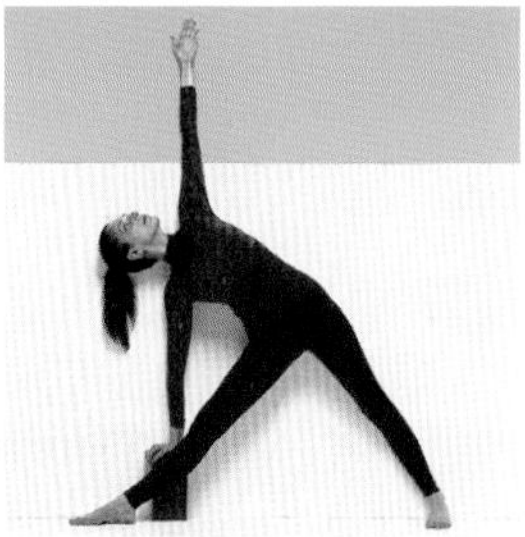

Stretch the left arm up, turning the palm to face forward. Turn the neck and head and look up at the hand. Breathe evenly. Stay in the pose for 20 to 30 seconds. Inhale and come up. Turn the feet to the front and rest the arms, then repeat on the other side. Exhale and bring the feet together, simultaneously bringing the arms down.

To Progress

Turn each leg from the top of the thigh, so that the whole leg is active. Turn the right leg outward, following the direction of the foot. Turn the left leg outward, in the opposite direction to the foot.

Lift the hips, and move the underside (right side) of the pelvis and rib cage away from the wall and the top (left) side toward it.

पार्श्वकोणासन *Pārśvakoṇāsana*

Side Angle Pose

Stabilized by the wall support, the legs become a firm pivot on which the trunk turns.

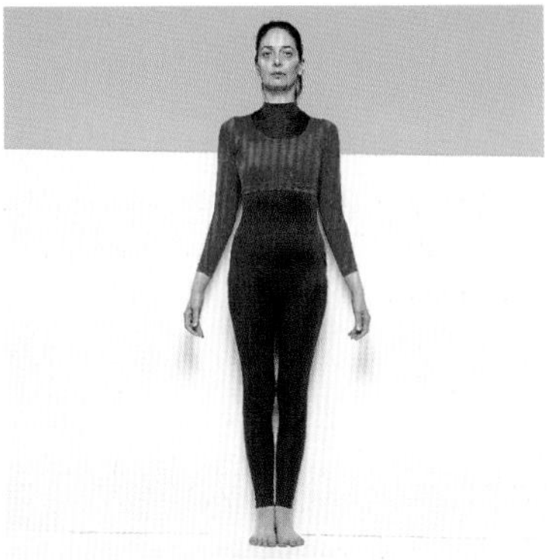

Stand in *Tāḍāsana* (see page 53) against a wall or ledge.

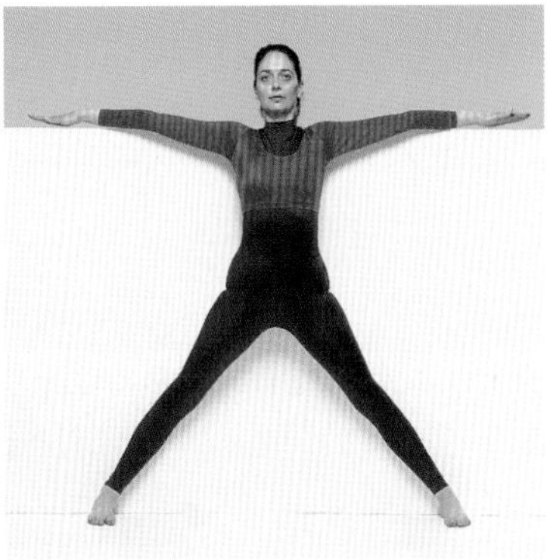

Inhale and jump or step the feet 4–4½ feet apart, extending the arms sideways to shoulder level with the palms facing down. Align the feet and make them parallel.

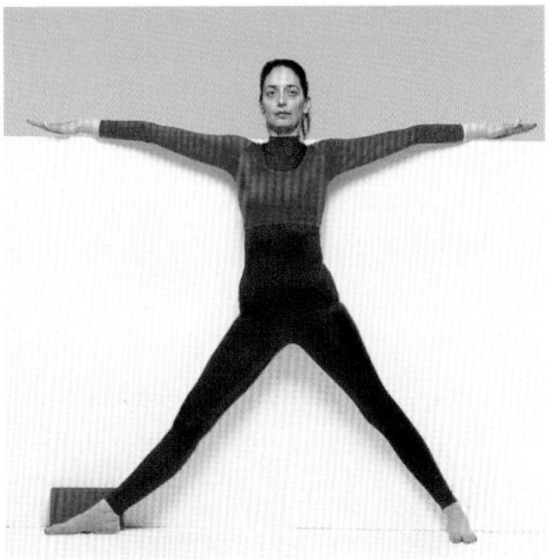

Turn the left foot 15 degrees in and the right foot 90 degrees out. Place a brick horizontally behind the right foot. Align the center of the right heel with the center of the left arch. (If possible, keep the left heel against the wall.) Revolve each leg outward. Tighten the kneecaps and pull up the thigh muscles.

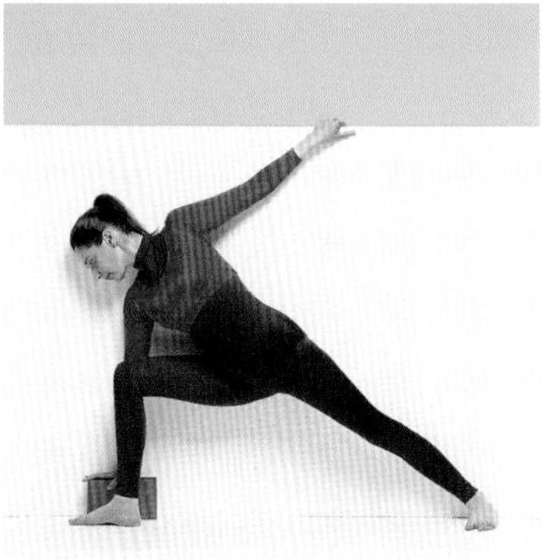

Exhale and bend the right leg to form a right angle, with the shin vertical and the thigh horizontal. Take the trunk sideways down toward the thigh, and place the right hand on the brick. The brick support gives the trunk height from the floor so that it does not collapse. Rest the left hand on the hip or ledge. Revolve the trunk toward the wall. Press the left shoulder back.

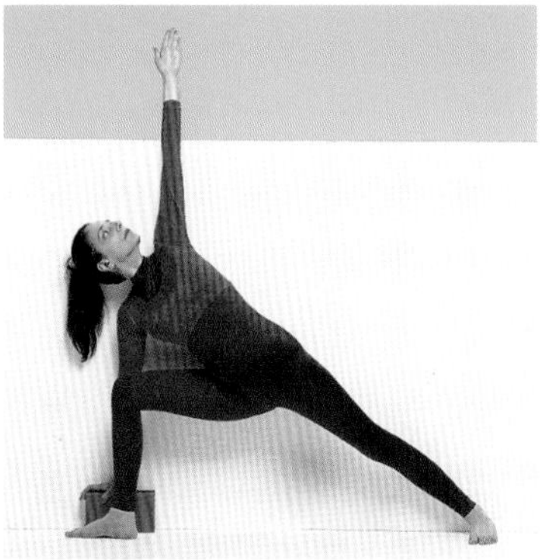

Take the left arm vertically up, and continue the upward rotation of the trunk. Turn the head and look up.

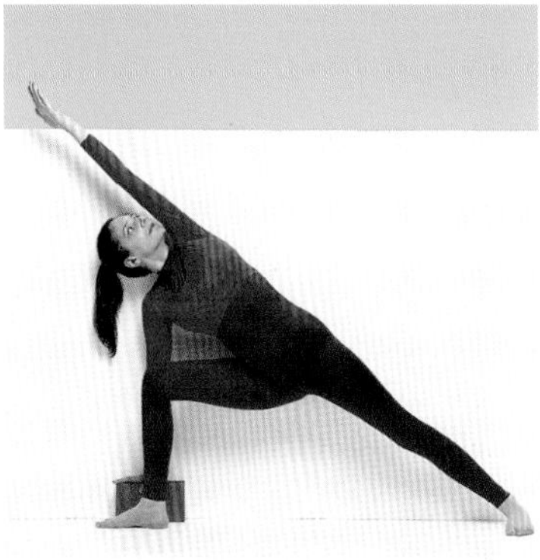

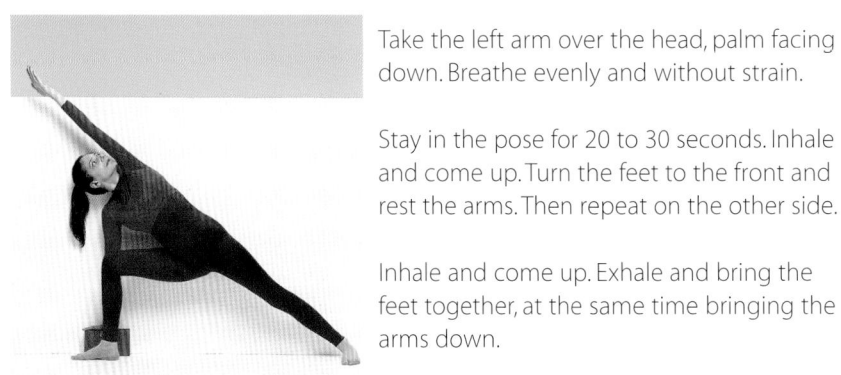

Take the left arm over the head, palm facing down. Breathe evenly and without strain.

Stay in the pose for 20 to 30 seconds. Inhale and come up. Turn the feet to the front and rest the arms. Then repeat on the other side.

Inhale and come up. Exhale and bring the feet together, at the same time bringing the arms down.

To Progress

Turn each leg from the top of the thigh, so that the whole leg is active. Turn the right leg outward, following the direction of the foot. Turn the left leg outward, in the opposite direction to the foot. When bending the right leg, do not allow the thigh to roll in.

Lift the left hip and press it toward the wall. Press the right knee and the left thigh toward the wall. Move the underside (right side) of the pelvis and rib cage away from the wall and the top (left) side toward it.

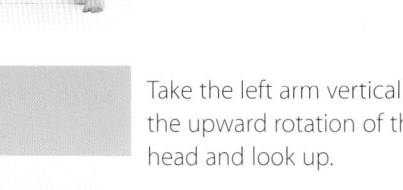

वीरभद्रासन २ *Vīrabhadrāsana 2*

Warrior Pose 2

Helped by the wall, the body is held in the vertical plane; as a result, energy is focused and does not dissipate in random directions.

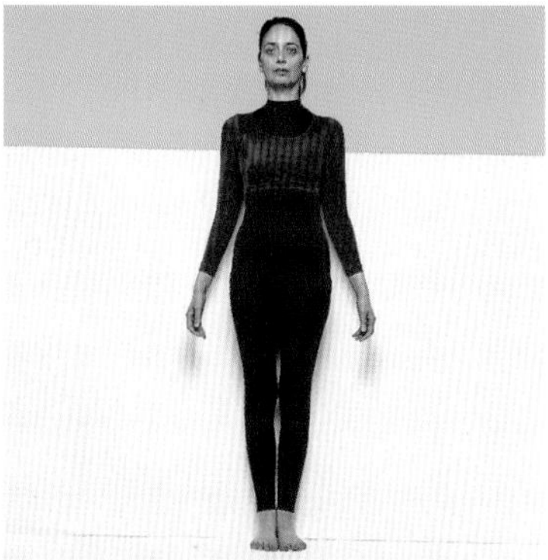

Stand in *Tāḍāsana* (see page 53) against the wall.

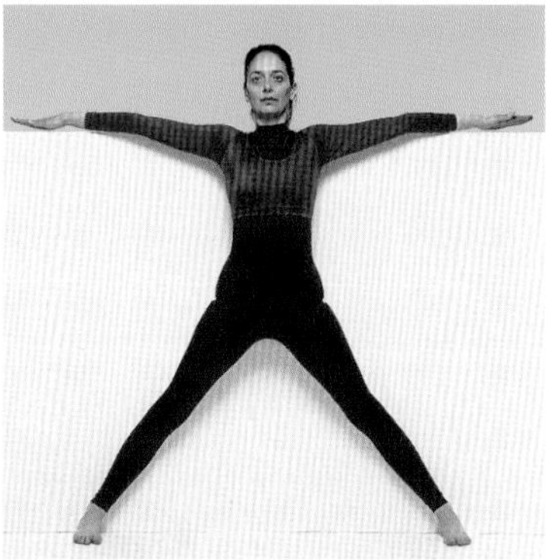

Inhale and jump or step the feet 4–4½ feet apart, extending the arms sideways to shoulder level with the palms facing down. Align the feet and make them parallel.

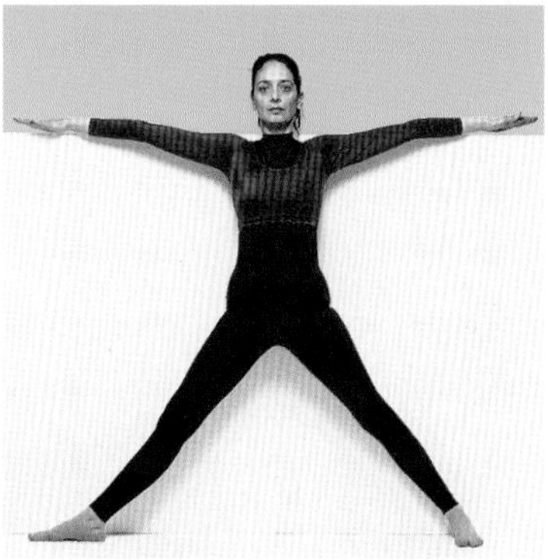

Turn the left foot 15 degrees in and the right foot 90 degrees out. Align the center of the right heel with the center of the left arch. (If possible, keep the left heel against the wall.) Revolve each leg outward. Tighten the kneecaps and pull up the thigh muscles.

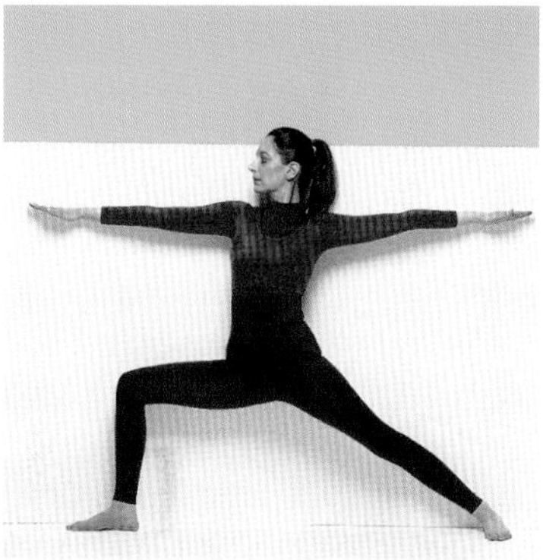

Exhale and bend the right leg to form a right angle, with the shin vertical and the thigh horizontal. Keep the trunk vertical and the arms parallel to the floor. Turn the neck and head, and look to the right. Breathe evenly and without strain.

Stay in the pose for 20 to 30 seconds. Inhale and come up. Turn the feet to the front and rest the arms. Then repeat on the other side.

Inhale and come up. Exhale and bring the feet together, simultaneously bringing the arms down.

To Progress

Turn each leg from the top of the thigh, so that the whole leg is active. Turn the right leg outward, following the direction of the foot. Turn the left leg outward, in the opposite direction to the foot. When bending the right leg, do not allow the thigh to roll in.

Move the left hip joint sharply in, so that the trunk lifts vertically up.

Press the right knee, left thigh and the left side of the trunk toward the wall.

अर्ध-उत्तानासन *Ardha-Uttānāsana*

Half Intense Stretch

Unless the legs are exactly vertical, the trunk does not get the maximum horizontal stretch.

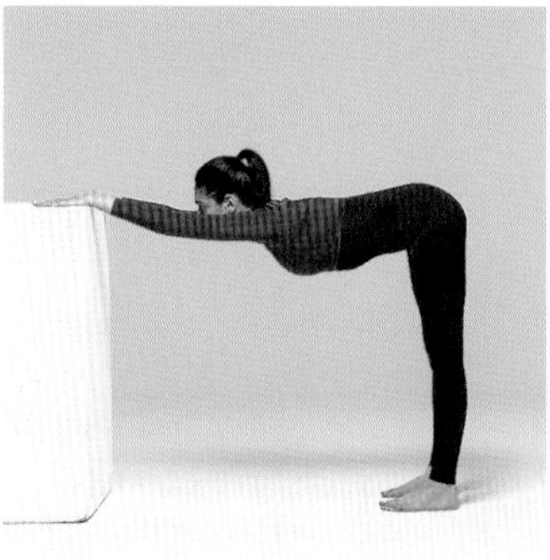

Follow the method given in Unit 2 (page 41).

To Progress

Move the tops of the thighs back so that the thighs remain in the vertical plane; this creates space in the hip joints. Stretch forward from the hips and lower back.

अधोमुख-श्वानासन

Adho-Mukha-Śvānāsana

Dog Pose, Head Down

The separate stretches of the limbs and trunk integrate to make the hips the apex of the body.

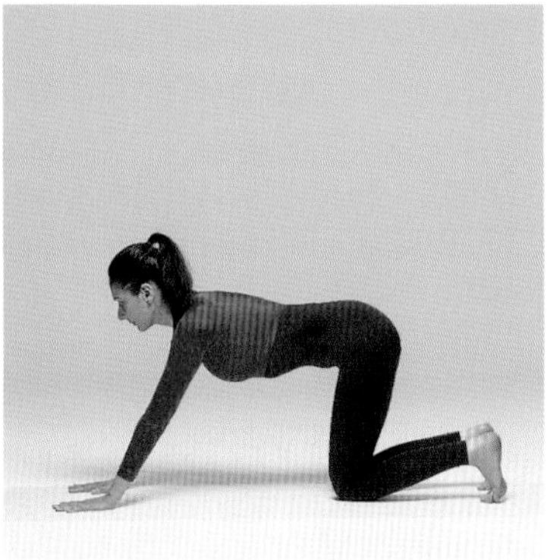

Kneel on the floor. Lift the hips, and place the hands about 2 feet in front of the knees. Spread the fingers, with the middle finger facing forward. Straighten the arms and stretch them towards the shoulders. They should be slanting. Curl the toes under.

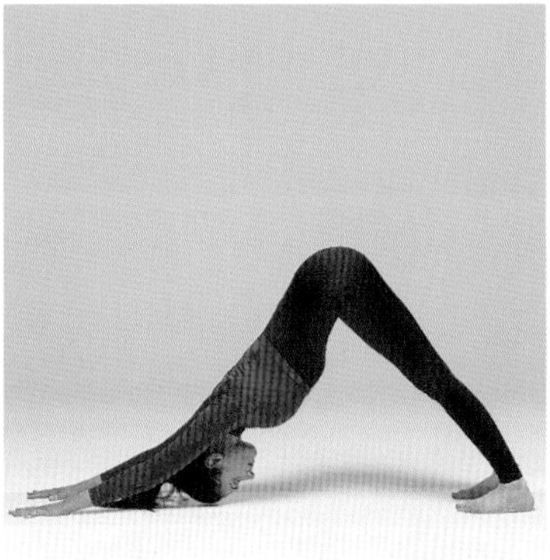

Raise the hips and straighten the legs. Move the trunk toward the legs so that the body forms an inverted "V" shape. Breathe evenly.

Stay in the pose for 30 seconds to 1 minute. Bend the knees and come down.

Kneel and bend forward in *Adho-Mukha-Vīrāsana* (see Unit 2, page 42), then come up.

To Progress

Keep the knees tight. Press the legs back, transferring the weight from the front to the back of the legs. Lower the heels without collapsing the legs.

Keep the elbows tight and stretch the arms up. Lift the shoulders, move the shoulder blades in, and stretch the trunk up. Raise the hips higher and higher.

पर्वतासन *Parvatāsana*

Mountain Pose

Height and firmness characterize mountains; so it is with this stretch of the arms and trunk.

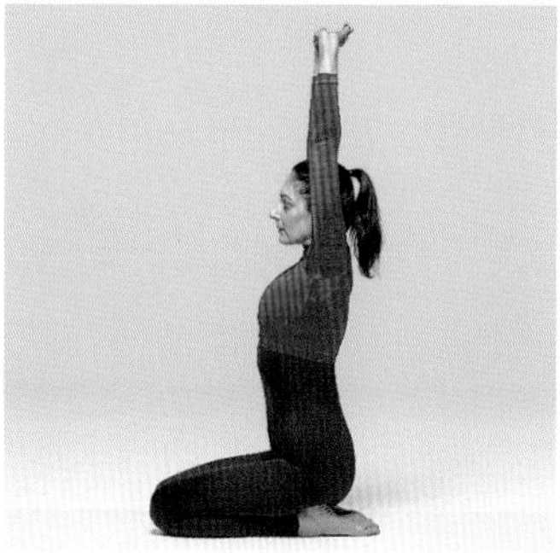

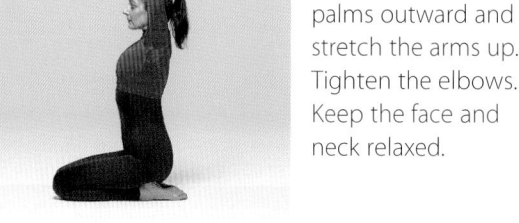

Sit on the heels. Interlock the fingers. Turn the palms outward and stretch the arms up. Tighten the elbows. Keep the face and neck relaxed.

Stay in the pose for 20 to 30 seconds. Bring the arms down, change the interlock of the fingers, and repeat.

To Progress

Begin the stretch from the hips and lower back. Extend the waist and sides of the rib cage. Move the shoulder blades in, and lift the upper trunk without compressing the shoulders and neck. Extend the armpits and take the arms back, into the vertical plane. Make the upper arms firm and lift them strongly up. Then stretch the forearms.

गोमुखासन *Gomukhāsana*

Cow-Head Pose, Arms Only

Vertical alignment here is in the arms: the elbows point up and down, and the upper arms find the vertical plane.

Sit on the heels, with the knees together. Lift the trunk and sit erect. Take the right arm behind the back, and move the right forearm and hand up the spine as high as possible. To position the right arm well, push the elbow up with the left hand. Take the left arm forward and stretch it up. Turn the arm so that the palm faces back; bend the elbow and catch the right hand. Keep the trunk facing forward. Relax the head and neck. Breathe evenly.

Stay in the pose for 20 to 30 seconds. Release the arms and repeat on the other side. Then bring the legs forward.

To Progress

Take the right arm back to make the upper arm vertical. Take the left shoulder and elbow back to make the left upper arm vertical. Catch the hand farther.

Help

- **If the hands cannot catch, hold a belt.**

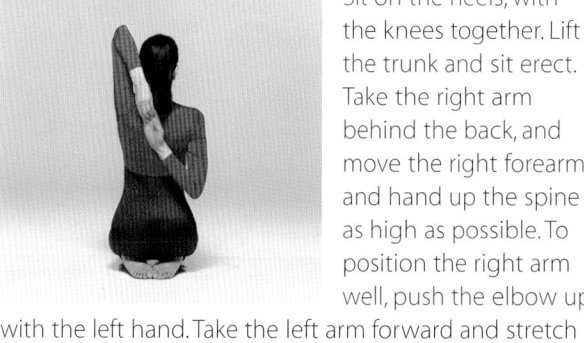

सर्वाङ्गासन *Sarvāṅgāsana*

Shoulder Balance

Literally meaning "Pose for the Whole Body," this is known as the mother of postures, because it soothes and nourishes the entire being.

Cautions

Do not do this pose during menstruation or if suffering from hypertension (high blood pressure), a neck injury, or a detached retina or other eye problems. If there is pressure in the head, eyes, neck, or throat, come down, readjust the head, neck, and shoulders in the starting position, and try again. If the pressure persists, seek the advice of a teacher.

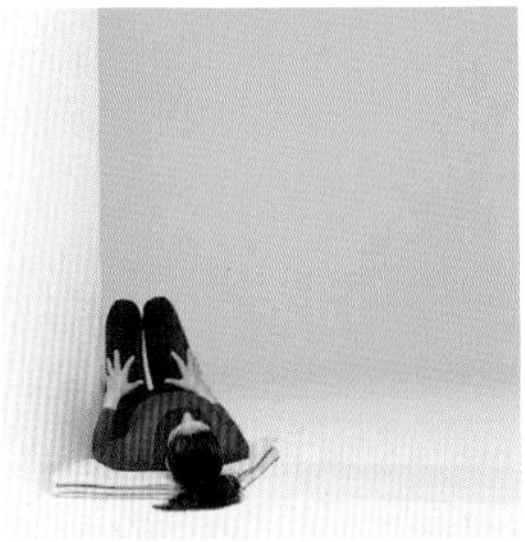

Place three or four folded blankets against the wall, with the neat folded edges facing into the room. Lie down sideways against the wall so that the shoulders are on the blankets. Press the shoulders down, and keep the knees bent.

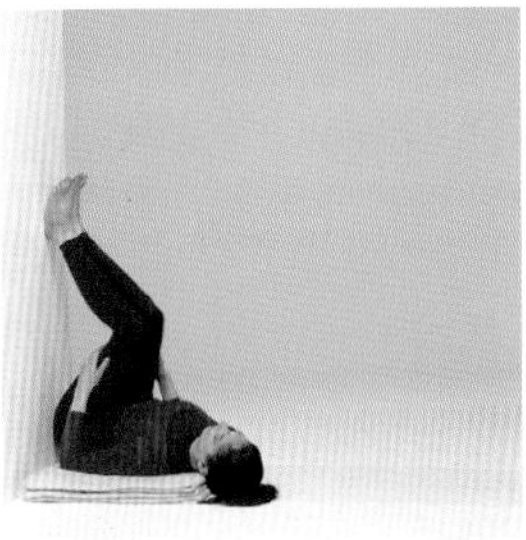

With the help of the hands, raise the feet onto the wall, and simultaneously swivel the body around until the trunk is at right angles to the wall. Keep the shoulders and trunk on the blankets and the head on the floor.

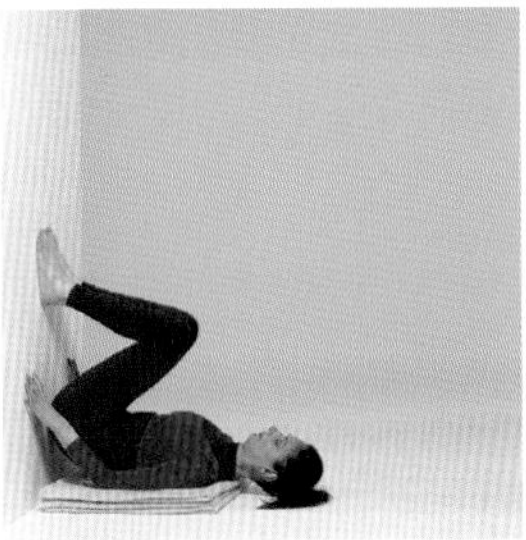

Align the body at right angles to the wall. Move the shoulders away from the neck, press them down, and move the shoulder blades in.

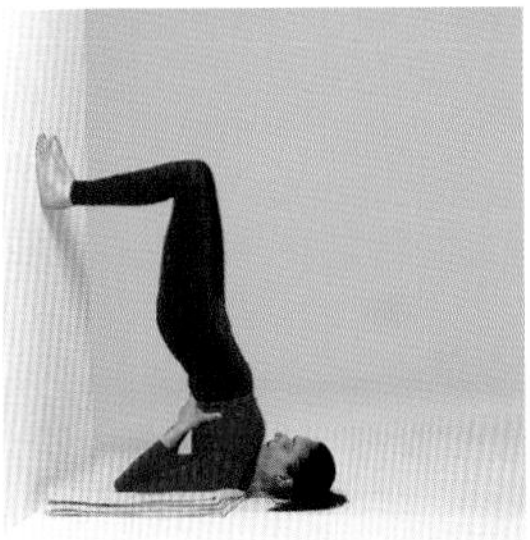

Lift the trunk, place the hands on the back, and take the feet higher up the wall. Move the elbows in. Move the rib cage and buttocks forward.

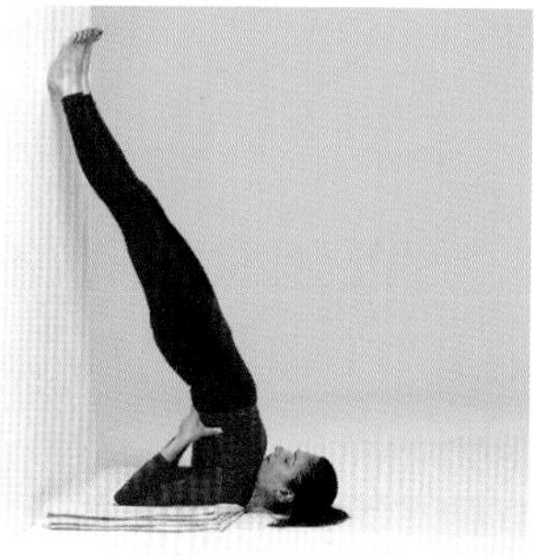

Straighten the legs, keeping the heels supported against the wall. If possible, move the hands farther down the back (toward the shoulders). Breathe evenly.

Stay in the pose for 1 to 3 minutes. Bend the knees to come down. Roll to the side to get up.

To Progress

Alternate between the bent-leg and straight-leg positions in order to build up stamina. When the legs are straight, tighten the knees and stretch the legs up.

Help

- **If there is pressure on the neck or throat, increase the height of the support.**
- **If there is pressure in the face or eyes, come down and try again after altering the height of the support. Pay attention to positioning the shoulders well. If the problem persists, seek advice.**

शवासन *Śavāsana*

Corpse Pose

The horizontal plane is the guide for this pose as the body levels out and relaxes.

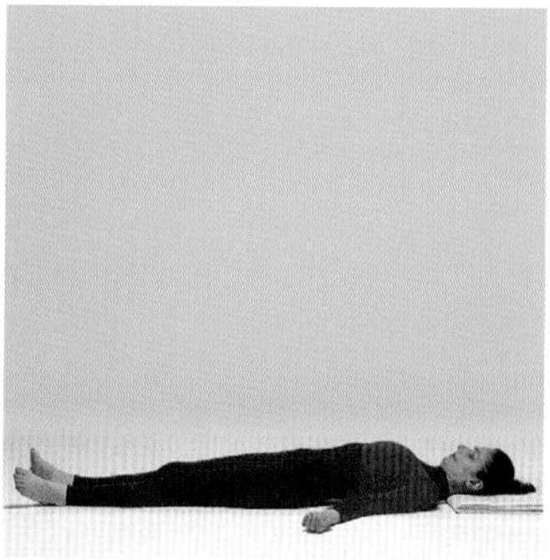

Follow the method given in Unit 1 (page 26).

To Progress

Observe the shape of the back of the body in relation to the flatness of the floor. Where the body projects downward, make it flatter: move the thoracic spine in, particularly between the shoulder blades, and smooth the lower back away from the waist with the help of the hands. Where the body tends to lift or project, move it downward: press the shoulders down, and relax the waist, thighs, feet, abdomen, neck, throat, and eyes.

The sources of yoga philosophy

KEY CONCEPT

School of philosophy An outlook toward philosophical issues determined by the priority it gives to the means of knowledge—mainly perception, inference, and scripture—on which it bases its doctrines. Such a school offers its views on (a) the world, (b) the soul, (c) God, and (d) the relationship between them.

To understand the philosophical underpinnings of Yoga, it is helpful to have a broad knowledge of the Indian philosophical tradition. This tradition has its roots in the oldest Sanskrit literature and continues to exert its influence today.

Vedic Literature

The oldest body of Sanskrit literature is known as Vedic literature. The basic meaning of the word "Veda" is "knowledge"; it is traditionally believed to be God-given. By common consent, it is accepted as the oldest in the world that deserves the name "literature." Scholars' opinions vary as to its precise age, but the oldest layer cannot reasonably be later than 3000 B.C. This literature contains the contributions of many authors over many centuries. It was transmitted orally, with the teacher reciting phrases and the student repeating them until he became word perfect (conventionally, seven times).

Vedic literature portrays the life and culture of the Aryans, an adventurous people who fought their way into the Land of Seven Rivers, now called India, leaving behind a group that settled in Iran. Their society was divided initially into two broad groups: priests and warriors. The four-caste system came later. Early Vedic religion was characterized by the worship of nature deities, fire, and heroes. This developed into an elaborate system of sacrifice and ritual.

Vedic "books of knowledge" have four divisions: chants addressed to deities (*Ṛg-Veda*), recitations for use in sacrifices (*Yajur-Veda*), songs for use in sacrifices (*Sāma-Veda*), and formulas for magic and witchcraft, both black and white (*Atharva-Veda*). The *Ṛg-Veda* and the *Atharva-Veda*, representing the religion and culture, respectively, of the educated classes and the masses, are basic texts. The remaining two, relating mainly to ritual, are secondary, as they assume the existence of the former.

To each of these collections are assigned various groups of works: commentaries on sacrifices and rituals (*Brāhmaṇas*), musings of forest hermits (*Āraṇyakas*), and knowledge passed on in intimate meetings (*Upaniṣads*).

The *Upaniṣads*

The *Upaniṣads* are works devoted to philosophy and esoteric knowledge, dating from 1500 B.C. According to them, the performance of ritual leads merely to heaven, while philosophy, when lived, brings liberation from worldly bonds, including heaven and hell. Though philosophical in content, many of the *Upaniṣads*, or sections within them, are presented in a framework of stories. They are the ultimate sources of ideas that have influenced Indian thought through the ages down to our own times.

There are ten very ancient, and six slightly less ancient, *Upaniṣads*. The high esteem in which they are held has inspired the composition of imitative works, including some devoted exclusively to Yoga.

The central stream of *Upaniṣadic* thought centers around the concept of an all-pervading principle (*brahman*) underlying the universe, characterized by existence, consciousness, and bliss. In the created world, it is the soul in the bodies of all creatures. The soul suffers from worldly woes, as it does not know that it is one with the all-pervading principle. However, the realization that it is so frees it from worldly suffering and restores it to its real nature. This is called liberation, the highest goal of human life. It is the fourth of a quartet of goals recognized by Indian philosophy. The other three—piety, prosperity and pleasure—are worldly aims that reflect basic human inclinations; they suffer from the drawback of impermanence. The philosopher opts for liberation because, once attained, it is permanent. Yoga shares this view with the philosopher.

Of particular importance to Yoga are the *Kaṭha* and the *Śvetāśvatara Upaniṣads*. The other major *Upaniṣads* cited in this book are the *Chāndogya* and the *Bṛhadāraṇyaka*.

The philosophical content of the *Kaṭha Upaniṣad* is presented in a dialogue between the god of Death and a precocious, inquisitive boy. It deals with the nature of the soul and the state of liberation. As part of his instruction, the boy is taught the entire subject of Yoga. The framing story and thrust of the teachings of this *Upaniṣad* are given in Unit 2.

The *Śvetāśvatara Upaniṣad* reveals familiarity with Yoga concepts and terminology. Several Yoga topics figure: the selection of a place for practicing Yoga, the proper posture for meditation, breath control, indications of the success of the practice, and the ultimate goal of attaining immortality in the *Haṭha* Yoga sense.

The *Bhagavad-Gītā*

The *Bhagavad-Gītā* is the most popular philosophical work in India, because it caters for the average person who also has a philosophical inclination. Consisting of 700 couplets spread over 18 chapters, it was originally part of the great epic, the

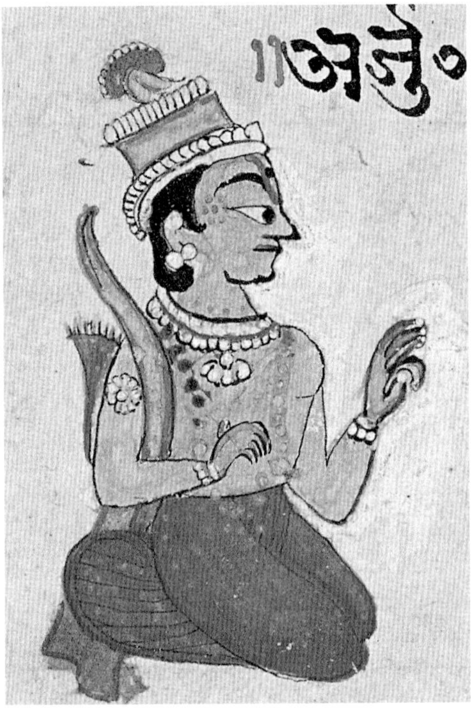

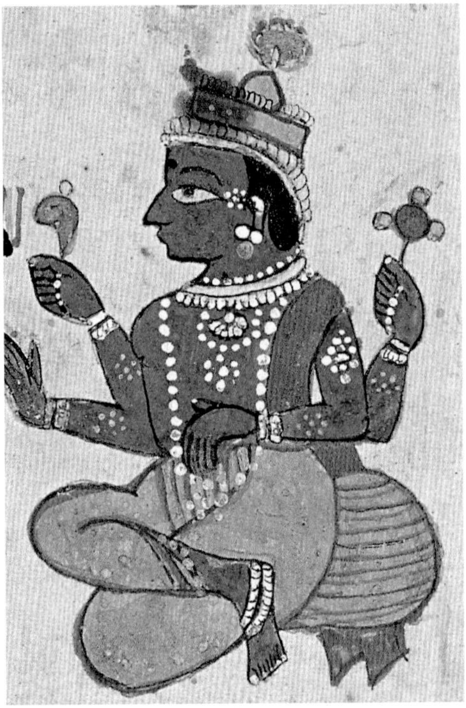

Illustrations of Arjuna (left) and Kṛṣṇa (right) from an undated *Bhagavad-Gītā*, kept at the Bhandarkar Institute in India.

Mahābhārata (400 B.C.–400 A.D.). It is presented against the background of a great war, which forms the central theme of the epic, and it takes the form of a dialogue between two major characters, Kṛṣṇa and Arjuna.

Kṛṣṇa is charioteer to Arjuna, a prince of the Pāṇḍava clan. War is about to begin between the Pāṇḍavas and their cousins, the Kauravas. Arjuna is sunk in gloom at the thought of being party to the mass slaughter of the imminent war. He announces his decision not to fight. Kṛṣṇa, as friend, philosopher, and guide to the Pāṇḍavas, discourses on all the reasons why he should fight, including the famous argument that we do not destroy the soul by killing the body. At the end of the work we find Arjuna restored to his warrior spirit.

The *Bhagavad-Gītā* presents many important concepts: action without selfish motive, knowledge of Reality, Yoga, selfless devotion, and renunciation in thought as well as deed. All are viewed as means of spiritual development.

In its explanation of Yoga, this work describes a sitting posture suitable for meditation, the ideal routine and observances for a Yogin, the supreme state of meditation, the ways to control the mind, and the fruition of Yoga practice through several incarnations. The topic of a Yogin voluntarily leaving his mortal body through breath control corresponds to concepts found in *Haṭha* Yoga that also date back to *Upaniṣadic* times.

Indian Philosophical Schools

The Indian philosophical tradition encompasses a wide range of schools, or systems, both orthodox and heterodox (such as Materialists and Buddhists). The orthodox schools recognize Vedic literature as the ultimate authority on matters beyond worldly means of knowledge. There are six orthodox schools, as follows:

Vedānta (meaning "the conclusion of the Vedas"—that is, the *Upaniṣads*). This school is founded on, and champions, the concepts found in the *Upaniṣads*.

Mīmāṃsā (meaning "the desire to discuss"). This school believes ritual to be the essence of the Veda, and develops a logical system of interpretation of texts dealing with ritual.

Nyāya (meaning "rule"). This school is mainly a system of logic; it borrows philosophical views mostly from the *Vaiśeṣika* school.

Vaiśeṣika (advocating the concept of "particularity," *viśeṣa*). The *Vaiśeṣikas* were, in essence, ancient physicists who analyzed the world into six categories: substance, quality, action, genus, and particular and inherent relation. To these was later added a seventh concept, that of nonexistence. The soul in this scheme is included in the category of substance. The *Vaiśeṣikas* do not accept the existence of God.

Sāṃkhya (from *saṃkhyā*, meaning "number" or "intellect"). Though conventionally the name of this school refers to its numbered list of basic principles, it more appropriately (taking the second meaning) refers to its insistence on intellectual discipline in presenting its theories. It analyzes the universe into 25 principles (the 24 products of Primordial Matter, plus Spirit or soul) and explains how the material world evolved out of Primordial Matter (see Unit 7, page 128). The entire philosophy presented in this book as Yoga philosophy—the nature of the soul, suffering rooted in ignorance, liberation through discriminating knowledge—comes in fact from *Sāṃkhya*. The sole exception is the concept of God, which is a Yoga view.

Yoga (from *yuj*, which has a number of meanings, including "to meditate"). The basic meaning of Yoga is "a means," out of which other meanings seem to have evolved. This school studies the mind and the ways to control it, as this subject is crucial to the concepts of liberation and how to attain it. It analyzes the mind into several modes (valid knowledge, mistaken knowledge, verbal knowledge, or conceptualization, deep sleep, and memory), explains how it causes worldly sufferings, and puts forward an eightfold plan to eliminate and transcend it.

The basic texts of all these schools belong to the beginning of the Christian era. They are traditionally viewed in three pairs: *Vedānta* with *Mīmāṃsā*, *Sāṃkhya* with *Yoga*, and *Nyāya* with *Vaiśeṣika*. *Vedānta*, *Sāṃkhya*, and *Vaiśeṣika* are philosophical systems, in the sense that they deal with metaphysics. The remaining three are disciplines that contribute to their counterparts either by developing the intellectual infrastructure of all the systems (*Mīmāṃsā* and *Nyāya*) or by methodically exploring their practical aspect (*Yoga*).

In the Sanskrit philosophical tradition, three trends are visible: monism, dualism, and pluralism. Monism characterizes *Vedānta* (including the *Upaniṣads*), which advocates a single, conscious principle as the essence of the whole world. Dualism is the standpoint of the *Sāṃkhya* school, which advocates insentient Matter and conscious Spirit as the two ultimate principles. Pluralism characterizes the *Vaiśeṣika* school, which advocates an infinite number of insentient atoms as the ultimate, eternal principle of the material world. Yoga accepts the *Sāṃkhya* view on philosophical matters. Of the six orthodox systems, we are concerned mainly with *Sāṃkhya* and Yoga, and with *Vedānta* to a limited extent. Although having different views (monism versus dualism) on the nature of Reality, the *Sāṃkhya-Yoga-Vedānta* triad forms a close group because of their agreement on other points, such as the nature of the soul, its liberation through knowledge, and so on.

All the orthodox schools, including theistic sects, recognize Yoga as a discipline crucial to the realization of the ultimate truth as viewed by them, the controlled mind being the sole means of experiencing this. For the same reason, Yoga is also adopted in the heterodox systems.

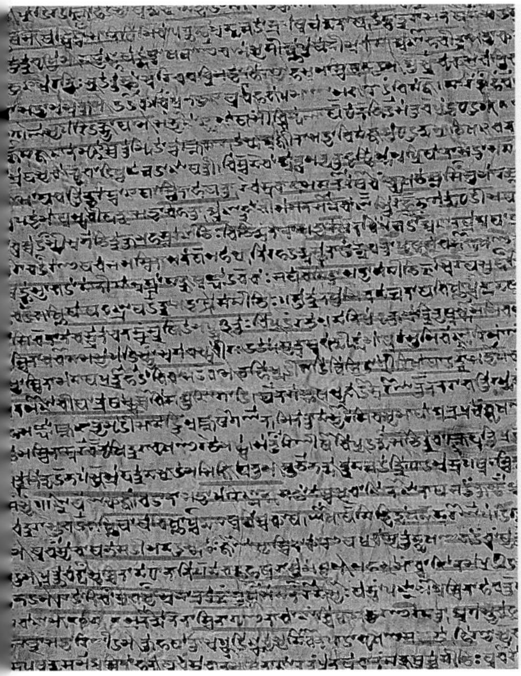

A *Ṛg-Veda* birch bark manuscript from the collection at the Bhandarkar Institute. It is undated, but Vedic literature is said to go back as far as 3000 B.C.

In Brief

Vedic literature has come down through an oral tradition;
Its oldest portion dates back more than five millennia.

The early Vedic people were priests and warriors.
Some worshiped deities such as Indra; others pursued magic.

Then emerged most complex sacrificial systems;
For their sake came two more Vedas and the literature on sacrifice.

Then books called *Upaniṣads* were created by seekers of Reality;
From them emerged philosophical systems, orthodox and heterodox.

Of the four goals of human life, liberation is the highest,
Since from it there is no return; it is obtained by knowledge.

Knowledge is gained by mind control. Mind control and its procedure
Are the sphere of Yoga. Yoga is valued by all philosophies.

For a wider perspective...

Schools of Indian Philosophy

A school of philosophy in the Indian tradition seeks answers to four basic questions: (a) What is this world? (b) What am I? (c) What is God? (d) What is the relationship between them? The answers to these questions depend upon another set of questions: (i) What are the means of knowledge? (ii) Which of them is superior or inferior to which?

Each school attempts to understand the outer and inner worlds by three principal means of knowledge: perception, inference, and scriptures, or revealed literature. Perception is the knowledge of objects directly through the sense organs (for example, we see a book, smell an odor, and so on). Inference is the knowledge of the unknown by means of perceptible or known indications closely associated with it (for instance, we see smoke and infer the existence of fire). Scriptures are said to contain the intuitive knowledge of seers or prophets preserved orally or in writing, or both. Orthodox schools of Indian philosophy class Vedic literature (including the *Upaniṣads*) as scripture.

Unit 4

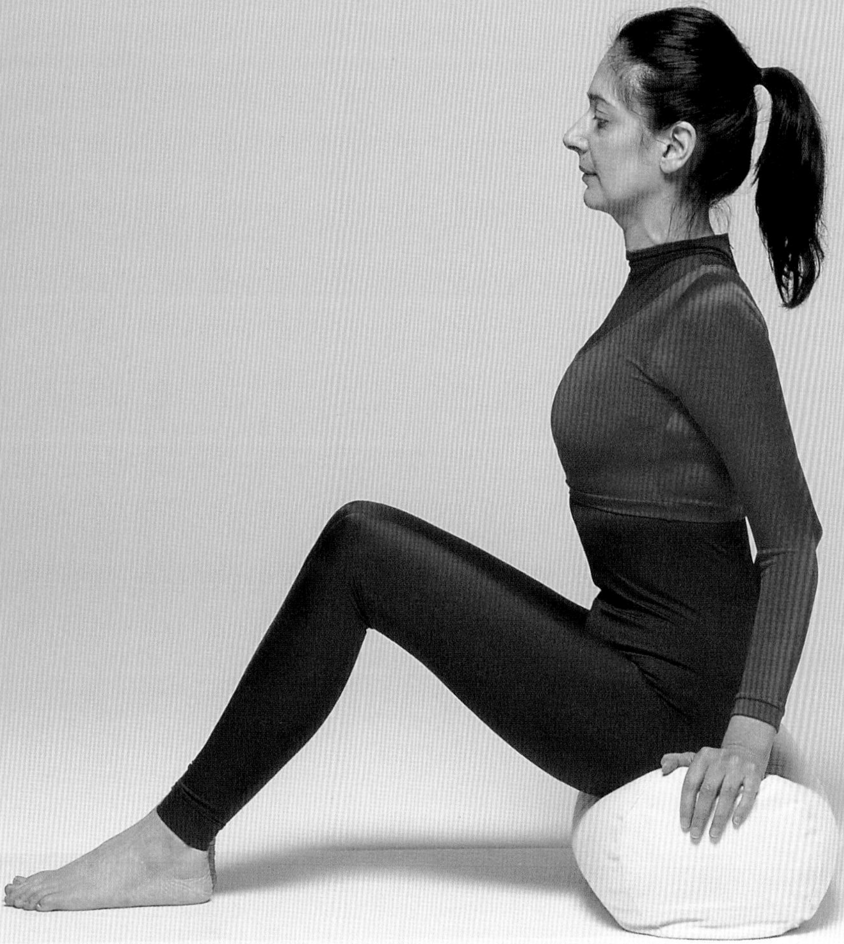

"People kill one another because of hunger," from an illustrated manuscript dated A.D. 1648

Yoga in life

CAUSE AND EFFECT

The jar of the Genie, once unstoppered,
Released its pent spirit, which expanded
Exponentially upward and outward
Into freedom coterminous with space.

No coercion, cajoling, or trickery
Could return the escapee to confinement;
But were the air sucked out of its sky-room
Would it not shrink back in the vacuum?

It is evident in everyday living that causes have effects and effects arise from causes.

Yoga philosophy takes this reasoning further and states that the effect lies dormant in the cause, and that something cannot arise from nothing. In terms of the created world, existence cannot arise from nonexistence. As the created world is material, all actions and consequences occur within the flow of the forces of nature.[1]

When an effect comes into being, it is not a new creation, but emerges from what preceded it, because the material barriers to its existence are removed. We cannot force water to penetrate the roots of a crop choked by weeds, but if the weeds are pulled out, the water flows to the roots automatically.[2]

This reasoning is applied also at the psychological level, for the mind is part of nature and follows its laws. Good and bad actions do not create consequences but enable them to occur. However, the mind is complex, and unless it is fully understood it can be unpredictable. Unknown factors can lead to unknown effects.

[1] *Yoga Sūtra 4.2*

[2] *Yoga Sūtra and Commentary 4.3*

Relaxing the body

The tensions of life are absorbed by the body and mold it into characteristic shapes: round shoulders, tight abdomen, and caved-in chest, to cite some examples. Injuries, habits of movement, and wear and tear also take their toll. When the body is under such stress, it is difficult for the mind to find freedom and tranquillity. Relaxation, therefore, starts with the body.

Profound physical relaxation does not occur merely by "letting go," as in sleep or slumping, as in an armchair after a day's work. These are temporary respites which leave the long-term imprints of tension in the body basically unchanged.

The principle of relaxation in Yoga is to eradicate these imprints of stress. This is achieved by bolstering the body in various postures so that the areas that are strained can find ease. With the comfort of a corrective support, the shoulders can straighten, the abdomen can relax, and the breastbone can lift. Gradually this postural freedom becomes habitual, and the body retains the feeling of ease during everyday activities.

A passive practice of restful poses complements an active practice, in much the same way as the daily life cycle needs to include rest as well as activity. Without sufficient daytime activity, the quality of sleep deteriorates; without adequate rest, energy levels dwindle and body and mind are not refreshed. Too much or too little of either exertion or sleep leads to imbalance. Thus, restorative poses should be done regularly.

The simplest restorative poses are supine. They involve lying down with a support under the back and head while the legs are bent in different positions. This back support encourages the chest to lift and the lungs to open and receive an increased intake of oxygen: a key factor in the recovery of energy.

Nervous energy abounds in the brain, however, its unceasing buzz of thoughts is stilled by resting the head on a support. This can be done in various poses. The light pressing of the head produces a soothing effect, similar to that felt when the head is pressed by the hands. In this way the constant release of mental energy is minimized. By staying in these poses, the mind becomes calm and collected.

Both body and mind need time to unwind. For this reason, all these poses need to be maintained for a length of time, often minutes. This is not difficult, because the body is supported. With practice it becomes possible to stay longer and longer, thereby increasing the benefits.

As with vigorous practice sessions, a session of passive poses includes inverted poses. Here a simple, supported version of Shoulder-Balance Bridge (*Setu-Bandha-Sarvāṇgāsana*) is introduced. In it, that great storehouse of tension, the throat, is rested.

The cumulative effect of all these quiet poses is a profound Corpse Pose (*Śavāsana*), which itself is done with the back supported so that breathing becomes deep and easy.

मत्स्यासन *Matsyāsana*

Fish Pose

A light, floaty feeling is enjoyed in this pose when the back is lifted on a support.

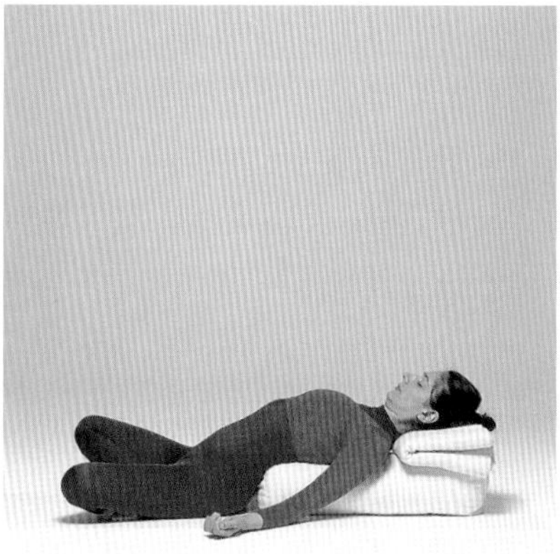

Place a bolster on the floor. Sit with the back against one end and cross the legs simply. Lie back on the bolster. Place a folded blanket under the head and neck. Rest the arms beside the trunk. Breathe evenly and relax.

Stay in the pose for 2 to 3 minutes. Come up and repeat with the legs crossed the other way.

Help

- **If the hip joints or groins feel strained, place supports under the thighs (see Unit 2, page 44).**
- **If the bolster feels too high, use one or two blankets folded lengthwise instead.**

To Progress

Be careful to place the trunk evenly on the bolster. Press the shoulders down and lengthen the neck. Turn the upper arms so that the palms face up.

सुप्त-बद्धकोणासन

Supta-Baddha-Koṇāsana

Supine Bound-Angle Pose

A feeling of space and freedom in the abdomen brings a revelation of relaxation.

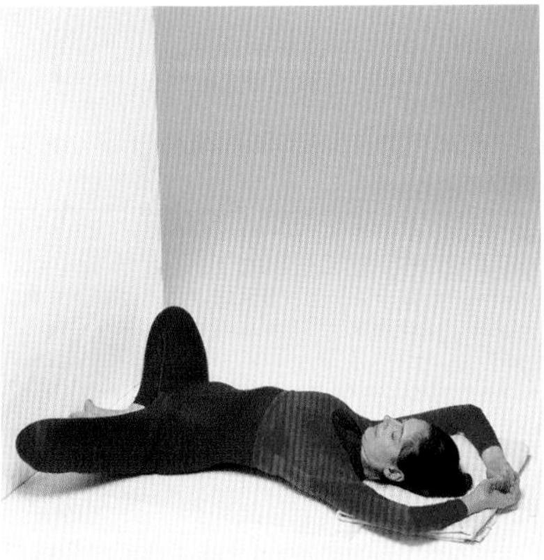

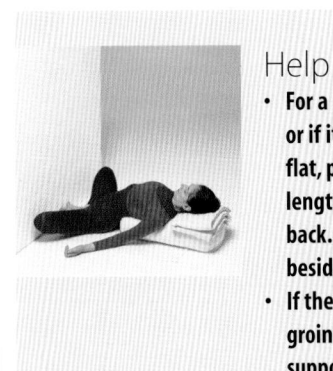

Sit facing a wall. Bend the knees out to the sides, and join the soles of the feet. Turn the toes outward and press them against the wall. Move the body toward the legs, so that the heels are as close as possible to the pubis. Lie back. Place a folded blanket under the head and neck. Take the arms over the head. Breathe evenly and relax.

Stay in the pose for 2 to 3 minutes. Bring the knees together, turn to the side, and come up.

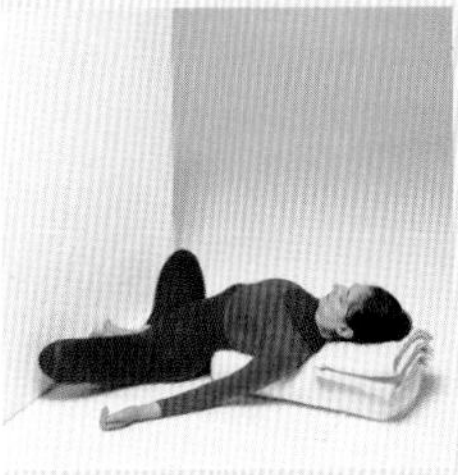

Help

- **For a deeper relaxation, or if it is difficult to lie flat, place a bolster lengthwise under the back. Keep the arms beside the trunk.**
- **If the hip joints or groins feel strained, place supports under the thighs.**

To Progress

Move the trunk closer to the legs. Make the knees level.

अधोमुख-श्वानासन
Adho-Mukha-Śvānāsana

Dog Pose, Head Down

While the body stretches, the head relaxes; this potent combination of active and passive is remarkably effective.

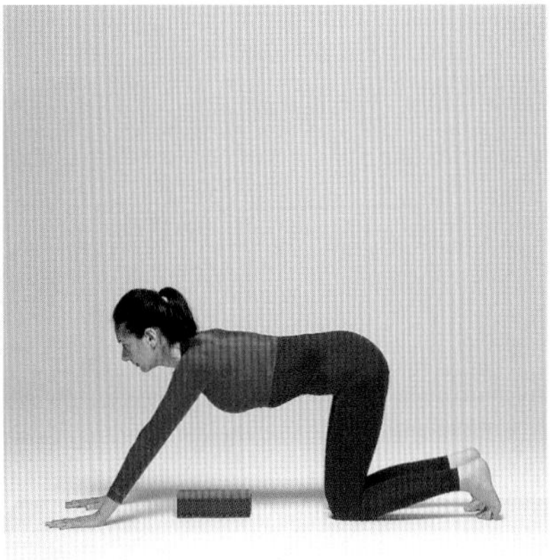

Kneel in front of a bolster, block, or other support. Lift the hips and place the hands on the floor about 2 feet in front of the knees. Spread the fingers, straighten the arms, and stretch the arms toward the shoulders. They should be slanting. Curl the toes under.

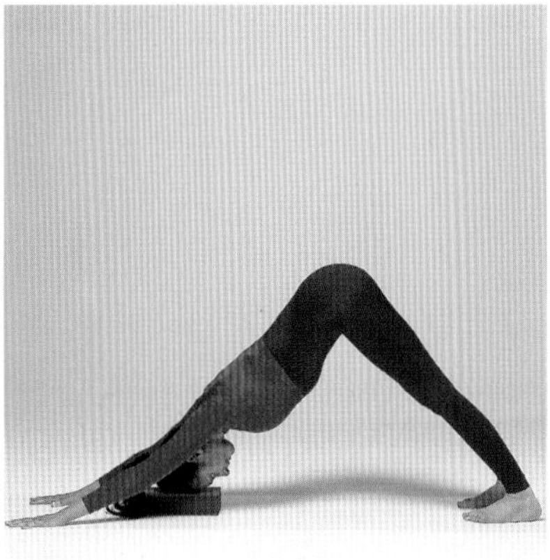

Raise the hips and straighten the legs. Move the trunk toward the legs, so that the body forms an inverted "V" shape. Rest the head on the support. Breathe evenly.

Stay in the pose for 30 seconds to 1 minute.

Bend the knees and come down. Kneel and bend forward. Come up.

To Progress

Keep the knees and elbows tight. Stretch the arms and trunk up, so that the head does not bear their weight. Bring the weight of the body onto the legs.

Help

- **Adjust the height of the support so that the head rests on it lightly and comfortably.**

उत्तानासन *Uttānāsana*

Intense Stretch

Held between two firm supports—stretched legs and a seat—the body and head relax.

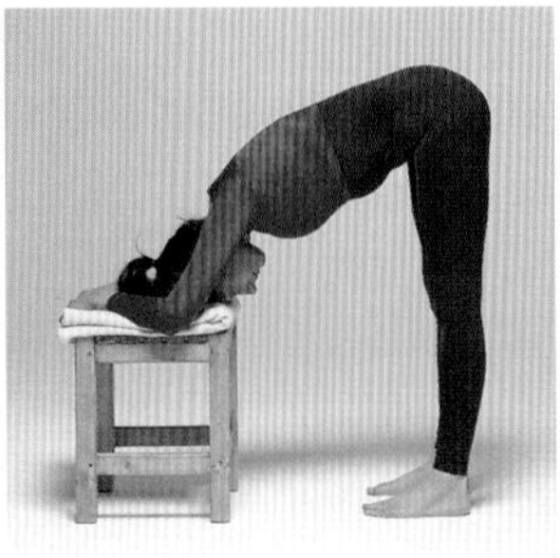

Place a folded blanket on a chair or stool. Stand in *Tāḍāsana* (see Unit 1, page 19) about 1 foot in front of it, the feet hip-width apart. Exhale, bend forward, and rest the head and arms on the seat. Keep the legs vertical. Breathe evenly and relax.

Stay in the pose for 1 to 2 minutes. Inhale and come up. Bring the feet together.

To Progress

Keep the knees tight and stretch the legs up.

Help

- **If the back is stiff, take the legs farther apart and adjust the height of the support—for example, with some folded blankets.**

अधोमुख-सुखासन *Adho-mukha-Sukhāsana*

Comfortable Pose, Head Down

Such a simple forward bend, yet it has a huge relaxing effect!

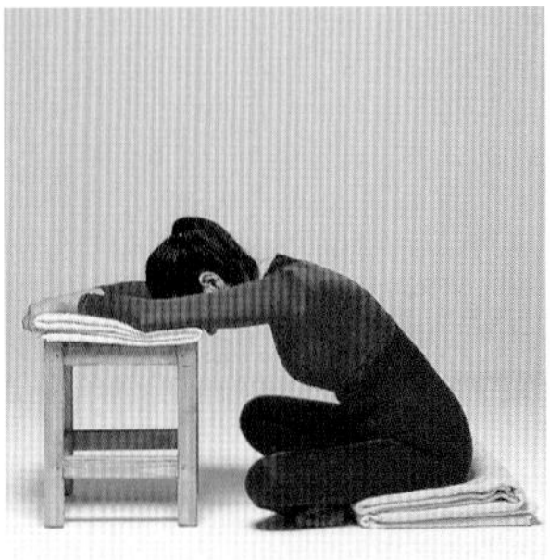

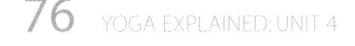

Sit on one or two folded blankets in front of a chair or stool. Bend the knees and cross the legs simply. Bend forward and rest the head and arms on the chair. Breathe evenly and relax.

Stay in the pose for 1 to 2 minutes. Cross the legs the other way and repeat.

Help

- **If the pose is not comfortable, adjust the height of the support under the head or buttocks.**
- **If the hip joints or groins feel strain, support the thighs.**

To Progress

Move the chair a little farther away, so as not to compress the front of the body.

सेतुबन्ध-सर्वाङ्गासन

Setu-Bandha-Sarvāṅgāsana

Shoulder-Balance Bridge

With the lower back raised on a support and a gentle incline of the trunk, relaxation comes surprisingly easily.

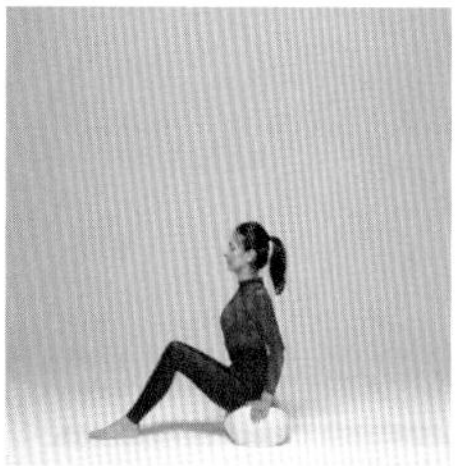

Sit on top of a bolster placed horizontally. Hold the ends.

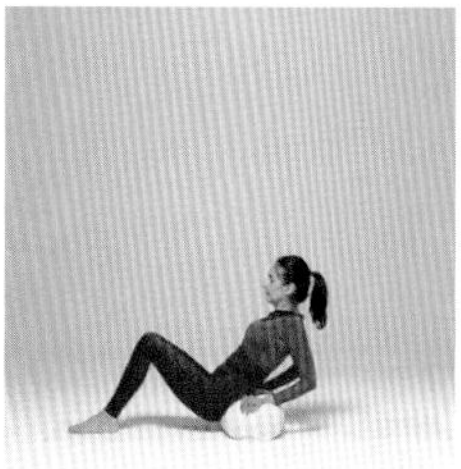

Move forward until the coccyx (tailbone) is off the bolster, and lean back.

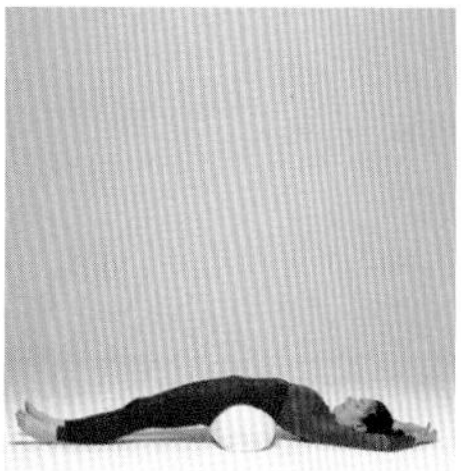

Lie down so that the lower back is supported on the bolster and the head and shoulders are on the floor. Stretch out the legs. Take the arms over the head. Breathe evenly and relax. Stay for 2 to 5 minutes.

To come down, slide backward off the bolster. Bend forward in simple cross-legs, resting the head on the bolster.

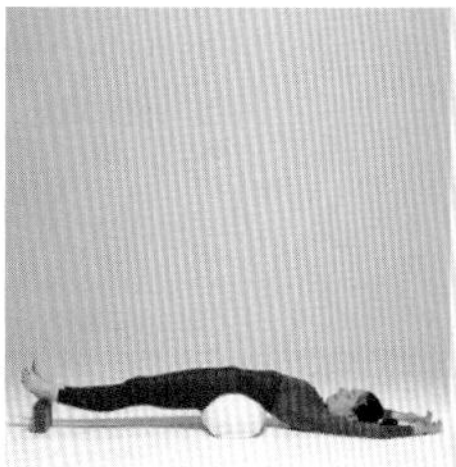

Help

- **Move backward or forward on the bolster to get a comfortable position.**
- **If the back feels strain, raise the feet on a support.**

To Progress

Increase the height of the support under the back.

विपरीत-करणी-मुद्रा *Viparīta-Karaṇī-Mudrā*

Reverse-Action Position

For recovery from fatigue, nothing can beat this pose.

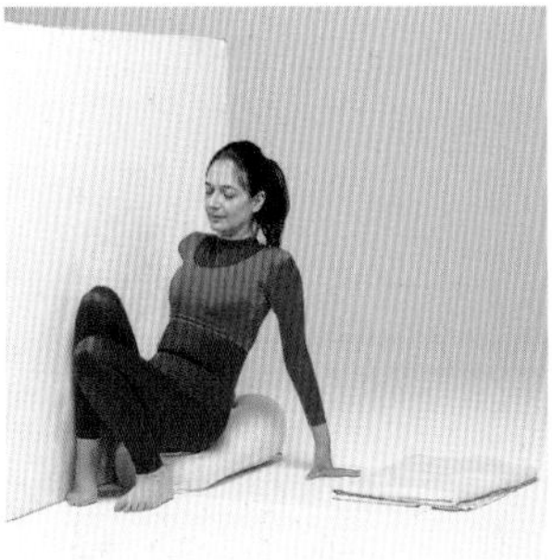

Place a bolster lengthwise against a wall. Keep a blanket nearby. Sit sideways on the bolster, with the right buttock against the wall.

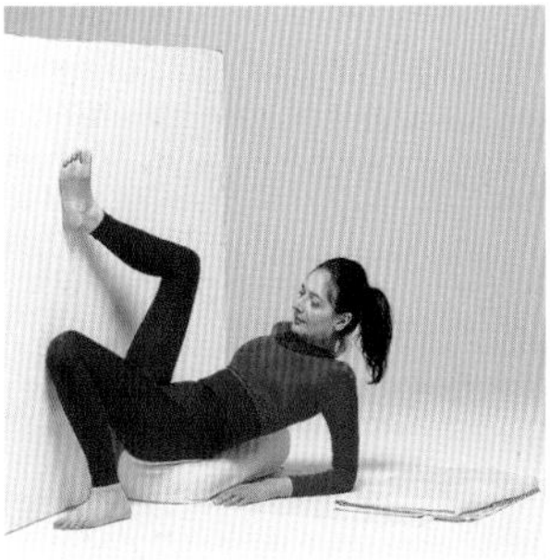

Lean back and raise one leg at a time onto the wall, simultaneously swiveling the body around to be perpendicular to the wall.

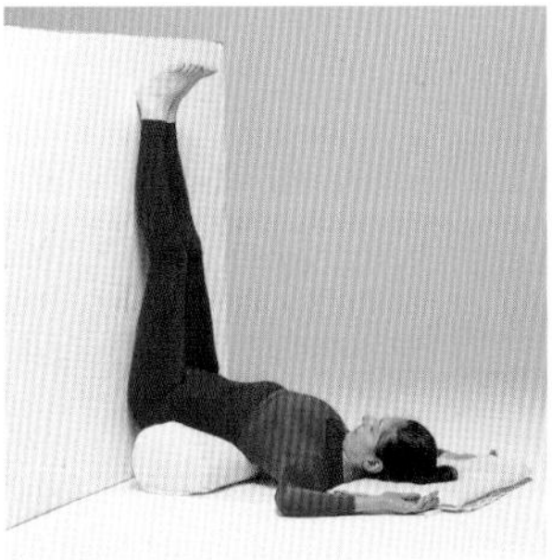

Lie down so that the lower back and waist are on the bolster and the head and shoulders are on the floor. Straighten the legs up. Place the blanket under the head and neck. Take the arms over the head. Breathe evenly and relax.

Stay in the pose for 5 to 6 minutes. To come down, slide backward off the bolster and turn to the side.

To Progress

Press the hips down, so that the lower abdomen tilts slightly toward the wall.

Place a folded blanket or two on top of the bolster, so that the chest expands more.

Help

- **Tall people may need to move the bolster a little away from the wall and place blankets on top of the bolster.**

शवासन *Śavāsana*

Corpse Pose

Relaxation is fast and deep when the back is raised on a support.

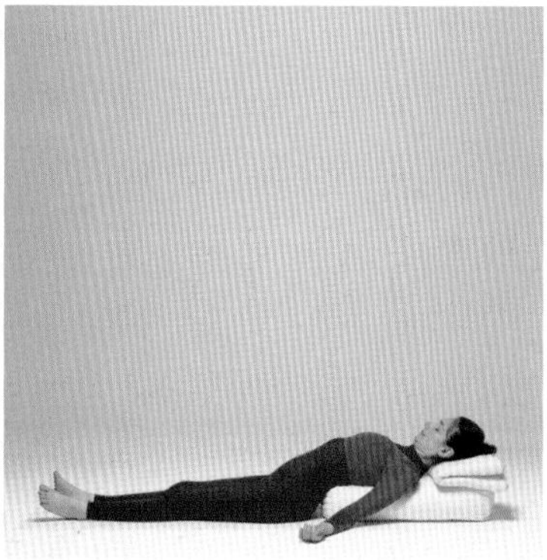

Sit on the floor with a bolster behind the back. Lie back on it, making sure the body is in a straight line. Place a folded blanket on the bolster under the head and neck. Stretch the legs and then let them drop to the sides. Press the shoulders down and move the shoulder blades in. Turn the upper arms so that the biceps face the ceiling. Stretch the arms and let them drop to the sides. Relax the hands, allowing the fingers to curl. Close the eyes and relax the face.

Stay in the pose for 5 to 10 minutes. Turn to the side, roll off the bolster, and get up.

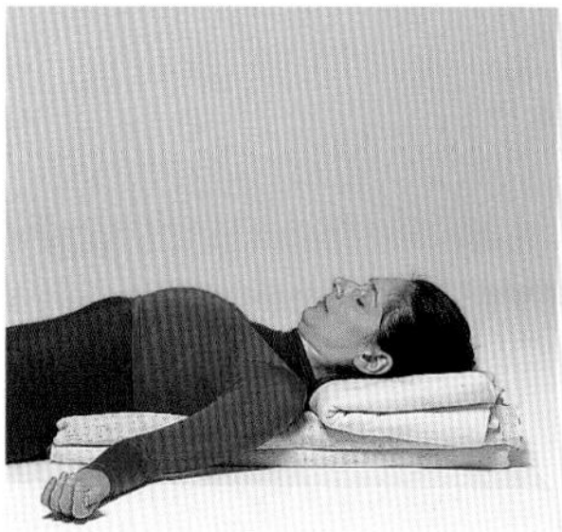

Help

- **If the bolster is too high for comfort, use one or two blankets folded into a narrow strip.**

To Progress

Do not sink into the bolster; make the back slightly concave so that the chest lifts.

Continuously relax the face and the sense organs: eyes, ears, nose, tongue, and skin. Relax the throat.

The major schools of yoga

KEY CONCEPT

Immortality In the *Haṭha* Yoga tradition, this means escaping death while retaining the very body with which we are born. This can be achieved, maintains the school, by imprisoning the breath in the body, mainly through the practice of breath control (*prāṇāyāma*), as death implies the departure of the breath from the body. In *Upaniṣadic* literature, however, "immortality" is generally used in the sense of liberation.

In the previous Units we saw how the philosophical search begins and how its field of inquiry can be divided into the outer and inner worlds.

Through such a search, the ancient Indian thinkers arrived at the conclusion that the principle underlying both the worlds is the same. What is within is also without. This outlook is known as monistic. However, the philosophical outlook of Yoga is dualistic: it regards the principles underlying the two worlds to be basically different – the inner principle is essentially consciousness, the observer, the subject, the soul; the outer principle is material, the observed, the object, Matter. Yoga seeks to find out the causes of the sufferings of the soul and the way to eradicate them. It is in the second aspect, the removal of suffering, that the contribution of Yoga to philosophy lies.

The concept of Yoga has come down to us through two main streams, *Rāja* Yoga and *Haṭha* Yoga. The first represents Yoga as conceived by Patañjali, and the second as conceived by masters like Matsyendra and others known only through legends. The names by which the two schools are recognized today are not found in older works, though traces of both the schools are found in *Upaniṣadic* literature, as already pointed out. The name *Haṭha* Yoga probably came into being from its characteristic outlook and practices (outlined below); the name *Rāja* Yoga presumably came into vogue to contrast its character with the *Haṭha* school. A third branch, *Tantra*, overlaps *Haṭha* Yoga to some degree.

Rāja Yoga

The *Yoga Sūtra* of Patañjali is the definitive source work on *Rāja* Yoga. Dating from the second century B.C., it consists of 194 aphorisms (195 according to some) and is divided into four chapters, dealing broadly with meditation (*samādhi*), aids to Yoga (*śādhana*), powers (*vibhūti*), and liberation (*kaivalya*).

The first chapter defines basic concepts of Yoga and gives an overall picture of the Yoga course from beginning to end.

The second chapter specifies eight aids of Yoga (see Unit 12) and details the first five of these.

The third chapter discusses the final three aids and the miraculous powers attained as the practice advances. Patañjali, however, warns the yoga disciple against being lured by these powers and missing the main object of Yoga, namely, liberation.

The last chapter explains the concepts of bondage to the world, liberation, actions, and the memory imprints associated with them. It concludes with the *Sāṃkhya*-Yoga view regarding the nature of the soul, and an examination of the opposing views of rival philosophical schools, mainly the Buddhists.

Though aimed at the purity and control of the mind, Patañjali's Yoga has to deal with such physical aspects as contribute to the control of mind. This makes room for Yogic postures and breath control, the third and the fourth of the aids of Yoga in Patañjali's scheme. These aids gained extreme importance in the other school, *Haṭha* Yoga.

Haṭha Yoga

The major text of *Haṭha* Yoga is the *Haṭhayoga-Pradīpikā* by Svātmārāma (fifteenth century A.D.). Written in lyrical Sanskrit verse (389 in number), the work is divided into four chapters.

The first chapter deals with postures (*āsanas*). After giving guidance regarding a suitable place for Yoga practice and naming 34 masters, it gives detailed instructions for 15 postures and refers to 84 in passing.

The second chapter is devoted to breath training (*prāṇāyāma*). It describes eight varieties of this (such as deep breathing and alternate nostril breathing) and six cleansing processes as preparatory practices for people with excess body fat.

The third and longest chapter deals with positions (*mudrās*). It includes some sexual and occult practices aimed at awakening the spiritual energy known as *kuṇḍalinī*, which lies dormant at the base of the spine like a sleeping snake. Once roused, this energy is channeled to the crown of the head, a process that is believed to make the practitioner immortal. The warning that this doctrine is a guarded secret and must be obtained from an authoritative teacher recurs in this text almost as a refrain.

The fourth chapter deals broadly with meditation—concentration of the mind on a selected mental object. This implies continuous thinking on the chosen object to the exclusion of other objects. The practice here can be equated with that explained by *Rāja* Yoga. It is said that with progress in breath training comes the awareness of an inner sound (*nāda*). The simplest introduction to this concept is the sound we hear on closing the ears with the hands. Listening to it helps develop the habit of concentration. The inner sound resembles progressively that of a cloud, sea, drum, conch, bell, flute, bee, and so on. The practitioner is advised to concentrate on subtle sounds in preference to loud ones. This stops the mind from jumping from object to object.

Svātmārāma attempts to relate *Haṭha* Yoga to the *Rāja* Yoga of Patañjali by considering it as a pathway to the latter.

However, his work is practical rather than philosophical, and it is therefore difficult to make a comparison of doctrines. Of major interest in this text is the detailing of *āsana* and *prāṇāyāma*, beyond what Patañjali has to say about them.

This school aims to achieve immortality by preserving the body through occult practices; ancient masters of *Haṭha* Yoga are believed to defy death and to be still "moving about" in this world, implying in the very bodies they were born with. This contradicts Svātmārāma's initial statement that the object of *Haṭha* Yoga is to pave the way for *Rāja* Yoga.

Tantra Yoga

There is a third branch of Yoga that can be traced to equally ancient times. It is known as Tantra, meaning "doctrine," and is characterized primarily by magic and mystic practices. Many schools in this branch borrow concepts—for example, energy channels (*nāḍīs*)—from the *Haṭha* Yoga theory about human physical structure, and superimpose on them their own devices of body control. These include the worship of friendly and ferocious gods, involving mystic diagrams, and the muttering of chants with sacred syllables and sounds believed to possess magic potency. To these devices are added mystical concepts such as energy centers (*cakras*) in the body situated along the length of the spinal column. These are imagined in the shape of lotuses with varying numbers of petals. These centers are important in the *Haṭha* Yoga ideal of awakening the "serpent power" (*kuṇḍalinī*). Some *Tantra* schools include in their sacred rites occult practices that are not accepted by mainstream society. Some of these practices are also found in *Haṭha* Yoga, showing that there is an overlap or unclear boundary between the two.

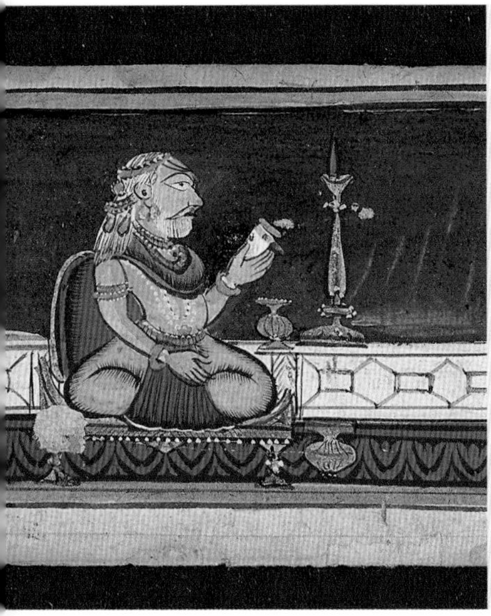

Vyāsa, the author of the *Bhagavad-Gītā* and commentator on the *Yoga Sūtras*.

In Brief

The seed of Yoga is the *Upaniṣads*. It became a tree in Patañjali's aphorisms.
It flowered and bore fruit in Vyāsa's commentary and in elucidations and dissertations.

Climbing the tree called *Rāja* Yoga, a Yogin, through meditation,
Merges his mind in Primordial Matter and attains liberation.

The Yogin intent on breath training, who climbs the tree called *Haṭha* Yoga,
Moves in the world and enjoys immortality.

Both these paths are spoken of in the scriptures; through one of them, the Soul
Is released from Matter; through the other, it is the lord of Matter.

Whether the Soul is the lord or vassal of Matter, there is
Contact with mind; being contact-free, liberation is the supreme way.

For a wider perspective ...

Verse Form in Sanskrit Literature

In the Sanskrit scholarly tradition it is not unusual to find serious works in verse form, meaning compositions containing four-line units of regular rhythmical patterns. A work in verse, therefore, need not be poetic in content. The reason for the use of verse is that it makes memorization of the text easier. The *Bhagavad-Gītā*, some *Upaniṣads*, the *Haṭha* Yoga *Pradīpikā*, and other *Haṭha* Yoga texts are in verse.

The Aphoristic Style in the Sanskrit Tradition

The aphoristic style, consisting of concise statements about a subject, developed uniquely in the Sanskrit literary tradition. Basic works in this style in all major subjects known to the contemporary world of scholars were written from the eighth century B.C. onward, most of them toward the beginning of the Christian era. Patañjali's *Sūtras* on Yoga belong to this time.

Sūtra is the Sanskrit word for "aphorism." Its primary meaning is "thread," and the role of a *sūtra* text in the presentation of a subject is compared to that of a thread in the weaving of a garland. It gives the core teachings and linking arguments. The garland is the principal commentary on the core text. It is an explanatory work that is indispensable for a full understanding of the subject. Such commentaries have given rise to successive subcommentaries explaining words, phrases, and points in the principal commentaries. The *sūtra* text can be committed to memory with minimum effort. This method of memorization is still in vogue today (although threatened by the modern educational system), representing an unbroken tradition of learning.

The Major Works on *Rāja* Yoga

AUTHOR, DATE, AND WORK

Patañjali (150 B.C.), *Yoga Sūtra* (*YS*)
Vyāsa (A.D. 300–400), Commentary (*Bhāṣya*) on *YS*
Vācaspati-miśra (A.D. 850), Commentary on Vyāsa's *Bhāṣya*
Bhoja (A.D. 1050), Commentary on *YS*
Vijñāna-bhikṣu (A.D. 1550), Commentary on *YS*
Nāgeśa-bhaṭṭa (A.D. 1725), Commentary on *YS*
Anonymous, *Yoga Upaniṣads* (various)

The Major Works on *Haṭha* Yoga

AUTHOR, DATE, AND WORK

Gorakṣanātha (12th–13th c. A.D.?), *Gorakṣa Śataka*
Svātmārāma (15th c. A.D.), *Haṭha Yoga Pradīpikā*
Gheraṇḍa (17th c. A.D.?), *Gheraṇḍa Saṃhitā*
Anonymous, *Śiva Saṃhitā*
Anonymous, *Yoga Upaniṣads* (various)

Unit 5

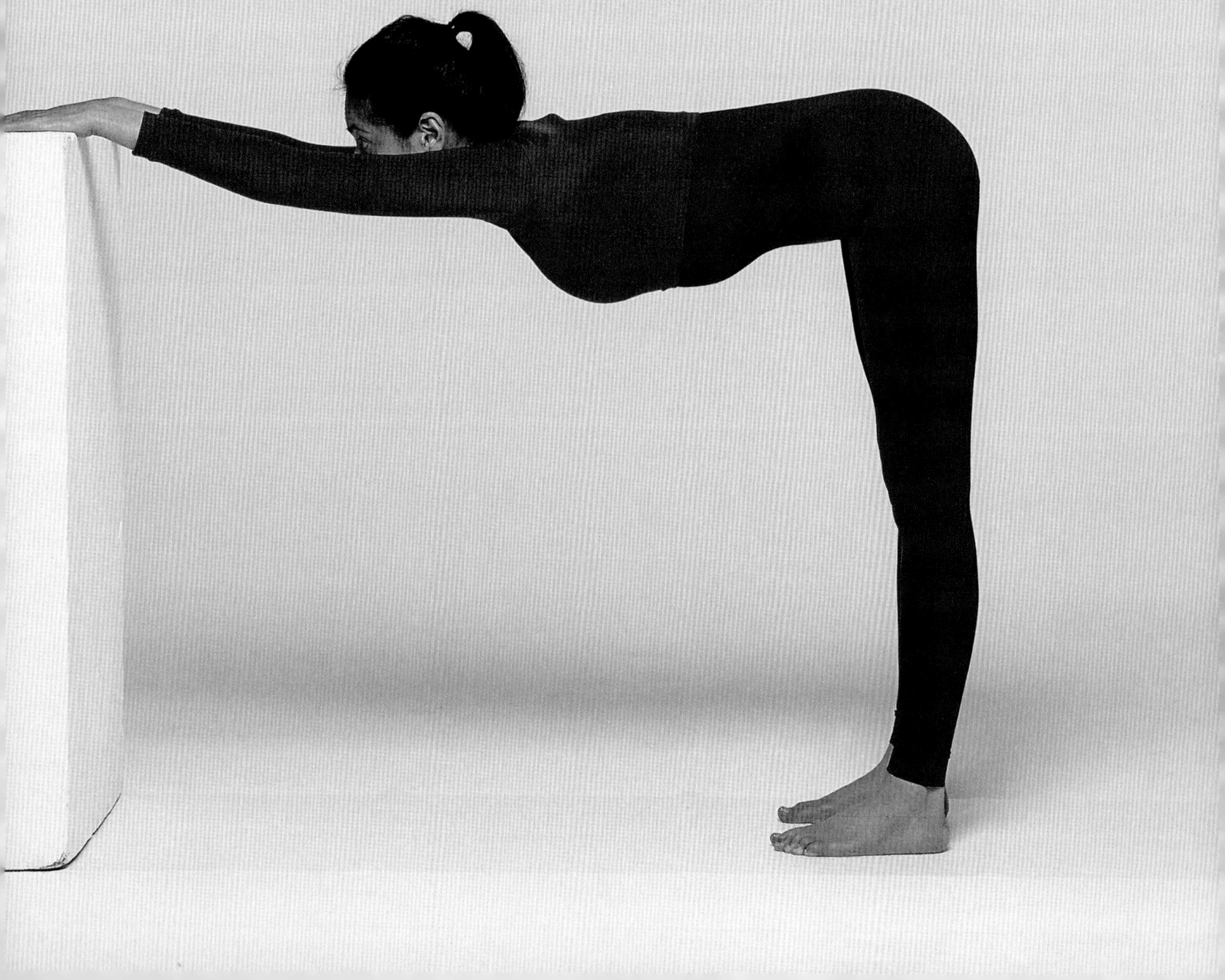

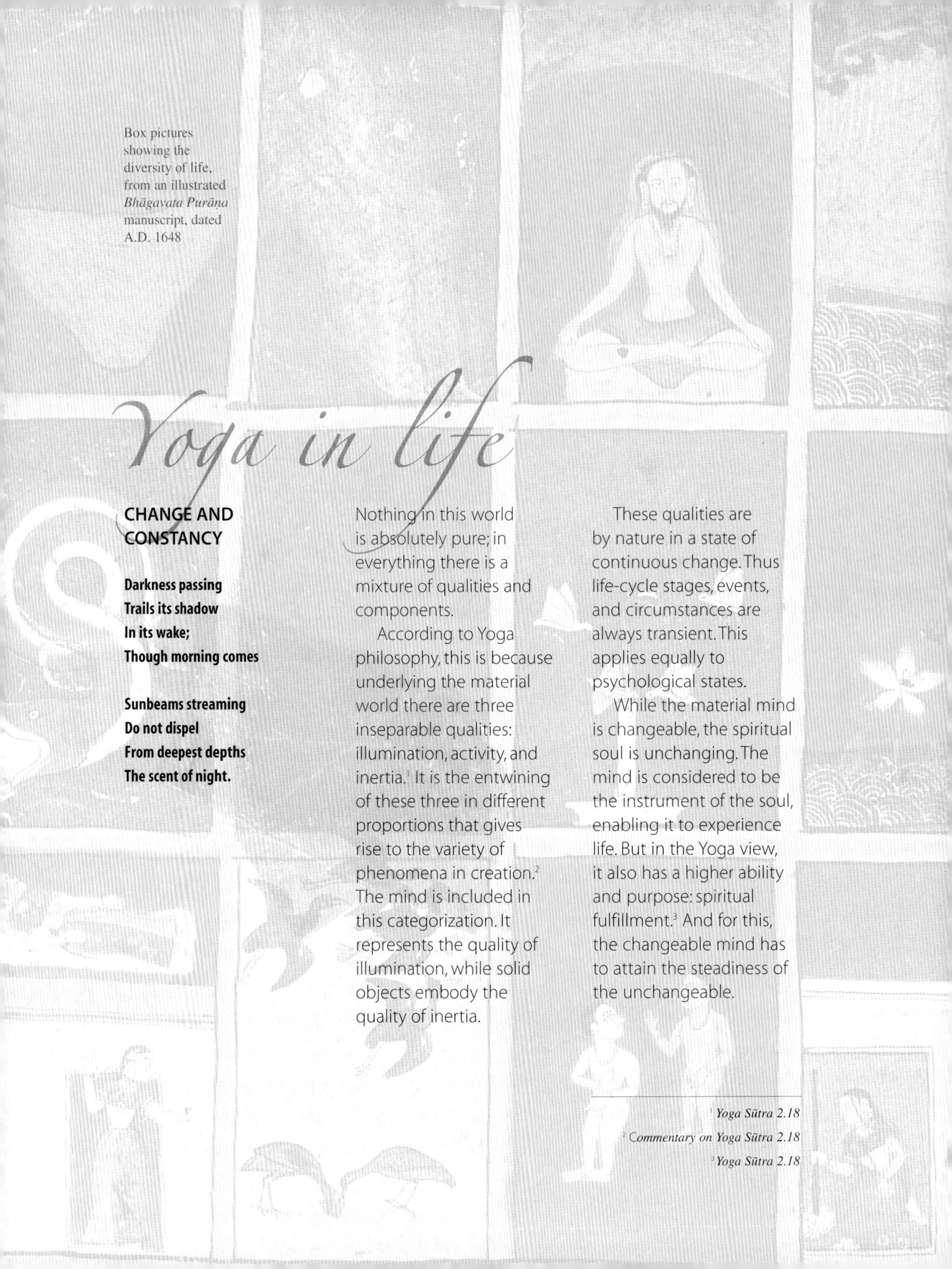

Box pictures showing the diversity of life, from an illustrated *Bhāgavata Purāna* manuscript, dated A.D. 1648

Yoga in life

CHANGE AND CONSTANCY

Darkness passing
Trails its shadow
In its wake;
Though morning comes

Sunbeams streaming
Do not dispel
From deepest depths
The scent of night.

Nothing in this world is absolutely pure; in everything there is a mixture of qualities and components.

According to Yoga philosophy, this is because underlying the material world there are three inseparable qualities: illumination, activity, and inertia.[1] It is the entwining of these three in different proportions that gives rise to the variety of phenomena in creation.[2] The mind is included in this categorization. It represents the quality of illumination, while solid objects embody the quality of inertia.

These qualities are by nature in a state of continuous change. Thus life-cycle stages, events, and circumstances are always transient. This applies equally to psychological states.

While the material mind is changeable, the spiritual soul is unchanging. The mind is considered to be the instrument of the soul, enabling it to experience life. But in the Yoga view, it also has a higher ability and purpose: spiritual fulfillment.[3] And for this, the changeable mind has to attain the steadiness of the unchangeable.

[1] *Yoga Sūtra 2.18*

[2] *Commentary on Yoga Sūtra 2.18*

[3] *Yoga Sūtra 2.18*

Moving the hips

In daily movements the articulation of the legs within the hip joints is often limited. Standing, walking, running, kneeling, squatting, and sitting on chairs all require a front-facing position of the thigh bone within the joint. An outward rotation of the thigh is required only in sitting cross-legged on the floor and in deliberately cultivated movements, such as in dance or Yoga.

Yet the potential of movement in the hips is greater than routine motions would suggest, and the price of underuse is high. The hip joints form a complex unit with the pelvis, and the pelvis houses the base of the spine. When the hips become stiff, the lower back also becomes rigid. This is turn reduces the mobility of the whole spine and increases the likelihood of pain.

When the body changes position, it is usually the legs that give the impetus of movement and the pelvis that remains relatively static; this reinforces the tendency of the lower back toward inflexibility. Yoga has an innovative approach to this problem. In certain postures the pelvis has to move while the legs are held stable. This lessens tightness of the lower back and hips, thereby increasing movement.

Standing poses are particularly effective in this respect. In all of them the legs remain firm after being turned, especially the back leg which is always held straight. Some standing poses, such as Triangle Pose (*Trikoṇāsana*) and Side Angle Pose (*Pārśvakoṇāsana*), require movement of the hips laterally away from the upright position. In the second Warrior Pose (*Vīrabhadrāsana* 2), the pelvis is maintained upright deliberately in order to prevent collapse to the front or side.

In the first Warrior Pose (*Vīrabhadrāsana* 1) and Sideways Intense Stretch (*Pārśvottānāsana*) the hips are rotated 90 degrees from the front. This requires a strong turn of the pelvis against the legs. In the latter pose the pelvis also bends forward toward the legs.

Hand in hand with freedom in the hip joints comes relaxation of the groin area. Tight groins hamper an easy stride and are liable to become strained. Separating the legs wide in standing poses stretches this region. This is also achieved in Fish Pose (*Matsyāsana*), a supine pose in which the legs are simply crossed.

When the hips are moved in various directions, they become agile. Lightness of the hips is further developed in Shoulder-Balance (*Sarvāṅgāsana*), where the body is inverted and stretches up in a vertical line, supported by the upper arms and shoulders. The muscles of the lower back are trained to lift the trunk and legs against gravity, and thus they develop strength.

Maintaining the upward thrust of this pose requires time and practice. However, the back enjoys relief from the strain of having to hold itself upright. A pose that brings the benefit of spinal inversion without effort is the Half-Plow (*Ardha-Halāsana*). In this, the legs are taken over the head and rested on a support. The head, back, and legs all relax blissfully, preparing the body and mind for deep relaxation in Corpse Pose (*Śavāsana*).

तडासन *Tāḍāsana*

Mountain or Palm Tree Pose

Firmly held hips are a key to this pose; unless the hips are activated, they become slack, as well as stiff, and the body goes out of alignment.

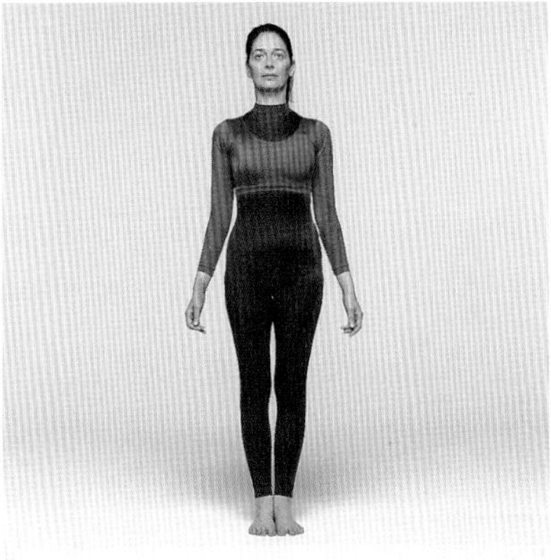

Follow the method given in Unit 1 (page 19).

To Progress

Contract the hips (the sides of the pelvis) and draw the pelvis up. At the same time lengthen the lower back away from the waist and draw the coccyx (tailbone) in.

त्रिकोणासन *Trikoṇāsana*

Triangle Pose

The use of a brick support in this pose helps the trunk to lift up, rather than collapse toward the floor. This is turn gives room for the hips and trunk to turn effectively.

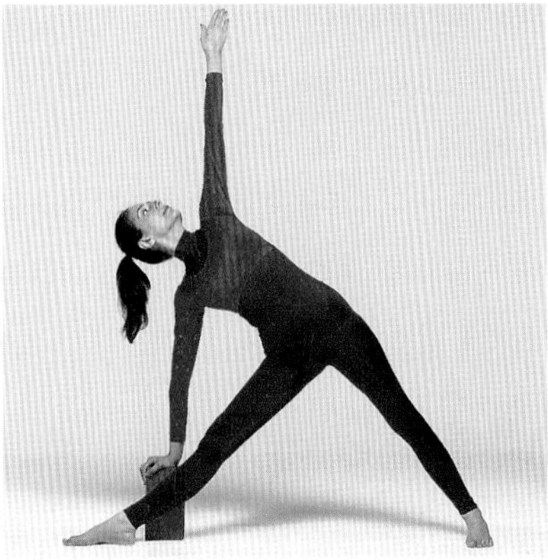

Follow the method given in Unit 2 (page 36).

To Progress

Revolve the right leg outward from the ankle to the thigh. Move the right buttock forward, and take the head back to bring the body into a plane. Lift the left hip strongly upward so that the pelvis and rib cage rotate to the same degree.

पार्श्वकोणासन *Pārśvakoṇāsana*

Side Angle Pose

The brick gives height to the supporting arm, and therefore lift and lightness to the trunk. With more space in which to maneuver, the hips and rib cage can turn better.

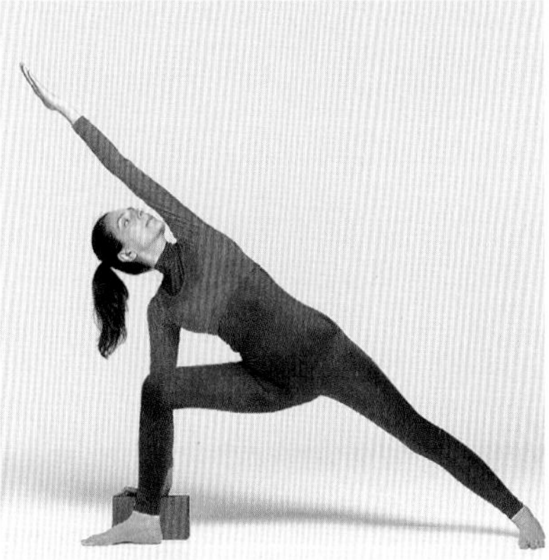

Follow the method given in Unit 2 (page 38).

To Progress

Move the right buttock forward, and press the right knee against the right arm. Press the left thigh back. With the help of the right arm and shoulder, bring the right side of the trunk forward. With the help of the extended left arm, take the left side of the trunk back.

वीरभद्रासन २ *Vīrabhadrāsana 2*

Warrior Pose 2

Like the stance of a warrior poised for action this pose conceals dynamism while appearing static.

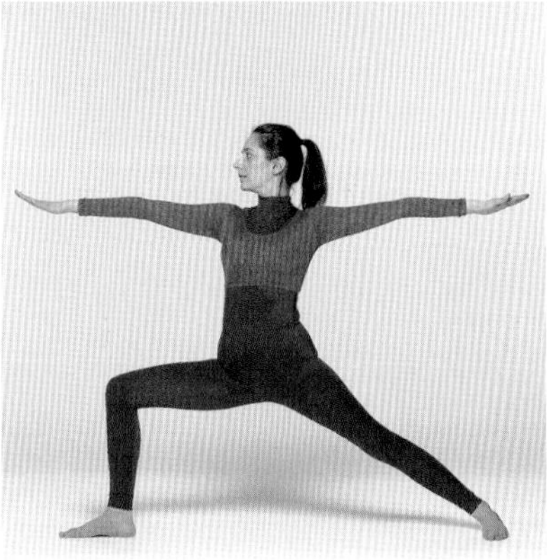

Follow the method given in Unit 2 (page 40).

To Progress

Move the right buttock forward and the right knee back. Make the back leg poker-stiff. Lift the hips away from the legs. Keep the left hip pulled back and to the left, to stop the pelvis from tilting to the right or downward.

Lift the rib cage away from the waist.

वीरभद्रासन १ *Vīrabhadrāsana I*

Warrior Pose 1

This pose imitates a warrior who swings his torso around without losing stability and power in the legs.

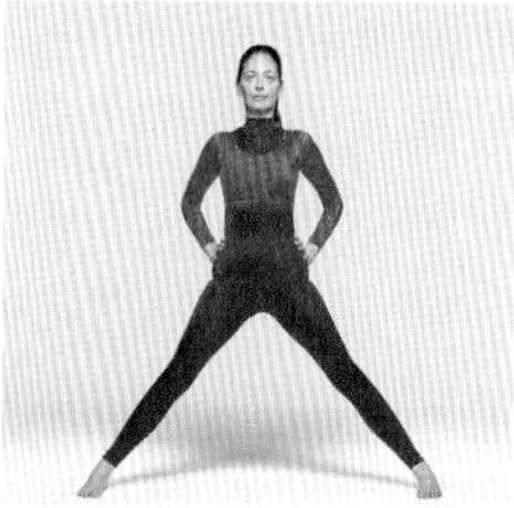

Stand in *Tāḍāsana* (see Unit 1, page 19). Take a deep inhalation and jump the feet 4–4½ feet apart, at the same time extending the arms sideways to shoulder level, with the palms facing down. Align the feet and make them parallel. Place the hands on the hips.

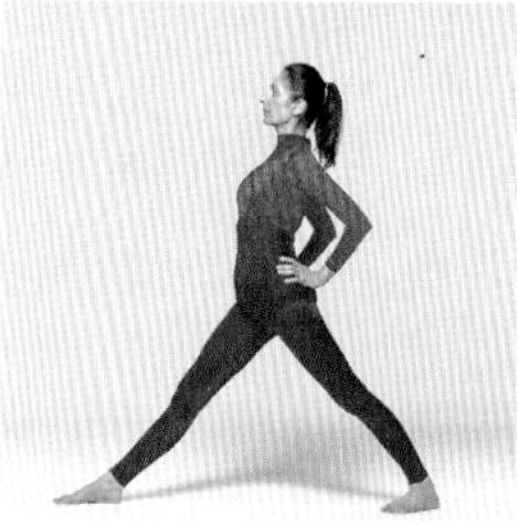

Turn the left foot 45–60 degrees in and the right foot 90 degrees out. At the same time, turn the trunk to the right. Align the center of the right heel with the center of the left arch. Revolve the left leg inward, in the direction of the foot. Tighten the kneecaps and pull up the thigh muscles.

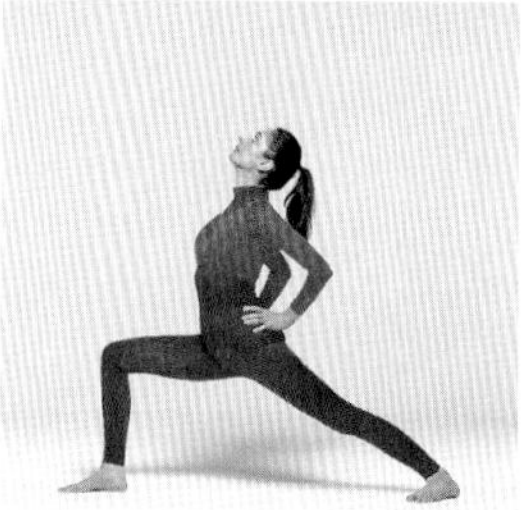

Exhale and bend the right leg to form a right angle, with the shin vertical and the thigh horizontal. Keep the trunk vertical. Take the head back and look up toward the ceiling. Breathe evenly and without strain.

Stay in the pose for 20 to 30 seconds. Inhale and come up. Turn the feet to the front and rest the arms. Then repeat on the other side.

Inhale and come up. Bring the arms to horizontal. Exhale, jump the feet together, simultaneously bringing the arms down.

To Progress

Press the outer edge of the left foot down. Lift and stretch the inner leg from the ankle to the groin.

Move the right knee further to the right, to bring it in line with the hip.

Move the pelvis back, so that the abdomen does not tilt toward the right thigh. Lift the hips, rib cage, and sternum (breastbone). Stretch the side ribs, but do not lift the shoulders.

उत्तानासन *Uttānāsana*

Intense Stretch

While the legs stretch, the head and heart rest as they are inverted, making this a restorative pose.

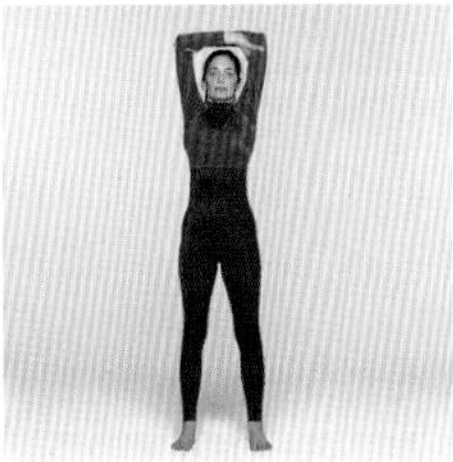

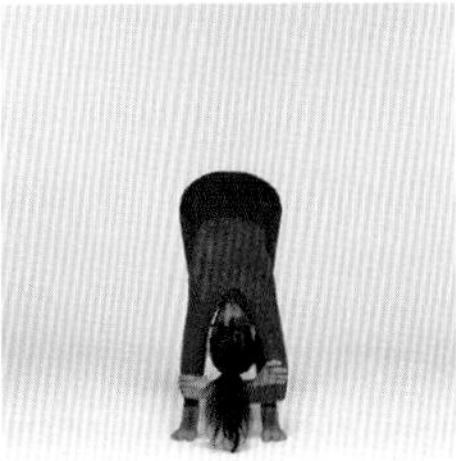

Stand in *Tāḍāsana* (see Unit 1, page 19). Take the feet hip-width apart, keeping them parallel. Catch the elbows. Inhale and take the arms over the head. Stretch the legs, trunk, and arms up.

Keeping the knees firm, exhale and bend forward from the hips, taking the trunk toward the legs. Relax the head.

Stay in the pose for 20 to 30 seconds. Inhale and come up. Release the arms and bring the feet together.

To Progress

Pull the thigh muscles strongly up toward the groins, in order to flex better at the hips.

Pull the elbows firmly down in order to lengthen the sides of the trunk.

अर्ध-उत्तानासन *Ardha-Uttānāsana*

Half Intense Stretch

The pelvis forms an exact right angle with the legs to create the optimal spinal extension.

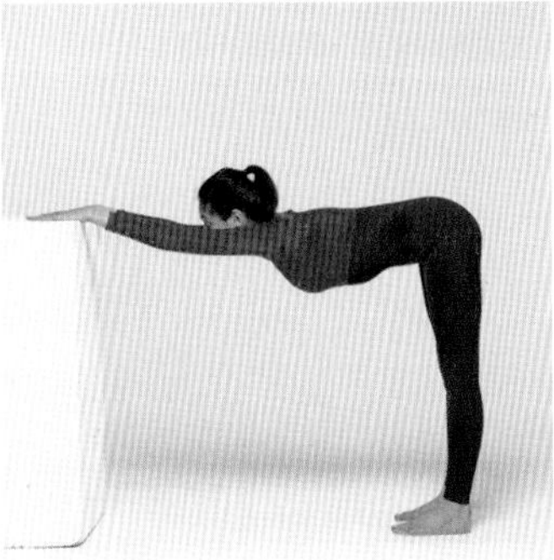

Follow the method given in Unit 2 (page 41).

To Progress

Pull the thigh muscles strongly up towards the groins. Lift the buttock bones and press the pelvis downward, without collapsing at the waist. Press the thoracic spine down, particularly between the shoulder blades. Lengthen the front of the body.

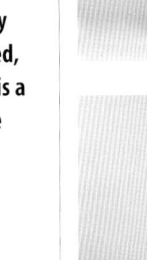

वीरभद्रासन ३ *Vīrabhadrāsana 3*

Warrior Pose 3

Balance and thrust are the hallmarks of this pose, even when supported.

Do *Ardha-Uttānāsa*, following the method in Unit 2, page 41.

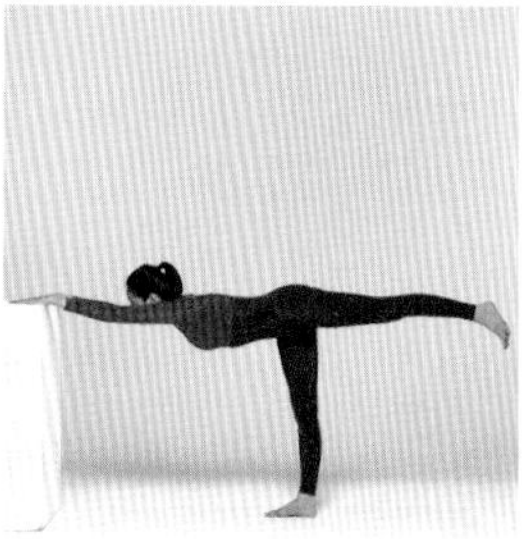

Raise the left leg back and up, keeping the knee firm and the foot extended, until it is parallel with the floor. Do not raise the left hip, buttock, or side of the trunk. Do not bend the elbows. Breathe evenly.

Stay in the pose for 20 to 30 seconds. Bring the leg down. Inhale and come up. Repeat on the other side.

To Progress

Pull the right thigh muscle strongly up. Control the left hip by moving the left buttock away from the spine. Make the left ankle firm.

पार्श्वोत्तानासन *Pārśvottānāsana*

Sideways Intense Stretch

A sideways direction is added to this stretch of the legs and spine.

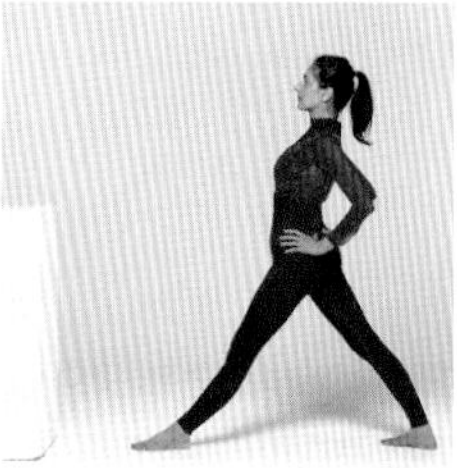

Stand about 3 feet away from a ledge of hip-height, with the right side facing it. Spread the legs 3½–4 feet apart. Place the hands on the hips. Turn the left foot 45–60 degrees in and the right foot 90 degrees out. Turn the hips so that the trunk faces the ledge.

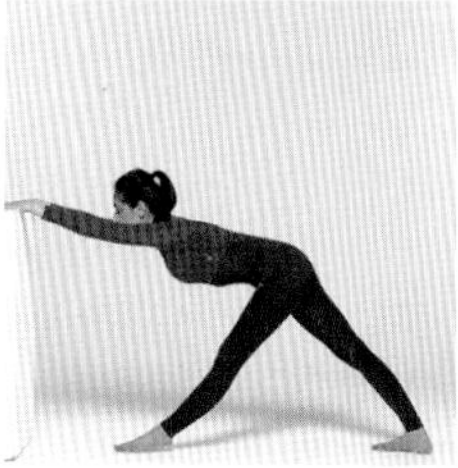

Bend forward from the hips, and place the hands on the ledge. Keep the knees tight, and stretch the legs up. Draw the hips slightly back, and move the trunk down without bending the elbows.

Stay in the pose for 20 to 30 seconds. Inhale and come up. Repeat on the other side.

To Progress

Pull up the thigh muscles of both legs. Take the left hip down to make the hips level. Move the pelvis slightly to the left, so that the spine is in a straight line.

अधोमुख-वीरासन *Adho-Mukha-Vīrāsana*

Hero Pose, Head Down

Flexing the hips is a key to this simple relaxing pose.

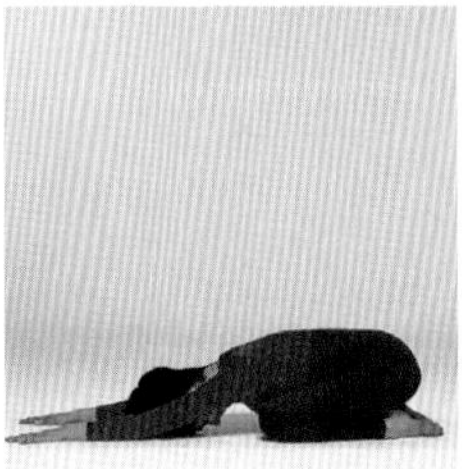

Follow the method given in Unit 2 (page 42).

To Progress

Press the hips down. Take the hands farther forward, and lengthen the sides and front of the body. Press the thoracic spine down, particularly between the shoulder blades.

शयित-ऊर्ध्व-हस्तासन *Śayita-Ūrdhva-Hastāsana*

Lying-Down Arm Stretch

The lower back lengthens along the floor in order to achieve the line of this stretch.

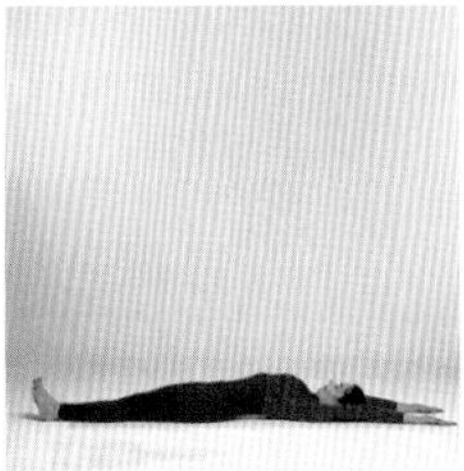

Follow the method given in Unit 2 (page 43).

To Progress

Before stretching, pass the hands under the buttocks and move them down away from the waist. Keep the hips down while stretching.

मत्स्यासन *Matsyāsana*

Fish Pose

The hips and groins open in this pose, bringing relaxation to the lower abdomen.

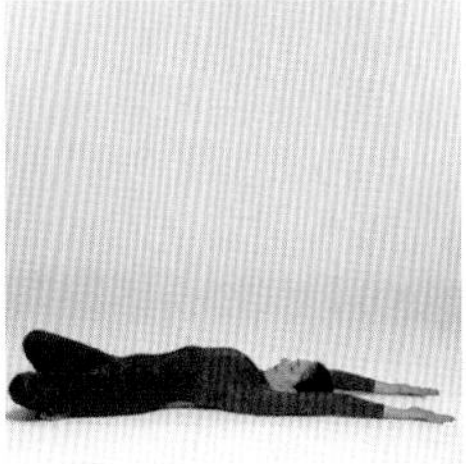

Follow the method given in Unit 2 (page 45).

To Progress

Stretch the arms from the shoulders.

सर्वाङ्गासन *Sarvāṅgāsana*

Shoulder-Balance

Surprise and pleasure are the usual reactions to inverting the body independently for the first time.

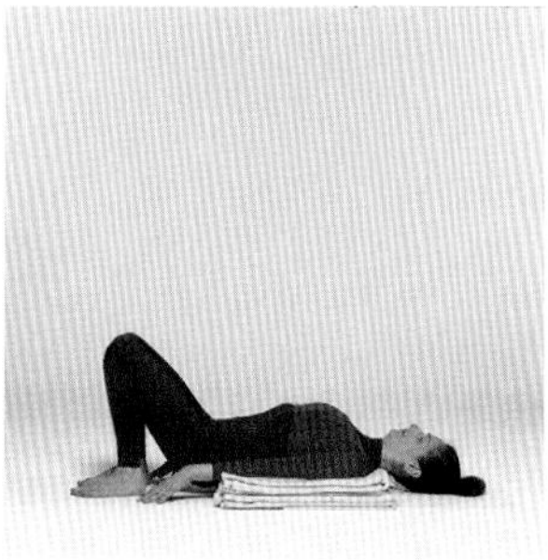

Fold three or four blankets and place them one on top of the other with the folded edges neatly on one side (see "Help," page 94).

Lie down with the shoulders on the folded edge of the set of blankets, and the head on the floor. Move the shoulders away from the neck and the shoulder blades in. Stretch the arms away from the shoulders. Bend the legs, keeping the feet on the floor.

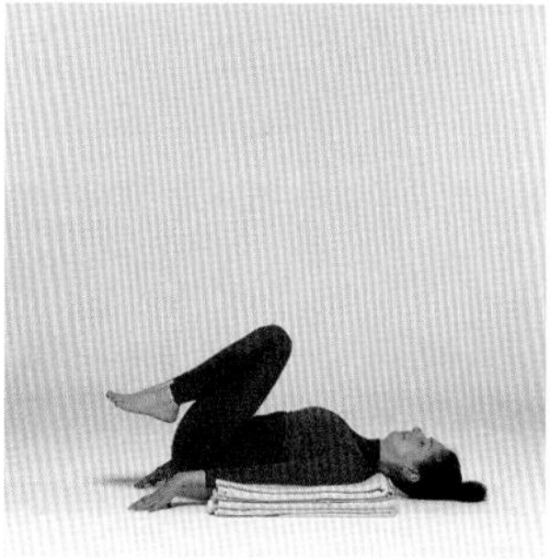

Bend the knees over the abdomen.

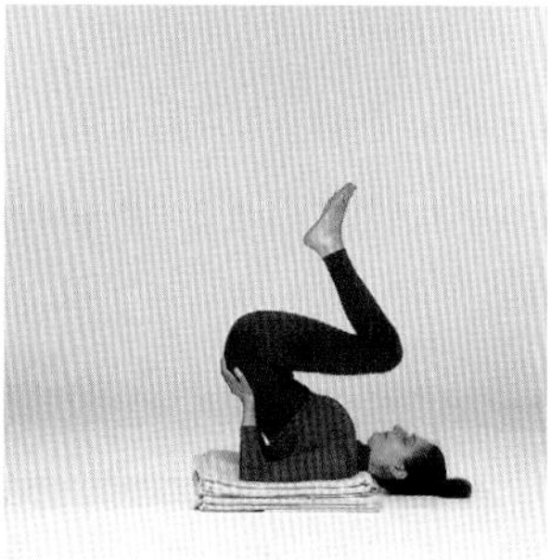

Lift the hips up and support the back with the hands.

Cautions

Do not do this pose during menstruation or if suffering from hypertension (high blood pressure), a neck injury, a detached retina, or other eye problems.

If there is pressure in the head, eyes, neck, or throat, come down, readjust the head, neck, and shoulders in the starting position and try again. If the pressure persists, seek the advice of a teacher.

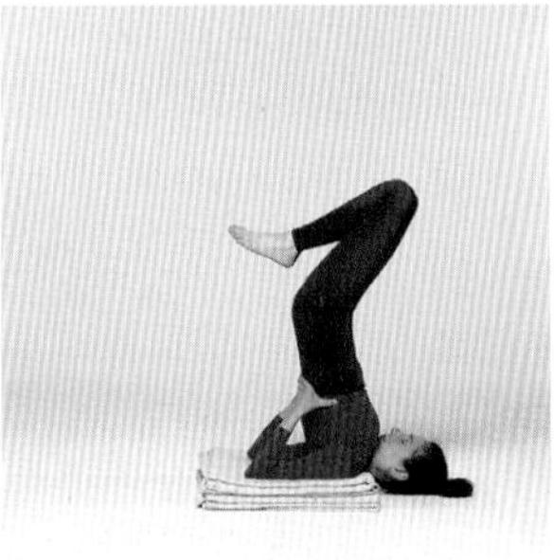

Lift the trunk higher, taking the hands lower down the back and bringing the elbows in to get a better support.

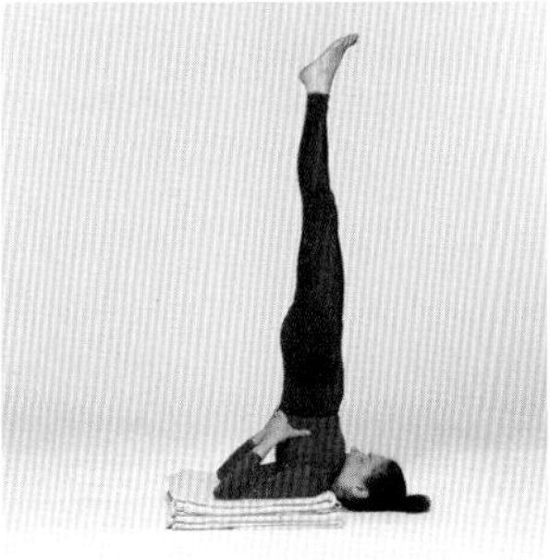

Straighten the legs up, and bring the whole body as much as possible toward the vertical.

Stay in the pose for 1 to 5 minutes. Bend the legs, exhale, and gently slide down.

Help

- **When folded, the blankets should be broader than the shoulders and longer than the upper arms. The blanket support prevents compression of the neck and throat.**

To Progress

Do not force the body into an upright position. This pose comes with time and practice.

अर्ध-हलासन *Ardha-Halāsana*

Half Plow Pose

When the thighs are rested on a stool in this pose, the spine is suspended upside down; relieved of its weight-bearing duties, it elongates and relaxes.

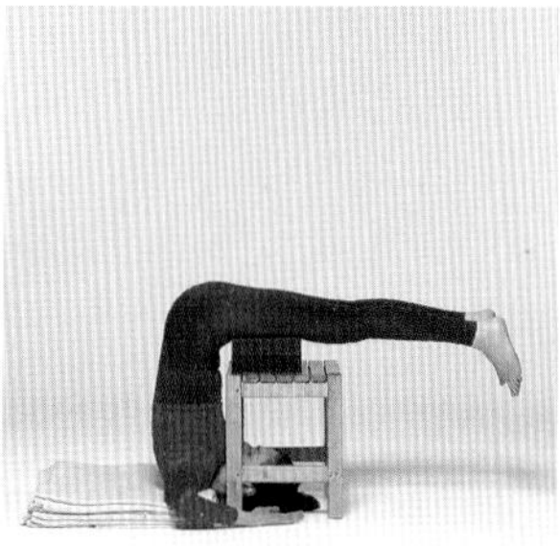

Do *Sarvāṅgāsana* (see pages 93–4), placing a medium-height stool a little beyond the head. Bend the legs and rest the thighs on the stool. If necessary, bring the stool closer in. Take the arms over the head. Relax.

Stay in the pose for 2 to 5 minutes. Bend the knees, ease the thighs backward off the stool, and push the stool away. Slide gently down.

Help

- **If the trunk feels compressed, raise the height of the stool support by placing folded blankets or a bolster on top.**

To Progress

Adjust the body so that the tops of the shoulders rest on the blankets. Lift the trunk up so that it does not collapse. Support the back with the hands if this is more comfortable.

शवासन *Śavāsana*

Corpse Pose

During this pose the fatigue of exertion is removed and the mind is refreshed.

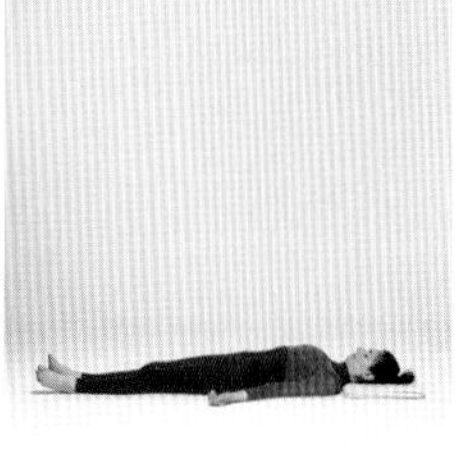

Follow the method given in Unit 1, page 26.

To Progress

Deliberately lengthen the legs away from the hips before relaxing them. Similarly lengthen the arms away from the shoulders. Do not let the limbs contract back into the trunk.

Ultimate reality

KEY CONCEPT

Knowledge In the philosophical context, the term "knowledge" in statements like "Knowledge leads to liberation" does not imply mere intellectual information, but actual experience, or "realization"—although information no doubt paves the way to experience. It is like the difference between understanding the sense of the word "sweet" and tasting something sweet.

Indian philosophical systems regard worldly life as a trap in which the soul is imprisoned, and they aim at finding a way for it to free itself. The trap functions because the soul does not know that the trap is outside itself; the mistaken notion that worldly life is intrinsic to the soul is due to its ignorance of its own nature. This ignorance leads the soul to consider as its own whatever mischief the trap causes. The moment it realizes Reality, it is freed from the trap. This, in brief, is what Indian philosophical schools endeavor to investigate and establish in a rational way.

Philosophy and the Highest Common Factor

The inquiry into Reality is, to borrow a term from mathematics, about finding the highest common factor of the world we live in. In other words, it aims to discover what is the common basis underlying all phenomena in the world. All analytical knowledge follows this formula. Oxygen and hydrogen constitute the highest common factor of water. Species of creatures emerge from or merge into others, depending on what is the highest common factor. Birds are separate from other species when wings form the highest common factor; they are not separate when life is the highest common factor. Life as the highest common factor distinguishes living forms from lifeless matter. Birth, growth, and death are characteristic of life; they are not found in earth and stones, which are part of inert matter.

Matter and Spirit

This analysis illustrates the process by which the twin-systems—the metaphysical system *Sāṃkhya* and its practical counterpart, *Yoga*—conceived Reality to be dual in nature, consisting of insentient (unconscious) Matter, *prakṛti*, and sentient (conscious) Spirit, *puruṣa*. What we have to note is that the concept of soul is not the same as that of life. Life, which is essentially breathing, pertains to the body, which is Matter and hence different from the Spirit. What is breathing, if not the commuting of air to and from the body? Modern science explains all bodily structures and functions in terms of the basic elements of nature like oxygen and hydrogen. What it cannot explain is the conscious "force" (Spirit) that makes these elements in the body function in a way they do not function elsewhere in the material world. The live body, for instance, moves and stops, grows and decays, but a stone is incapable of such internally generated operations or changes. This force, Spirit, defies all the laboratory skills man has developed through the centuries.

Analysis of States of Consciousness

It is here the philosopher steps in to say that this force (Spirit, or soul) is a distinct entity that cannot be equated with life. And he has reasons to maintain his stand. An analysis of the states of consciousness—waking, dreaming and deep sleep—shows that our worldly identities and experiences, existing in the first two states and leading us to pleasure and pain, are totally absent in the third. This fact, supported by everybody's experience, gives us an insight into the pure nature of the Spirit not enveloped by the body-mind complex. An insightful *Upaniṣadic* thinker compares this situation to that of a hawk who, after a long flight in the sky, becomes tired and heads for its nest. Likewise the soul, after roaming in the waking and the dreaming states, heads for the state of deep sleep, in which it does not act or dream, but crosses beyond worldly relations and experiences. Here a father is not a father, a mother is not a mother, a thief is not a thief, and a sinner is not a sinner.

This experience is terminated after some time, when we return to the two other states. These are likened to the banks of a river between which a fish swims.

Is it possible to make the transcendent but temporary experience of deep sleep permanent? Yes, says the philosopher, if we can succeed in severing our soul from the body-mind complex through which we experience the world. Such a possibility is known in philosophical terms as liberation. Liberation can be achieved during life—that is, before death—as it is the disowning of the body by the soul. It is like a snake casting away its skin, unaffected by its withering away. To cite a contemporary parallel: when we sell our car, we are no longer concerned if it meets with an accident.

The Intrinsic State of the Soul: Freedom

How can this state be attained? It is by discovering what we really are. Freedom is said to be the natural state of the soul; when the soul is liberated, it is merely restored to its real nature, of which it is unaware because of ignorance. We discover our worldly identity when a dream comes to an end and we enter the waking state; this restoration to the waking state puts a stop to the illusory experiences in the dream. A similar reasoning is applied to liberation. In our worldly identity, we seldom think of ourselves as distinct from our mind. When we realize that the mind is part of Matter, and hence we are at core unconnected with it, that puts an end to our worldly sufferings. The problem is that we are so overwhelmingly ruled by the mind that we are unable to discern our real self, the soul. Yoga makes this problem its sphere of inquiry, and, by means of a deep analysis of the mind, shows the ways to control it, thereby making it possible for us to look at our own soul.

Once it is realized that the soul is distinct from Matter, it follows that it is untouched by the properties of the latter. As the *Bhagavad-Gītā* says, the soul cannot be cut, burned, wetted, or dried—processes that affect all material objects. The mind, being formless, is also beyond the reach of these physical actions, but is affected when the body experiences them. The Self is eternal—continues the *Gītā*—it is everywhere, unmoved and unlimited by time. It neither kills, nor is killed; it is neither born, nor dies.

What is Matter?

God Brahman gives the branches of knowledge (the *Vedas*) to the primeval Sages.

The ultimate root of the material world is insentient Primordial Matter (*prakṛti*), as the *Sāṃkhya*-Yoga systems name it. All gross objects have their roots in subtle principles. Primordial Matter (*prakṛti*) is said to have three qualities (*guṇas*): illumination (*sattva*), activity (*rajas*), and darkness (*tamas*). The material world inherits these from the primordial cause, leading to light/knowledge, activity and delusion/ignorance, respectively, on the part of the soul.

Matter constantly undergoes the processes of evolution and involution. It lacks consciousness, whereas the soul is conscious. If Matter is insentient, how can it operate on its own towards these processes? Because of the mere presence of the conscious soul, maintain the *Sāṃkhyas*. They explain this phenomenon by the analogy of the movements of iron filings caused by the mere presence of a magnet.

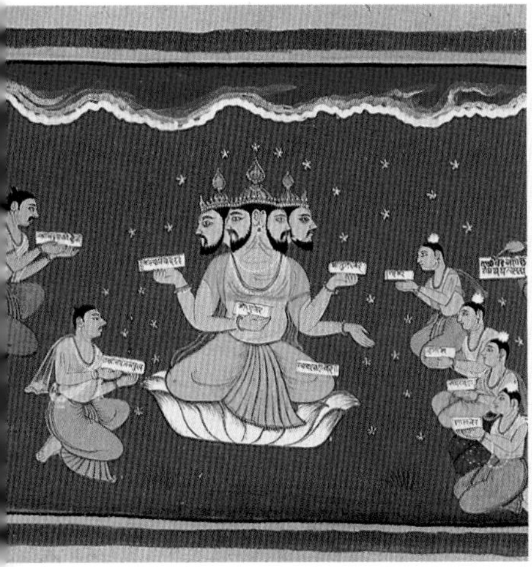

In Brief

If the quintessence of everything is determined on the basis of logic,
The distinction between insentient and sentient leads to the conclusion of duality.

Matter and Spirit: the qualities of light, activity, and darkness
Form Matter; Spirit is by nature free and inactive.

Insentient Matter acts due to the proximity of Spirit
As inert iron filings act due to the proximity of a magnet.

As long as the soul does not discern its distinctness from the mind
It experiences pleasure and pain; on discerning it, the soul attains liberation.

For a wider perspective ...

Existence

The analysis of water leads us to its components, oxygen and hydrogen. In the same way, everything in the material world is reduced by scientists to a limited number of elements. Elements consist of molecules, molecules of atoms, atoms of electrons, protons, and neutrons—each stage being subtler than the last. For the scientist, components at the final stage are the ultimate reality, and the earlier stages consist of combinations of the ultimate reality. This logic, if pursued further, may lead to the philosopher's concept of Ultimate Reality, as illustrated in the dialogue from the *Chāndogya Upaniṣad* cited in Unit 1. In contrast to the search for subtler components in science, philosophy seeks a wider and wider principle underlying phenomena until it arrives at the Infinite, also known as Existence. This is the highest flight of philosophical thinking.

Approaches to the Truth

Man's adventures in the world of spirituality reveal two basic trends: faith and reason. Of these, faith claims the largest portion of human society; all religions are based on it. Differing in details and practices, religions are unanimous in conceptualizing a supreme power controlling the world. This power is called God. Faith implies the surrender of reason.

Philosophies, on the other hand, are founded on reason and secular means of knowledge, though they are not free from the element of faith influencing their followers. The proportion of faith and reason varies from tradition to tradition and from school to school, influencing their conceptions of ultimate reality and what they consider the concerns of philosophy. This gives rise to numerous outlooks toward philosophical issues, leading to a mixture of philosophical and religious ideas in certain schools. Thus, the philosophical concept of an Ultimate Reality is equated with the religious concept of a personal God in some schools of Indian philosophy. This is the case with Yoga schools whose followers worship a particular deity—for example, *Haṭha* Yogins traditionally worship Śiva as supreme.

Schools that rely exclusively on reason conclude that matter and spirit are contrastive principles and hence see Ultimate Reality as dual. These are the *Sāṃkhyas*. The Yoga school accepts this view, but includes God as a special Soul or Spirit. Those who, to some extent, place more importance on intuition than on reason conclude that spirit is the sole, eternal reality, since the destructibility of matter is commonly observed. This is the main *Upaniṣadic* tradition, which is founded on experience as well as reason. Others who also limit their search exclusively to reason arrive at the concept of indivisible atoms as the ultimate reality of the material world, at the same time maintaining the separate existence of the soul.

Unit 6

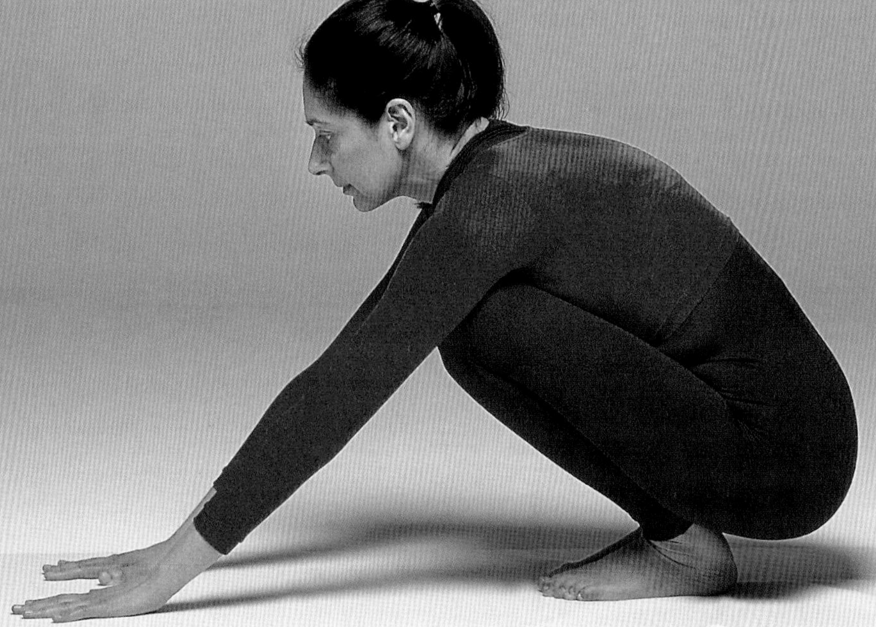

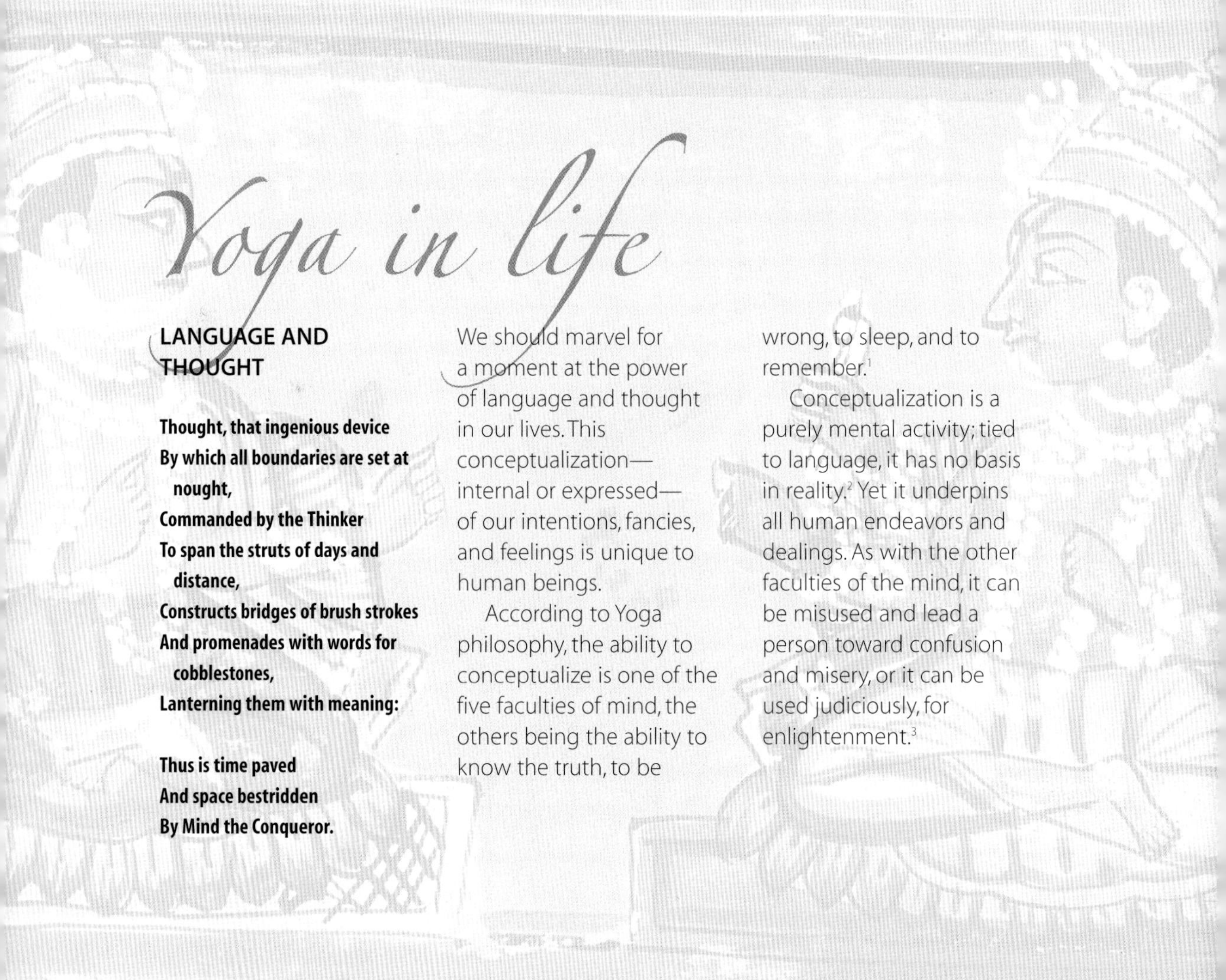

An illustration from the *Bhagavad-Gītā* (undated) showing a dialogue between Kṛṣṇa and Arjuna.

Yoga in life

LANGUAGE AND THOUGHT

Thought, that ingenious device
By which all boundaries are set at nought,
Commanded by the Thinker
To span the struts of days and distance,
Constructs bridges of brush strokes
And promenades with words for cobblestones,
Lanterning them with meaning:

Thus is time paved
And space bestridden
By Mind the Conqueror.

We should marvel for a moment at the power of language and thought in our lives. This conceptualization—internal or expressed—of our intentions, fancies, and feelings is unique to human beings.

According to Yoga philosophy, the ability to conceptualize is one of the five faculties of mind, the others being the ability to know the truth, to be wrong, to sleep, and to remember.[1]

Conceptualization is a purely mental activity; tied to language, it has no basis in reality.[2] Yet it underpins all human endeavors and dealings. As with the other faculties of the mind, it can be misused and lead a person toward confusion and misery, or it can be used judiciously, for enlightenment.[3]

[1] *Yoga Sūtra 1.6*

[2] *Yoga Sūtra 1.9*

[3] *Yoga Sūtra 1.5*

The arms and legs

Human limbs are capable of an extraordinary range of movements, over and above those needed for everyday activities. To keep joints mobile and muscle tone at its best, it is necessary to practice movements that take account of this potential, on the principle that by aiming for the maximum safeguards a minimum.

Bending the arms and legs in unaccustomed ways is the first step in the exploration of possible movements. This adds the power of flexion to that of stretching in the maintenance of a good physique.

Standing and sitting poses involve a wide range of limb positions. Tree Pose (*Vṛkṣāsana*) entails bending one leg out to the side and supporting it on the straight standing leg, as a branch is borne by the trunk of a tree. The upstretched arms help the body to maintain balance. In Eagle Pose (*Garuḍāsana*), another balancing posture, one leg is wound around the other and the arms are similarly entwined in front of the body. In Upraised-Hips Pose (*Utkaṭāsana*), the body stays stationary between standing and sitting, with the legs bent and the arms stretched up.

Among sitting poses, Hero Pose (*Vīrāsana*) involves folding the legs back so that the feet are beside the hips. In Bound-Angle Pose (*Baddha-Koṇāsana*) the legs are bent outward and the feet drawn in toward the body.

Mountain Pose (*Parvatāsana*) stretches the palms and fingers as well as the arms. In Cow-Head Pose (*Gomukhāsana*), the arms are taken behind the back from above and below so that the hands can catch. Another pose involves folding the hands behind the back in prayer position.

All these movements have an effect on a greater area than just the limb in question. The positioning of the legs has consequences for the hips, and therefore also the lower back. That of the arms affects the shoulders, and thus the upper back, neck, and head.

In all poses, in fact, the arms and legs play a crucial role. In Shoulder-Balance (*Sarvāṅgāsana*), the arms support the rib cage and help the trunk to lift. The legs stretch upward and pull the trunk erect from above. Similarly in Plow Pose (*Halāsana*), the action of the arms and legs prevents the collapse of the trunk.

In Corpse Pose (*Śavāsana*), the quality of relaxation depends in the first case on the limbs. If they hold tension, so does the whole body, and the mind cannot let go.

Thus, the arms and legs are active agents in shaping the postures, not passive appendages. They have specific functions: to bend, to stretch, to turn, to support, to hold, to connect, to anchor, to intensify actions, to empower other body parts. In this way coordination of all parts of the body is developed. At the same time, because this harmony cannot occur without the direction of the mind, there is integration of body and mind. It is this holistic approach that distinguishes postures from exercises.

ताडासन *Tāḍāsana*

Mountain or Palm Tree Pose

The joined legs give a strong base, and the arms give ballast to this vertical stretch of the body.

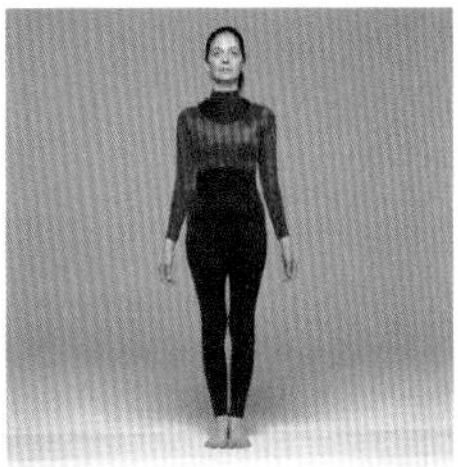

Follow the method given in Unit 1 (page 19).

To Progress

Synchronize the upward extension of the legs and the downward extension of the arms. Connect these two stretches with the lift of the trunk.

ऊर्ध्व-हस्तासन *Ūrdhva-Hastāsana*

Uplifted-Arm Pose

The fingers dovetail together, making the two raised arms a single powerful pulling device for giving traction to the trunk.

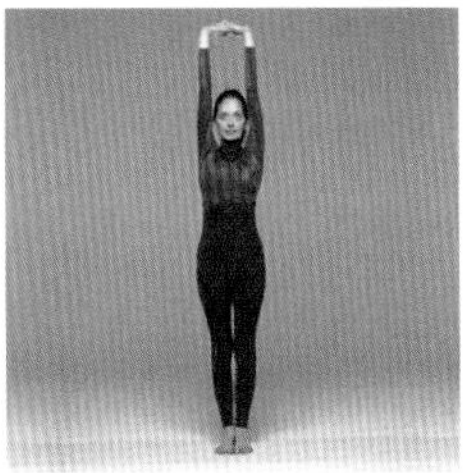

Follow the method given in Unit 2 (page 35).

To Progress

Maintain the firm upward stretch of the arms. Press the shoulder blades in, open the armpits, and take the arms farther back to make them vertical.

वृक्षासन *Vṛkṣāsana*

Tree Pose

The body imitates the shape and sturdiness of a tree, but not its tendency to sway in the wind!

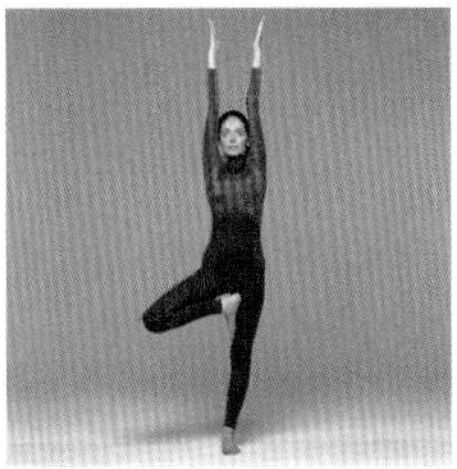

Stand in *Tāḍāsana* (see Unit 1, page 19). Bend the right leg outward, hold the bottom shin, and place the foot against the top of the inner left thigh. Fit the heel into the groove of the groin. Keep the left leg firm. Raise the arms out sideways to shoulder level, and turn the palms up. Tighten the elbows and stretch the arms and hands. Inhale and take the arms up, palms facing each other. Balance, breathing evenly.

Stay in the pose for 20 to 30 seconds. Exhale and bring the arms and leg down. Repeat on the other side.

To Progress

Press the left hip in to keep the vertical alignment of the standing leg and trunk. Press the bent knee back. Stretch the arms farther up and extend the sides of the trunk.

गरुडासन *Garuḍāsana*

Eagle Pose

Lightness and poised alertness characterize this pose, enabling a balance that depends delicately on flexed arms and legs.

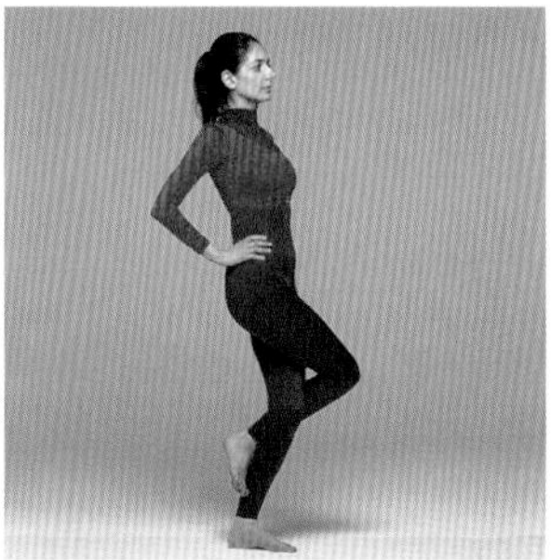

Stand in *Tāḍāsana* (see Unit 1, page 19). Place the hands on the hips and bend the legs a little. Lift the right leg a little, and take the right thigh across the left thigh. Take the right shin behind the left calf, and hook the foot against it just above the left inner ankle. Balance.

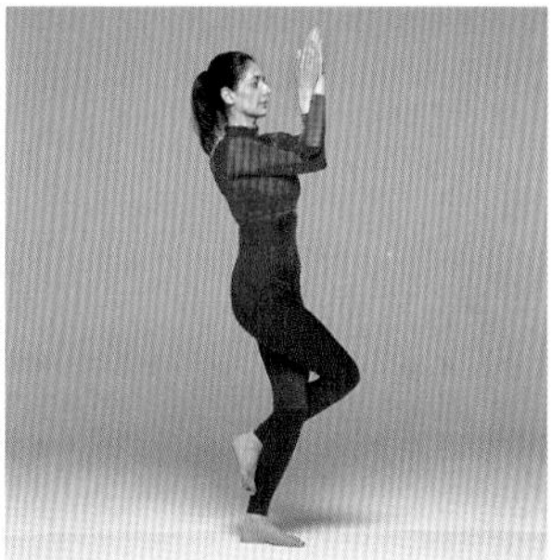

Raise the arms to the front, and bend them so that the upper arms are parallel to the floor and the forearms are vertical. Keep the palms facing each other. Bring the arms closer, and cross the left upper arm over the right. Take the left forearm in front of the right, and press the left palm against the right fingers. Keep the head straight. Balance, breathing evenly.

Stay in the pose for 20 to 30 seconds. Release the arms and legs and repeat on the other side.

To Progress

Press the standing shin back to maintain the upward energy of the standing leg. Stretch the trunk up. Raise the elbows slightly till the forearms are horizontal, and move the arms away from the chest.

उत्कटासन *Utkaṭāsana*

Upraised-Hips Pose

The upward thrust of the trunk and arms counterbalances the downward pull of the flexed legs to allow the hips to stay raised.

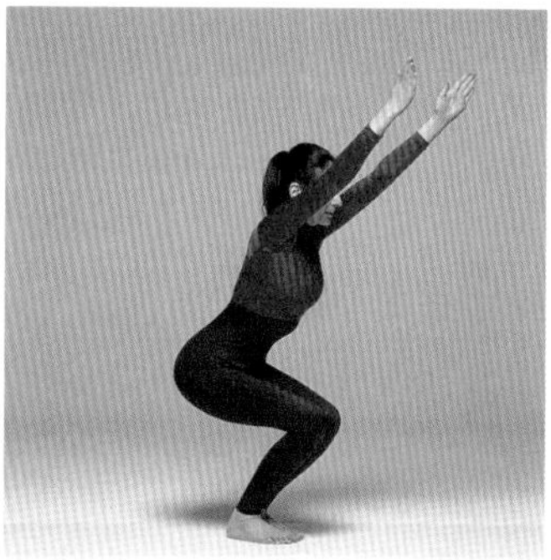

Stand in *Tāḍāsana* (see Unit 1, page 19). Inhale and raise the arms, keeping the elbows tight and palms facing each other. Extend the arms and trunk up. Exhale and bend the legs, taking the hips back until the thighs are almost parallel with the floor. Relax the head and neck. Look straight ahead and breathe evenly.

Stay in the pose for 15 to 20 seconds. Exhale, bring the arms down, and stand straight.

To Progress

Flex further in the ankles, knees and hips to sharpen the zigzag of the legs. Press the shoulder blades in and lift the front of the body.

पर्वतासन *Parvatāsana*

Mountain Pose

The arms stretch up and help the ribcage to lift; the legs press down and help the pelvis to lift.

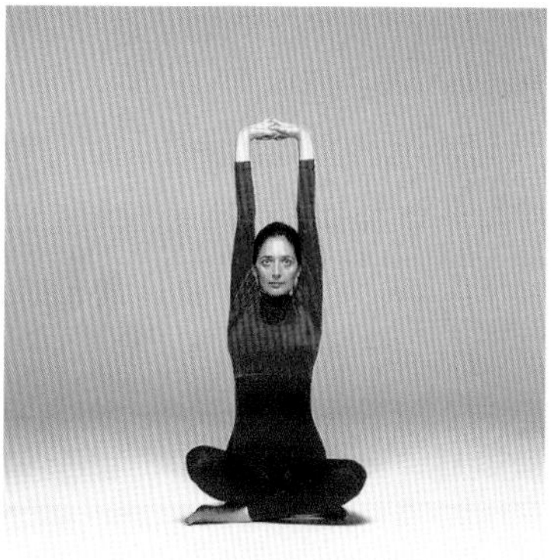

Follow the method given in Unit 1 (page 24).

To Progress

Make the following manual adjustments. Move the flesh of each buttock away from the other, and sit on the points of the buttock bones. Roll the thighs outward so that the inner thighs face the ceiling. Similarly roll the calves upward. These adjustments improve the lift of the lower back and relieve tightness in the groins and knees.

गोमुखासन *Gomukhāsana*

Cow-Head Pose, Arms Only

The full pose in profile resembles a horned bovine head; the upward-pointing elbow forms the cusp of the horn.

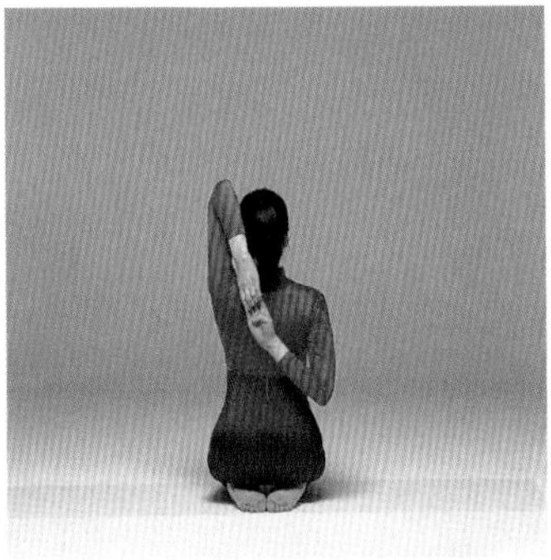

Follow the method given in Unit 3 (page 61).

To Progress

Stretch the left arm up and extend the armpit. Stretch the right upper arm downward and move the forearm away from the trunk.

Help

- **If the hands cannot catch, hold a belt.**

नमस्ते *Namaste*

Salutation

It's goodbye to stiff shoulders and sunken chest when the palms join in prayer position behind the back.

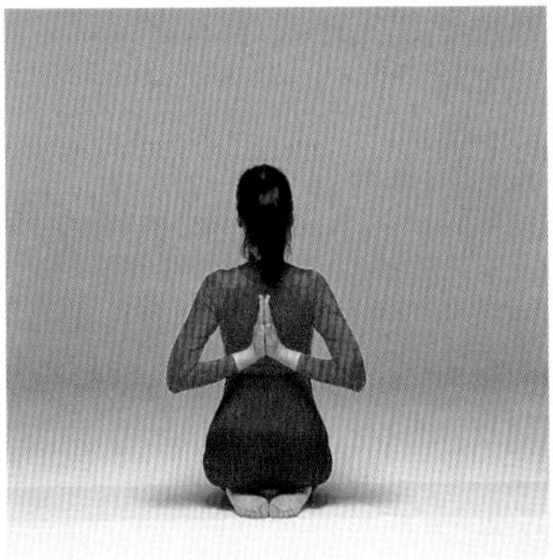

Kneel with the knees together. Lift the trunk and sit erect. Join the palms behind the back, turn the hands inward and upward and raise them as high as possible up the spine. Take the shoulders and elbows back. Breathe evenly.

Stay in the pose for 20 to 30 seconds. Release the hands and bring the legs forward.

To Progress

Stretch the arms and hands; try not to lose this extension while moving them into position. Move the hands higher.

Help

- **If this position is impossible, catch the elbows. Take the shoulders back and lift the chest. Repeat, catching the elbows the other way.**

वीरासन *Vīrāsana*

Hero Pose

A hero has a core of composure, which sustains his exploits; such composure is to be sought, and can be found, in this pose.

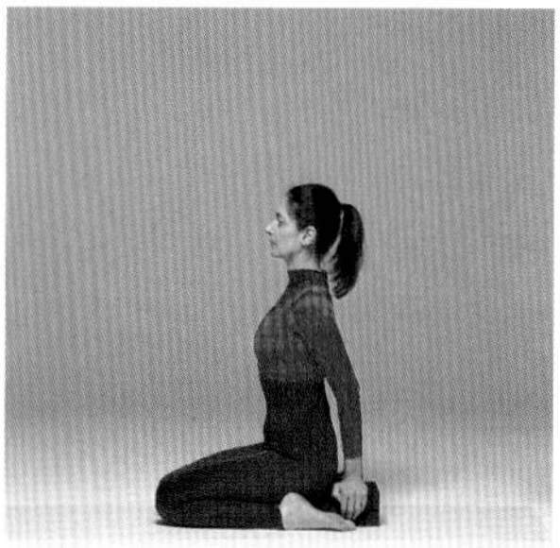

Sit on the heels with the knees together. Take the feet apart and insert a support, such as one or two folded blankets or a block, under the buttocks. Place the hands on the support. Roll the shoulders back and stretch the trunk up. Breathe evenly.

Stay in the pose for 1 or 2 minutes. Bring the legs forward.

Help

- **If the ankles are stiff, place a rolled blanket under the lower shins (see Unit 2, page 42).**
- **If there is tension in the knees, sit on a higher support.**

To Progress

Rotate the thighs outward, and press the outer shins down in order to keep the knees facing forward.

बद्धकोणासन *Baddha-Koṇāsana*

Bound-Angle Pose

The traditional sitting position for cobblers, this pose is beneficial during menstruation and for urinary disorders, as it features an open groin and an erect pelvis.

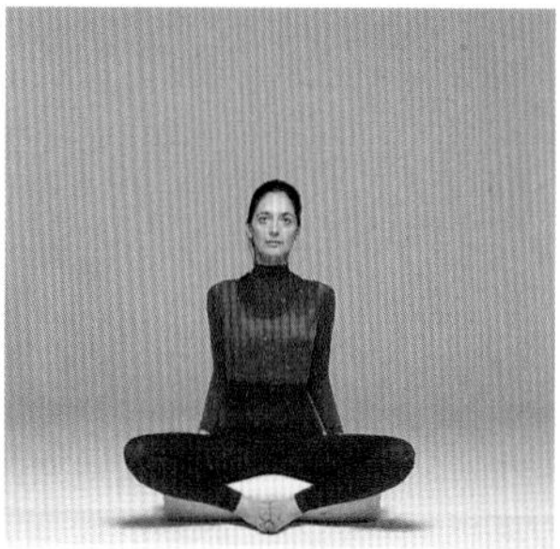

Sit against the wall on a support, such as a bolster or folded blankets. Bend the knees outward and bring the soles of the feet together. Bring the feet toward the pubis. Place the hands beside the hips and stretch the trunk up.

Stay in the pose for 30 seconds to 1 minute, or longer. Release the legs and bring them forward.

To Progress

Pressing down with the fingers, move the lower back forward and lift the abdomen up. Lift the rib cage and roll the shoulders back. At the same time open the groin and lengthen the thighs toward the knees.

मालासन *Mālāsana*

Garland Pose

This pose pays dividends by restoring the limberness of the natural human art of squatting; in the final pose, the arms encircle the legs and trunk.

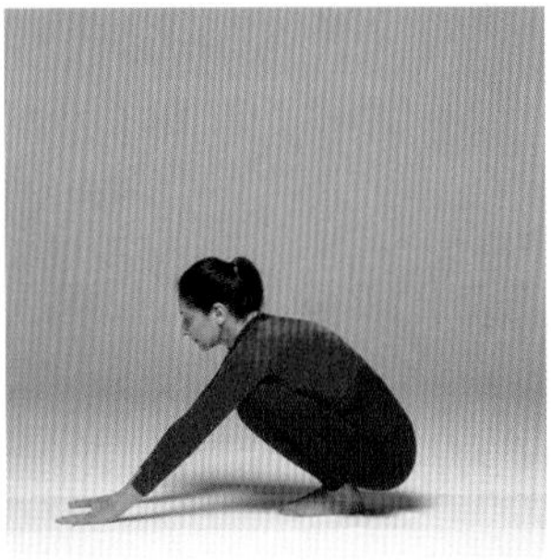

Squat with the feet and knees together. Keep the heels down. Stretch the arms forward. Breathe evenly.

Stay in the pose for 30 seconds to 1 minute. Release the legs.

To Progress

Bring the body weight forward while keeping the heels down.

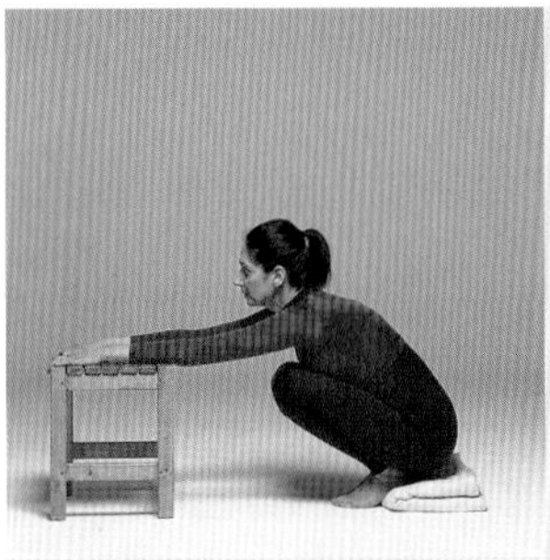

Help

- **Place a rolled blanket under the heels.**
- **Hold on to a support such as a stool or chair.**

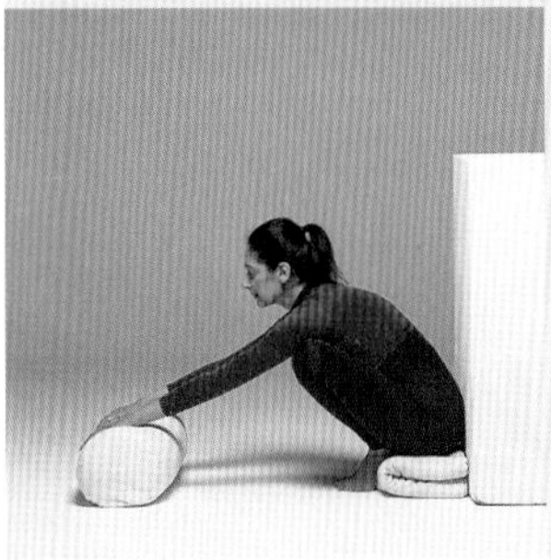

- **Rest the lower back against the wall, and rest the hands on a support.**

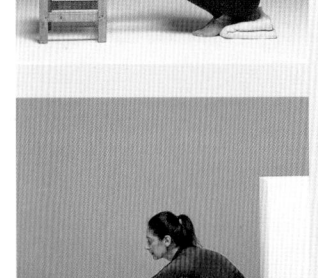

सर्वाङ्गासन *Sarvāṅgāsana*

Shoulder-Balance

As this pose becomes more familiar, it becomes like a trusty friend, reliably giving emotional support and calming the mind.

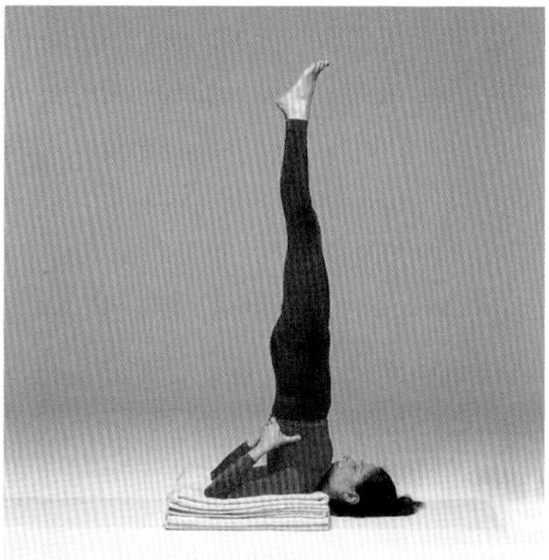

Follow the method given in Unit 5 (page 93).

To Progress

Keep the knees tight and extend the backs of the legs. Adjust the hands on the back from time to time to maintain a good support of the trunk.

Cautions

Do not do this pose during menstruation or if suffering from hypertension (high blood pressure), a neck injury, a detached retina, or other eye problems.

If there is pressure in the head, eyes, neck, or throat, come down, readjust the head, neck, and shoulders in the starting position, and try again. If the pressure persists seek the advice of a teacher.

हलासन *Halāsana*

Plow Pose

Taking the legs over the head is surprisingly restful for both body and mind.

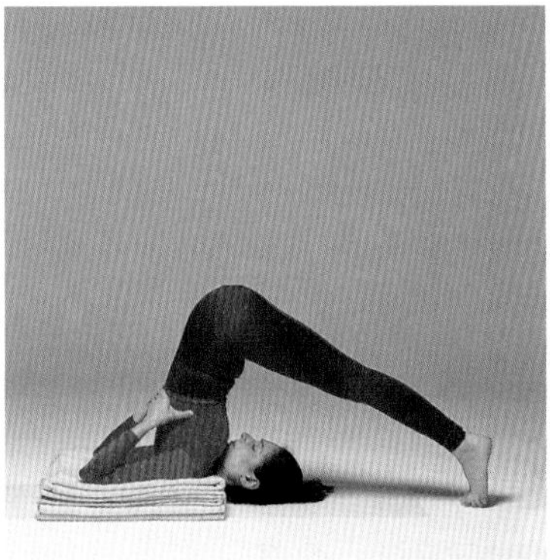

Do *Sarvāṅgāsana* (see Unit 5, page 93). Bend the legs and take the feet to the floor. Straighten the knees and lift the hips and trunk. Breathe evenly.

Stay in the pose for 30 seconds to 1 minute. Bend the legs and gently slide down.

Help

- **If the back and legs are stiff, raise the feet onto a support, such as a stool or block.**

To Progress

Go onto the tips of the toes and stretch the soles of the feet up. With the help of the hands on the back, lift the front of the body.

शवासन *Śavāsana*

Corpse Pose

The limbs must be made passive if the body is to relax; the body must be made passive if the mind is to relax.

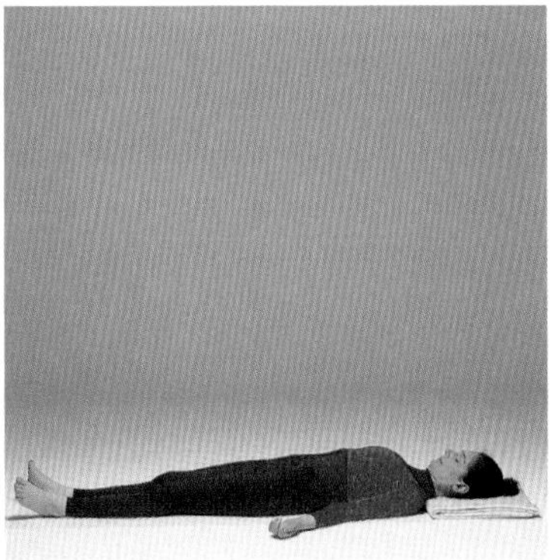

Follow the method given in Unit 1 (page 26).

To Progress

Pay attention to placing the limbs symmetrically. After relaxing them, keep them passive, and control any urge to fidget.

The workings of the mind

KEY CONCEPTS

Ignorance In the philosophical context, ignorance does not mean the absence of worldly information, but not knowing the intrinsic nature of the soul. Even a highly informed person, in the worldly sense, can be ignorant in the philosophical sense.

Instincts and memories Instincts belong to the same category of mental phenomena but differ in that they are deep-rooted, carried through many incarnations, and aroused by the circumstance of birth in a specific species. Memories do not depend on such conditions, as is shown by dreams, which are classed as memories.

We have seen that the philosopher views life as suffering and the mistaken identification of the soul with the nonspiritual mind as its cause. Although distinct from the mind, the soul considers itself one with it, and this involves it in the sufferings that really belong to the mind. To find out how to eliminate these sufferings, it is necessary to know what the mind is and how it works.

The Mind: the Object of Yoga Discipline

A Sanskrit philosophical treatise makes the following observation: "Nothing but the mind is the cause of the bondage and liberation of men. It leads to bondage when a person is attached to worldly objects, or to liberation, when freed from them."

Of the two properties of the mind mentioned in this passage, attachment to objects is instinctive, being a tendency from birth; freedom from them is to be sought through resolute efforts. What the direction of these efforts should be is the field of search for the *Yoga* system. It bases its findings in a logical analysis of the mind and its properties. These properties, being the causes of worldly sufferings, are themselves termed sufferings, *kleśas*. Patañjali identifies five causes of suffering: ignorance (*avidyā*), the soul-mind union leading to a sense of self (*asmitā*), attachment (*rāga*), aversion (*dveṣa*), and clinging to life (*abhi-niveśa*).

The Way the Mind Works

The *Sāṃkhya-Yoga* philosophy views the mind as the principal instrument of receiving, interpreting, and responding to the experiences of worldly events.

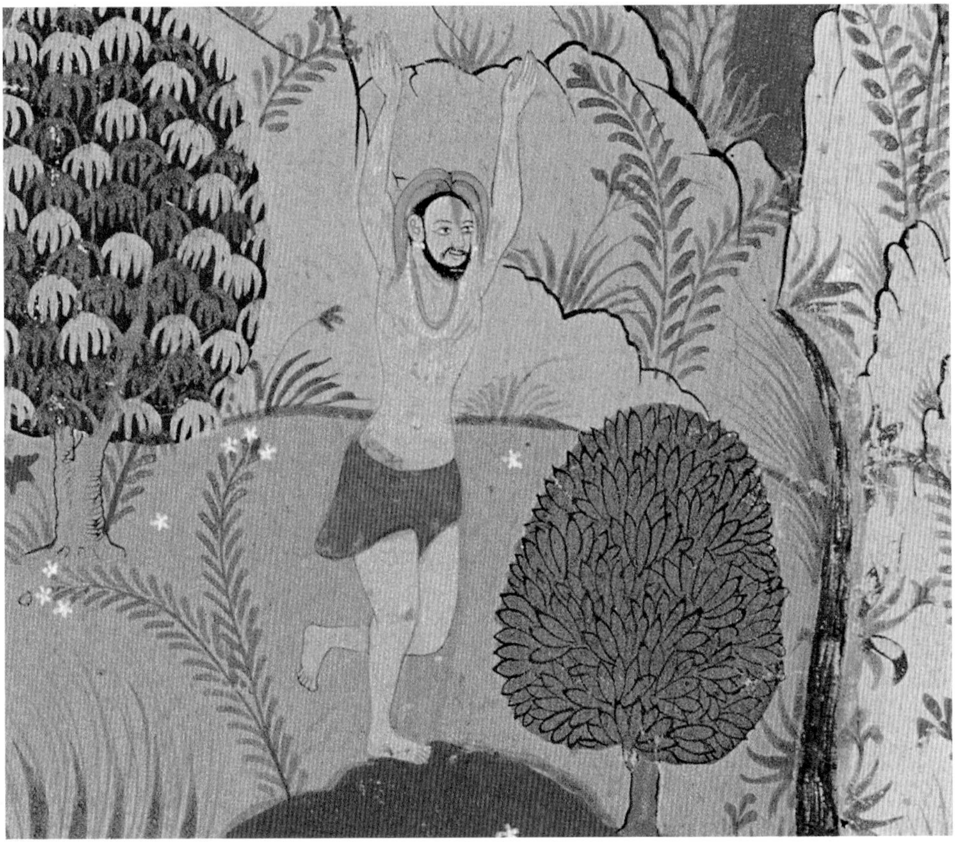

The Sage, Manu, stands on one leg as a way of practicing mind control.

It receives signals from the external world through the sense organs, and responds through the organs of actions. However, the interpretation of these signals is swayed by attachment and aversion, two of the causes of suffering. Underlying the mind's activities are the basic causes of suffering: ignorance, the apparent union of the mind and the soul, and clinging to life.

The activities of the mind are guided by memory records, such as instincts (*vāsanās*), which accumulate through a series of past lives and lie dormant till appropriate occasions prompt them to reveal themselves. For example, the instincts of a cat are aroused when the soul is born as a cat. The very sight of a mouse tempts a cat to pounce on it as if it were a sweet dish! A man would not do this, even if he had been a cat in an earlier birth. Even in our normal life we observe that responses are conditioned by upbringing and circumstances, despite the fact that all human beings are alike in their basic faculties. The factor of instincts is all the more decisive when it concerns behavior across lives in different species. This is what is meant by the stimulation of instincts in appropriate conditions. The mind, with countless instincts accumulated through past lives, is likened to a fishing net formed of innumerable knots.

Memory imprints of experiences (*saṃskāras*) are similar to instincts but have a more general application. They are reinforced by a person's interests and efforts —for example, what we call study is nothing but the strengthening of specific memory imprints. Although memory imprints entangle ordinary people in worldly life, their power enables a Yoga practitioner to strengthen his Yogic mind-set.

Ignorance and its Forms

The ultimate cause of sufferings, identified with its effects, is the ignorance (*avidyā*) or mistaken view of the soul in regarding what is not eternal as eternal, what is not pure as pure, what is painful as pleasing, and what is not the soul as the soul. This ignorance further leads to:

1. Sense of self (*asmitā*), which is the false identification of the power of consciousness (soul, Spirit—*puruṣa*) with the power of the intellect (*buddhi*).
2. Attachment (*rāga*) springing from an earlier experience of pleasure.
3. Aversion (*dveṣa*) springing from an earlier experience of pain.
4. Clinging to life (*abhiniveśa*), an instinct found in all creatures. When aware of an imminent danger, even a tiny insect attempts to escape it and save its life.

We may term these four root causes of suffering as attributes of the mind. They are merely manifestations of the primary force, ignorance.

Phases of the "Root Causes of Suffering"

These four attributes of the mind, the root causes of suffering, do not operate with the same intensity at all times: they may be dormant, reduced, interrupted, or operative. The first two phases relate to Yogins. They are "dormant" when a Yogin is perfected, and "reduced" when a Yogin is progressing. The practice of Yoga reduces the intensity of the root causes of suffering; in the case of perfected Yogins, they are so diminished that they have no effect on the Yogin, even in the presence of otherwise desirable objects. For a Yogin, something desirable to most people is essentially a cause of suffering, as it is short-lived. To take an example, a Yogin would be unmoved at the sight of gold, unlike an ordinary person. The remaining two phases (interrupted and operative) relate to people involved in the world. In their case, one root cause of suffering gets interrupted when another is in operation. For instance, a man's attachment to money would be suspended when his life is endangered. This does not mean that he has given up his love of money; it is only temporarily interrupted by a stronger concern.

Ignorance: a Positive Concept

Ignorance (*avidyā*), as defined in *Yoga*, does not merely mean the absence of knowledge, as is normally understood, but the opposite of knowledge, or that which obstructs knowledge. To cite a parallel from

English, "injustice" does not mean merely the absence of justice, but the opposite of justice. Similarly, *avidyā* is a fact that opposes knowledge; it is perverse knowledge. Thus, mistaking a rope for a snake is *avidyā*. It belongs to the mode of mind termed misperception or mistaken knowledge, which is countered by correct or valid knowledge.

The Root Causes of Suffering Breed Further Suffering

The root causes of suffering induce the embodied soul to perform actions which, in their turn, lead it to experience pleasure and pain. The basic principle of the theory of actions is that no soul can escape the result of its action. Since physical actions are momentary and perishable, they are said to have invisible forms that cling to the soul until they bear consequences. Therefore, the experience of pleasures and pains in our present life is the result of our actions performed in our past lives. In other words, the life we are currently leading is neither the first nor the last; this inevitably leads to the supposition of a chain of actions and incarnations that has no beginning. This supposition is validated by the inability of the human mind to determine the first of the pairs that perpetually follow each other, such as seed and sprout, egg and hen, and day and night. To designate these pairs as having no beginning is the philosopher's way of expression; in other words, it means that we have no answer to this question.

Thus, the chain of actions and incarnations has no beginning; but it certainly has an end, liberation, which is another name for release from suffering. The only means of liberation is the experiential knowledge that the soul is distinct from the mind. This puts an end to ignorance and what ensues from it—sense of self, and so on.

In Brief

What is called the mind is indeed a fisherman's net
Tied with the knots of countless instincts; it is this that binds the soul.

In appropriate conditions, various instincts surface
And spur creatures of diverse species to act.

From actions comes fate; from fate, the succession of births and deaths;
From that, fate, pleasure, pain; this is an everlasting wheel.

All this arises from ignorance, is strengthened by the sense of self, and so on,
And rests on the urge to live; it is ended only by discriminating between mind and soul.

For a wider perspective...

The Mind as the Instrument of the Soul

According to Yoga philosophy, the mind is the principal instrument of the soul in its experience of worldly pleasures and pains. It receives information (knowledge) from the sense organs (hearing, touch, sight, taste, and smell) and interprets it as welcome or not welcome, thereby leading the soul to the experience of pleasure or pain. At the same time, it is a huge storehouse of the imprints of these experiences, which are aroused in appropriate situations and cause memory. When deep-rooted, these imprints are carried over many incarnations of the soul. What are called instincts belong to this category. In addition, memories associated with earlier incarnations are also awakened. This hypothesis explains why some people are born as geniuses. The awakening of the imprints of the practice of Yoga in earlier incarnations is said to help the Yogin to carry it on further. The system of Yoga studies the mind and the ways to control it because it recognizes that the mind is the starting point of all philosophical search.

The Subtle Body

Indian philosophical schools consider that the soul possesses a subtle body besides the material body of flesh and blood, which perishes at the end of a life. The concept of this subtle body is in tune with, and an inevitable corollary of, the theory that the soul reincarnates appropriate to its fate, determined by its own actions, and which no one (unless they realize Ultimate Reality) can escape. Thus, the theories of action, transmigration, and subtle body are closely tied together.

The subtle body has the same faculties as the gross body; the difference is that it is not perceptible. Being subtle, it is not subject to the limitations of the gross body. Thus, it remains when the gross body perishes; it can move anywhere instantly; it can penetrate barriers; it associates itself with whatever species type the soul is allotted. It is said that when a Yogin, by virtue of his miraculous powers, assumes several gross bodies simultaneously, his subtle body is unchanged. This implies that a Yogin at this stage of practice is still a worldly soul, though at a higher level than others. This explains why **Patañjali** warns Yoga practitioners against being tempted by miraculous powers and losing sight of the ultimate goal of disjunction from worldly life—that is, liberation.

Unit 7

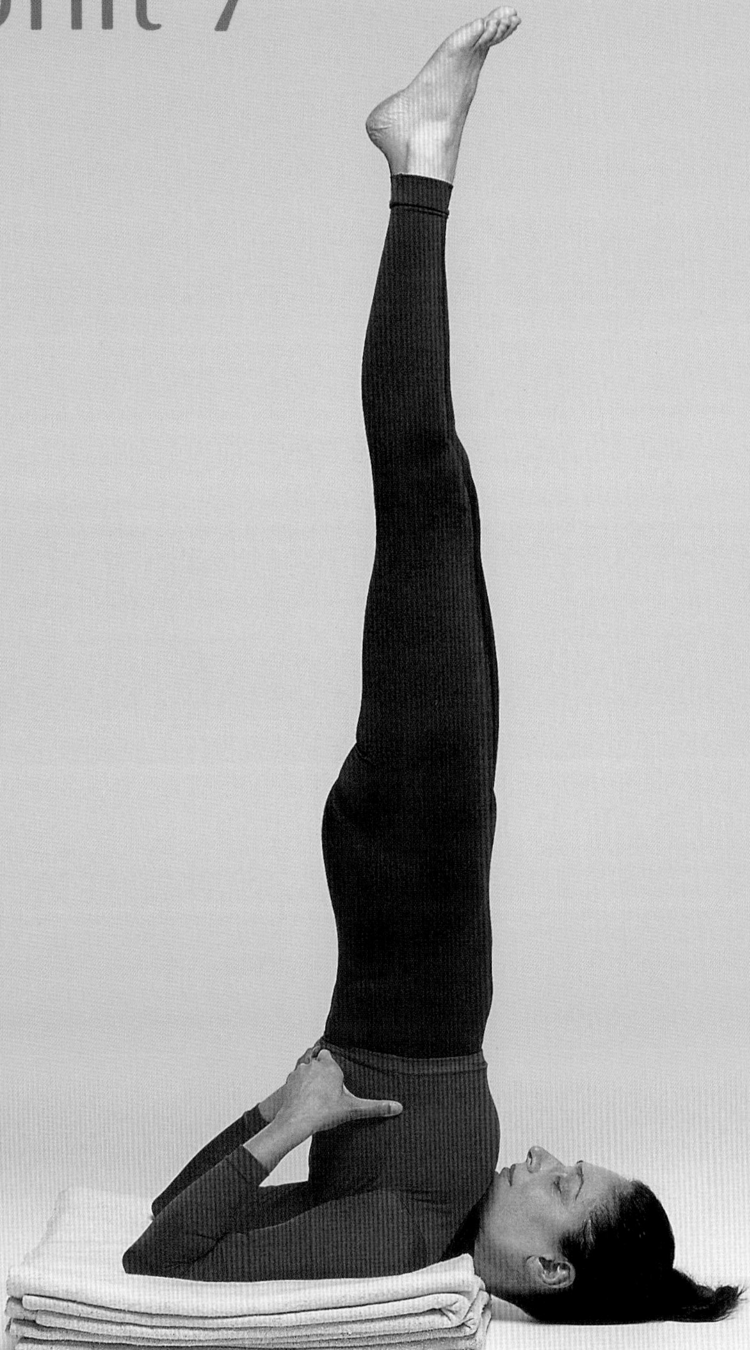

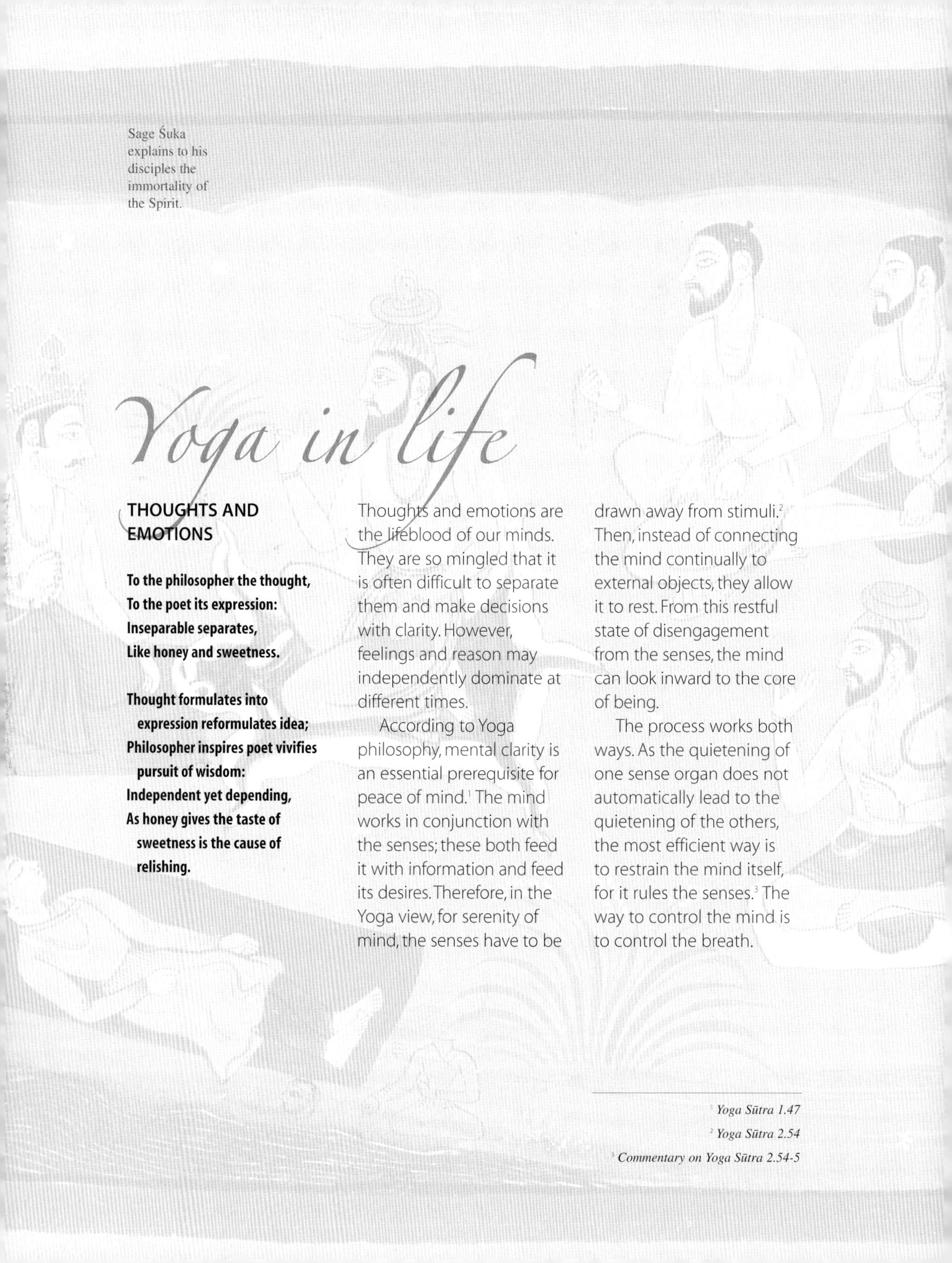

Sage Śuka explains to his disciples the immortality of the Spirit.

Yoga in life

THOUGHTS AND EMOTIONS

To the philosopher the thought,
To the poet its expression:
Inseparable separates,
Like honey and sweetness.

Thought formulates into
expression reformulates idea;
Philosopher inspires poet vivifies
pursuit of wisdom:
Independent yet depending,
As honey gives the taste of
sweetness is the cause of
relishing.

Thoughts and emotions are the lifeblood of our minds. They are so mingled that it is often difficult to separate them and make decisions with clarity. However, feelings and reason may independently dominate at different times.

According to Yoga philosophy, mental clarity is an essential prerequisite for peace of mind.[1] The mind works in conjunction with the senses; these both feed it with information and feed its desires. Therefore, in the Yoga view, for serenity of mind, the senses have to be drawn away from stimuli.[2] Then, instead of connecting the mind continually to external objects, they allow it to rest. From this restful state of disengagement from the senses, the mind can look inward to the core of being.

The process works both ways. As the quietening of one sense organ does not automatically lead to the quietening of the others, the most efficient way is to restrain the mind itself, for it rules the senses.[3] The way to control the mind is to control the breath.

---

[1] *Yoga Sūtra 1.47*

[2] *Yoga Sūtra 2.54*

[3] *Commentary on Yoga Sūtra 2.54-5*

The anchor of movement

Movement needs stability. If it is not to be unstable it must be anchored. If it is not to be random it must have a controllable source and a purposeful direction. To understand the movements and composition of Yoga postures—which follow principles of kinetics and statics—it is helpful to use a wall as an aid. This support reinforces and clarifies the various stretches, lifts, grips and rotations involved.

For example, Dog Pose (*Adho-Mukha-Śvānasana*), in which the body forms an inverted "V" shape, involves a simultaneous extension of the legs, arms, and trunk. For a part of the body to stretch, another part must be held firm. For the leg stretch, the anchor is the heel. When the heels press against the wall, their stamp becomes more powerful, resulting in a stronger leg extension. Similarly, with the hands braced against the wall, the arm stretch is intensified.

This principle applies even more to the back leg in the standing poses. This is the stable leg, whose main function is to counter-balance the movement and weight of the body over the front leg. When these poses are done in the middle of the room, the back leg is often unsteady. With wall support for the back foot, the leg becomes firm and can stretch and rotate without shaking. Once the legs are trained in this manner, they retain their strength even in the middle of the room.

Apart from enabling the body to move more vigorously and steadily, the wall also provides a reference point by which to navigate movements accurately. Limbs or muscles stretch away from the wall, rotate toward it, press against it, and so on. This sense of direction is retained in the body even when there is no wall support.

Other props also serve this purpose. In Half-Plow Pose (*Ardha-Halāsana*), by resting the feet on a stool, the knees can be held tight with greater ease, and the legs can lift up better and for longer.

The principle of support empowering the body applies to all postures. The prop, however, is not necessarily used for extra strength. In Supine Bound-Angle Pose (*Supta-Baddha-Koṇāsana*), the feet are placed against the wall in order to stop them from slipping and to achieve greater groin opening. This can also be effected by tying the legs in position with a belt. In both cases it is the stable support—the anchor, as it were—that allows more movement.

Another important function of props is to aid the release of tension. When Corpse Pose (*Śavāsana*) is done with the calves resting on a chair, the chair carries the weight of the legs. Because of this, the lower back, free of the pull of the legs and able to lie fully flat, relaxes. This enables the abdomen to sink down toward the spine and relax in its turn. Thus, by the simple expedient of stabilizing the lower back on the floor, the chair allows the passive realignment of muscles and soft tissue.

अधोमुख-श्वानासन

Adho-Mukha-Śvānāsana

Dog Pose, Head Down

By pressing hands and feet against the wall, one gives double strength to the stretches of the arms and legs.

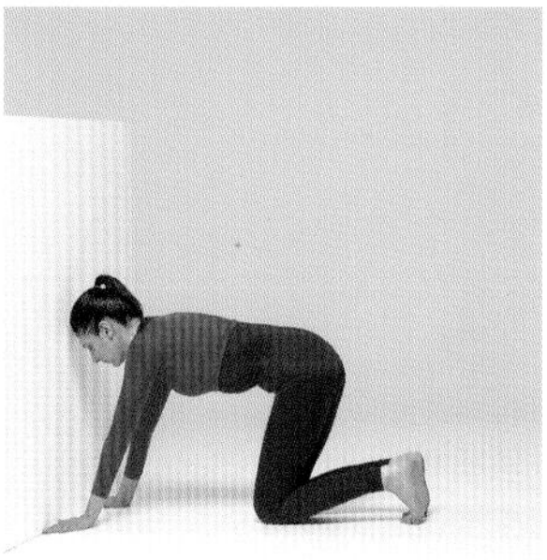

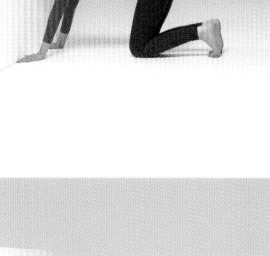

Method 1

Kneel about 2 feet in front of a wall. Lift the hips, and place the hands against the wall, with the thumbs and little fingers pressing against it. Make the span between thumb and forefinger as wide as possible, and keep the whole palm on the floor. Straighten the arms and stretch them toward the shoulders. Curl the toes under.

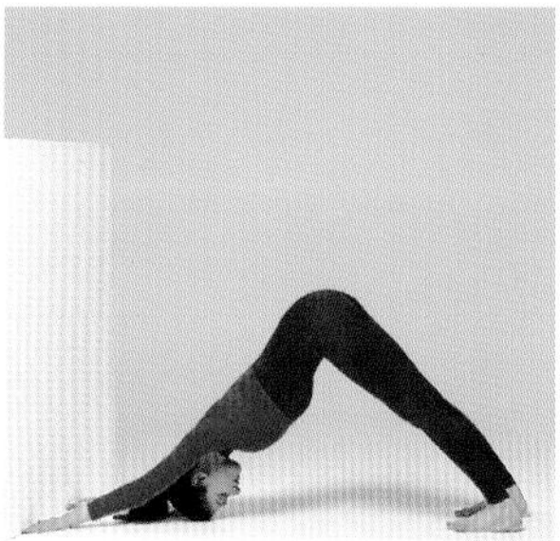

Raise the hips and straighten the legs. Lift the shins, press them toward the wall, and lower the heels. Move the trunk toward the legs so that the body forms an inverted "V" shape. Breathe evenly.

Stay in the pose for 30 seconds to 1 minute. Bend the knees and come down. Kneel and bend forward in *Adho-Mukha-Vīrāsana* (see Unit 2, page 42). Come up.

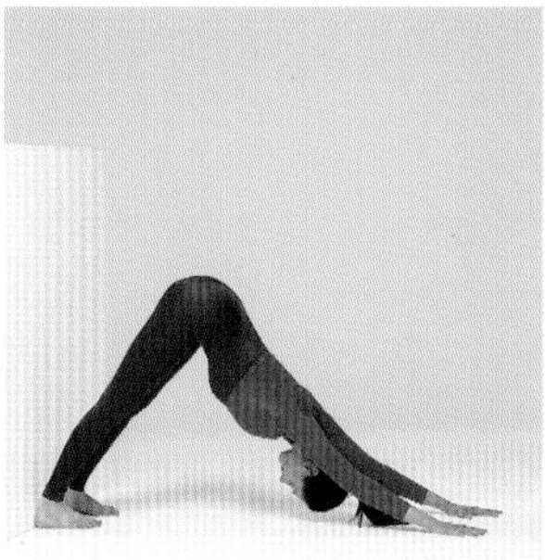

Method 2

Kneel with the back to the wall. Follow the method given in Unit 3 (page 60), placing the backs of the heels against the wall. Lift the shins and thighs toward the wall, and press the legs strongly back.

To Progress

As if pushing the wall away, stretch the arms and trunk strongly toward the legs. Do not bend the elbows.

त्रिकोणासन *Trikoṇāsana*

Triangle Pose

With wall support for the back foot, ricketiness is transformed into stability, an essential quality of all postures.

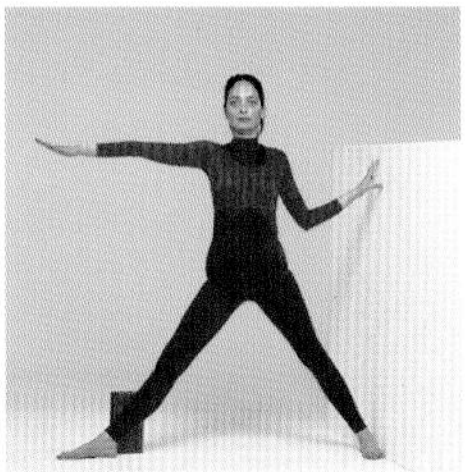

Stand in *Tāḍāsana* (see Unit 1, page 19) about 2 feet away from a wall, with the left side facing the wall. Take the left foot to the wall, placing the outer edge of the foot against it. Spread the legs 3½–4 feet apart. Place a brick behind the right foot. (This makes it easier to do the pose and concentrate on the back leg.) Turn the right foot 90 degrees out. Align the center of the right heel with the center of the left arch. Revolve each leg outward. Tighten the kneecaps and pull up the thigh muscles. Bend the left arm and place the fingertips on the wall in line with the shoulders. Stretch the right arm out to the right.

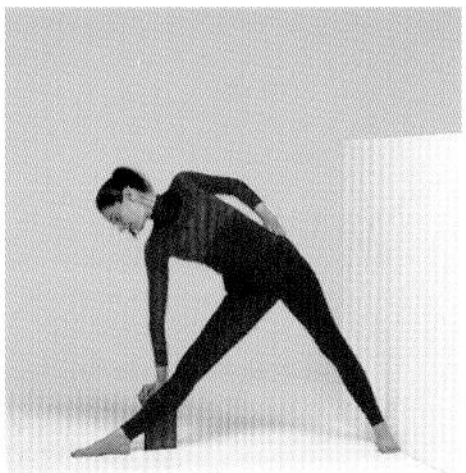

Exhale; take the trunk sideways down to the right, and rest the right hand on the brick. Rest the left hand on the hip, and revolve the trunk strongly upward.

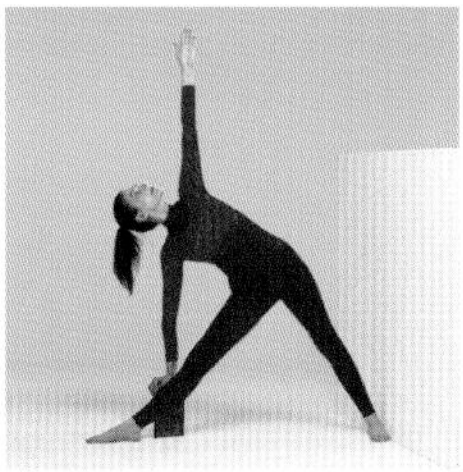

Stretch the left arm up and turn the palm to face forward. Turn the neck and head, and look up at the hand. Breathe evenly.

Stay in the pose for 20 to 30 seconds. Inhale and come up. Turn the feet to the front and rest the arms. Then repeat on the other side.

Inhale and come up. Exhale; bring the feet together and the arms down.

To Progress

Press the outer edge of the left foot down against the wall, and lift the instep and inner ankle. Make the inner leg firm, and move the leg strongly toward the wall. Revolve the right leg outward and press the right buttock in. Move the shoulder blades in, and take the shoulders and head back.

पार्श्वकोणासन *Pārśvakoṇāsana*

Side Angle Pose

Dynamic energy flows into the pose, as strength is drawn from the wall support.

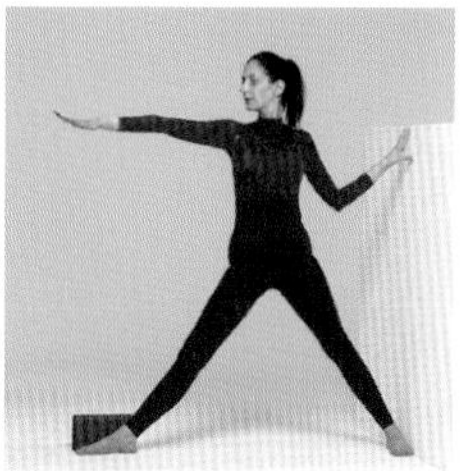

Stand in *Tāḍāsana* (see Unit 1, page 19) about 2 feet away from a wall, with the left side facing the wall. Take the left foot to the wall, placing the outer edge of the foot against it. Spread the legs 4–4½ feet apart. Place a brick horizontally behind the right foot. (This makes it easier to do the pose and concentrate on the back leg.) Turn the right foot 90 degrees out. Align the center of the right heel with the center of the left arch. Revolve each leg outward. Tighten the kneecaps and pull up the thigh muscles. Bend the left arm, and place the fingertips on the wall in line with the shoulders. Stretch the right arm out to the right.

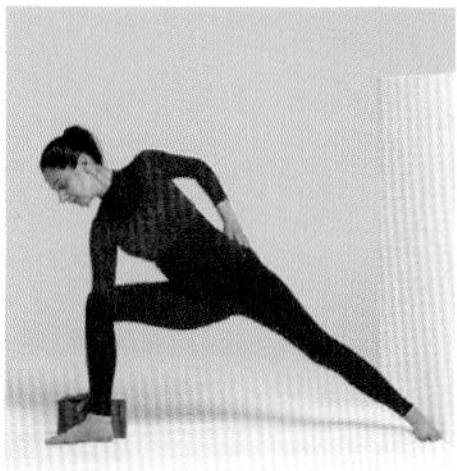

Exhale and bend the right leg to form a right angle, with the shin vertical and the thigh horizontal. Simultaneously take the trunk sideways down toward the thigh and place the right hand on the brick. Rest the left hand on the hip. Revolve the trunk upward.

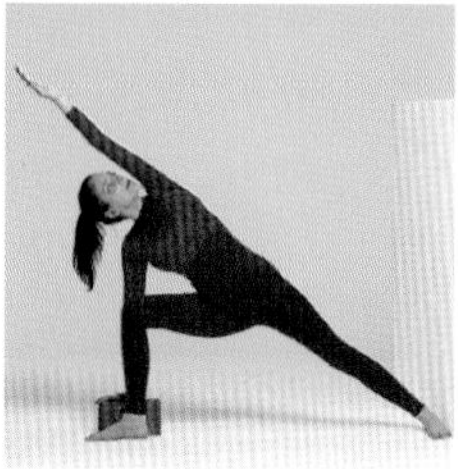

Take the left arm up and over the head, palm facing down. Turn the neck and head, and look up at the arm. Breathe evenly and without strain.

Stay in the pose for 20 to 30 seconds. Inhale and come up. Turn the feet to the front and rest the arms. Then repeat on the other side.

Inhale and come up. Exhale; bring the feet together and the arms down.

To Progress

Press the outer edge of the left foot down against the wall and lift the instep and inner ankle. Make the inner leg firm, and move the leg strongly toward the wall. Maintain the outward turn of the right leg while bending it; take the top of the thigh down. Press the right buttock in and the knee back. Move the shoulder blades in, and take the shoulders and head back.

वीरभद्रासन १ *Vīrabhadrāsana 1*

Warrior Pose 1

Stability of the back leg allows a powerful upward thrust of the arms.

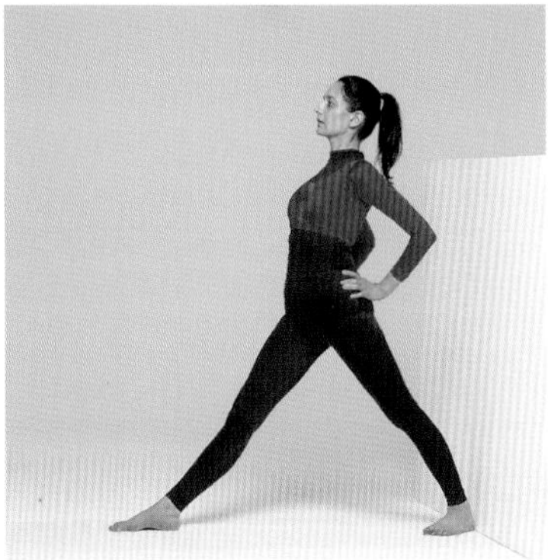

Stand in *Tāḍāsana* (see Unit 1, page 19) about 2 feet away from a wall, with the left side facing the wall. Take the left foot to the wall, placing the outer edge of the foot against it. Spread the legs 4–4½ feet apart. Turn the right foot 90 degrees out, and revolve the leg outward. Turn the left foot deep in (60 degrees), so that only the heel is against the wall. Revolve the left leg in at the same time. Align the center of the right heel with the center of the left arch. Place the hands on the hips, and turn the trunk to the right. Tighten the kneecaps and pull up the thigh muscles.

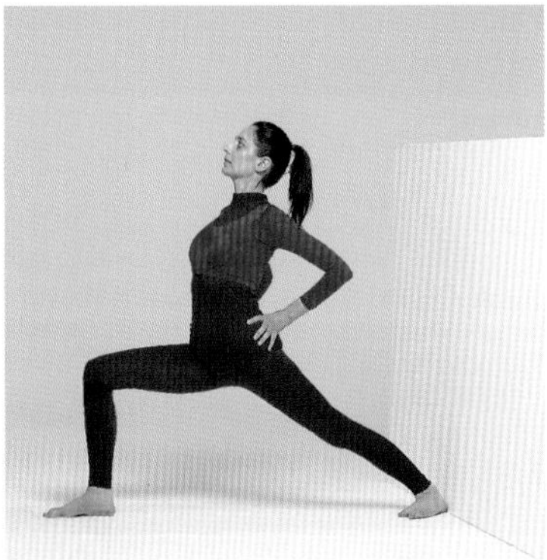

Exhale and bend the right leg to form a right angle, with the shin vertical and the thigh horizontal. Keep the trunk upright.

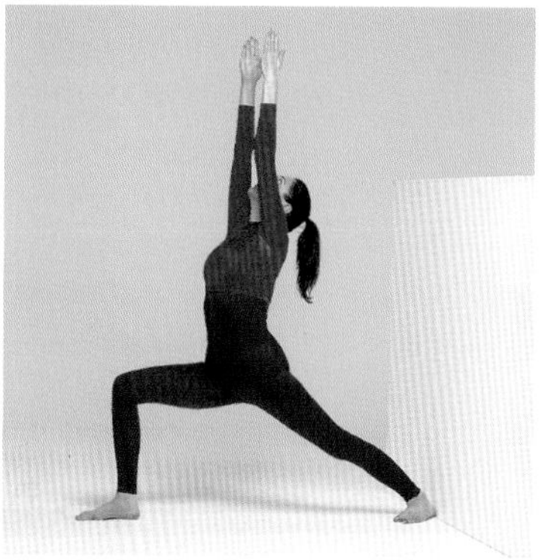

Raise the arms over the head, palms facing each other. Tighten the elbows and stretch the arms and trunk up. Take the head back and look up. Breathe evenly and without strain.

Stay in the pose for 20 to 30 seconds. Inhale and come up. Turn the feet to the front and rest the arms. Then repeat on the other side.

Inhale and come up. Exhale and bring the feet together and the arms down.

To Progress

Press the outer edge of the left foot firmly against the wall, and lift the instep and inner ankle. Make the inner leg firm, and move the leg strongly toward the wall. Turn the abdomen from left to right to help the turn of the hips. Take the top of the thigh down, and lift the pelvis and rib cage.

Help

- **To turn the hips more, place the sole of the back foot on the wall, keeping only the toes on the floor.**

उत्तानासन *Uttānāsana*

Intense Stretch

Extending the trunk and arms upward is strenuous for the heart; relaxing them downward removes strain.

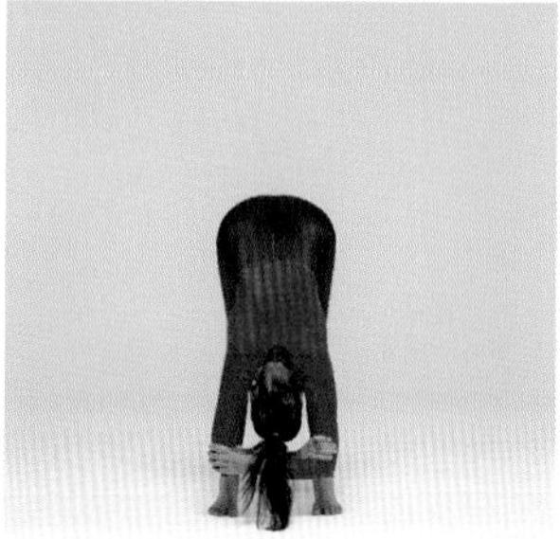

Follow the method given in Unit 5 (page 90).

To Progress

Stretch the soles of the feet to give a broader base to the pose. Extend the balls of the feet and the toes forward, and stretch the heels back.

Make the inner legs firm and move them away from each other. Separate the buttock bones.

Release the trunk downward from the hips, and release the arms downward from the shoulders.

वीरभद्रासन २ *Vīrabhadrāsana 2*

Warrior Pose 2

One half of the body counterbalances the other half to achieve equipoise.

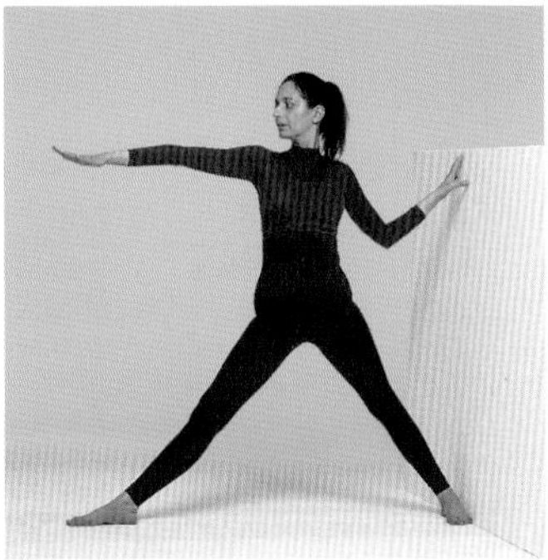

Stand in *Tāḍāsana* (see Unit 1, page 19) about 2 feet away from a wall, with the left side facing the wall. Take the left foot to the wall, placing the outer edge of the foot against it. Spread the legs 4–4½ feet apart. Turn the right foot 90 degrees out. Align the center of the right heel with the center of the left arch. Revolve each leg outward. Tighten the kneecaps and pull up the thigh muscles. Bend the left arm and place the fingertips on the wall in line with the shoulders. Stretch the right arm out to the right.

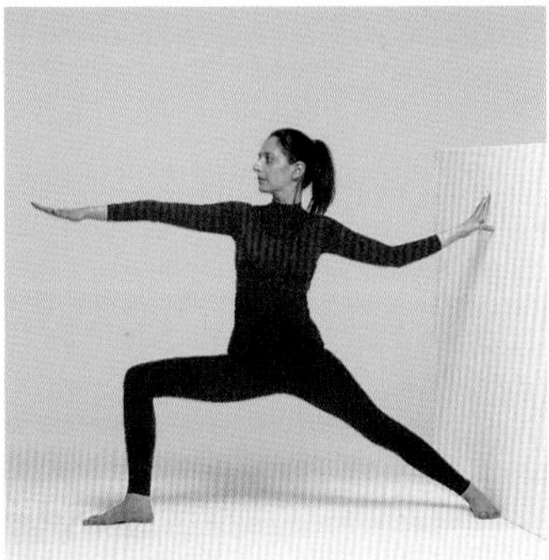

Exhale and bend the right leg to form a right angle, with the shin vertical and the thigh horizontal. Keep the trunk upright. Turn the neck and head to the right. Breathe evenly and without strain.

Stay in the pose for 20 to 30 seconds. Inhale and come up. Turn the feet to the front and rest the arms. Then repeat on the other side.

Inhale and come up. Exhale and bring the feet together and the arms down.

To Progress

Press the outer edge of the left foot down against the wall, and lift the instep and inner ankle. Make the inner leg firm, and move the leg strongly toward the wall. Maintain the outward turn of the right leg while bending it; take the top of the thigh down and the knee back.

पार्श्वोत्तानासन *Pārśvottānāsana*

Sideways Intense Stretch

The wall gives extra stability to this dynamic stretch of both legs.

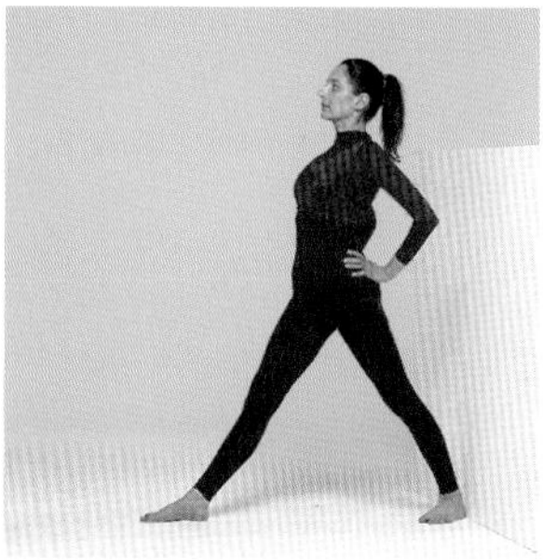

Stand in *Tāḍāsana* (see Unit 1, page 19) about 2 feet away from a wall, with the left side facing the wall. Take the left foot to the wall, placing the outer edge of the foot against it. Spread the legs 3½–4 feet apart. Turn the right foot 90 degrees out, and revolve the leg outward. Turn the left foot deep in (60 degrees), so that only the heel is against the wall. Revolve the left leg in at the same time. Align the center of the right heel with the center of the left arch. Place the hands on the hips, and turn the trunk to the right. Tighten the kneecaps and pull up the thigh muscles.

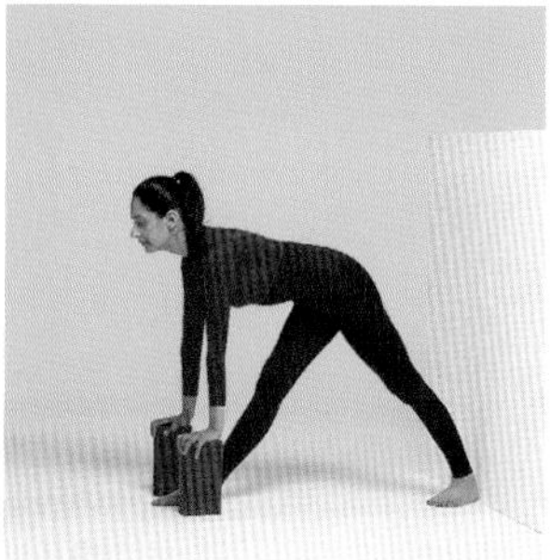

Place two bricks upright on either side of the right foot. Bend forward from the hips, and place the hands on the bricks, keeping the arms straight. Press the sacrum (lower back) and thoracic spine down, as if making them concave, and lengthen the front of the body. Lift the head.

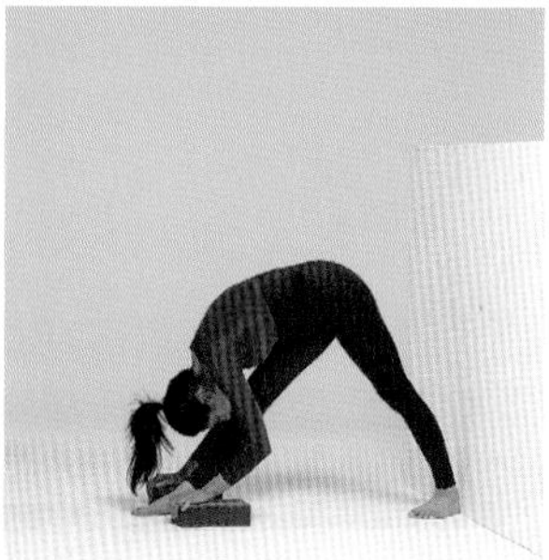

Bend the elbows and lower the trunk toward the right leg. Relax the head. Breathe evenly.

Stay in the pose for 20 to 30 seconds. Inhale and come up. Repeat on the other side.

To Progress

Take the left hip down to make the hips level. Move the pelvis slightly to the left, so that the spine is in a straight line. Release the trunk downward from the hips and extend the sides of the rib cage.

सुप्त-बद्धकोणासन
Supta-Baddha-Koṇāsana

Supine Bound-Angle Pose

After the hamstrings have stretched strongly, relief comes in the shape of bent legs.

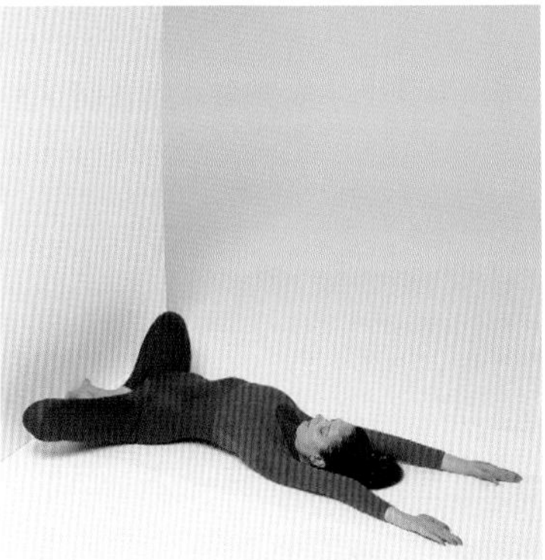

Follow the method given in Unit 4 (page 74). Stretch the arms over the head.

To Progress

Increase the length of time in the pose.

सर्वाङ्गासन Sarvāṅgāsana

Shoulder-Balance

Emotional calm, resulting from a sense of being nurtured, is the gift of this pose.

Cautions

See Unit 3 (page 62).

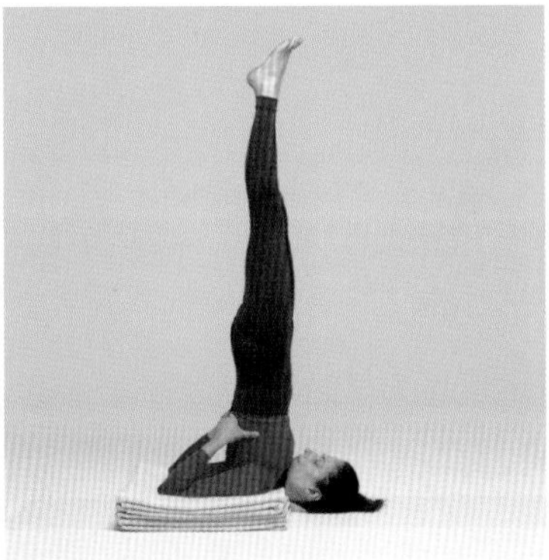

Follow the method given in Unit 5 (page 93).

To Progress

Lift the rib cage away from the shoulders. Maintaining the height of the upper trunk, lift the hips and stretch the legs. The better the position of the arms and shoulders, the better the lift in the pose.

हलासन *Halāsana*

Plow Pose

Being able to see only yourself and nothing else helps to quieten the senses and restore the mind to peacefulness.

Cautions

See Unit 3 (page 62).

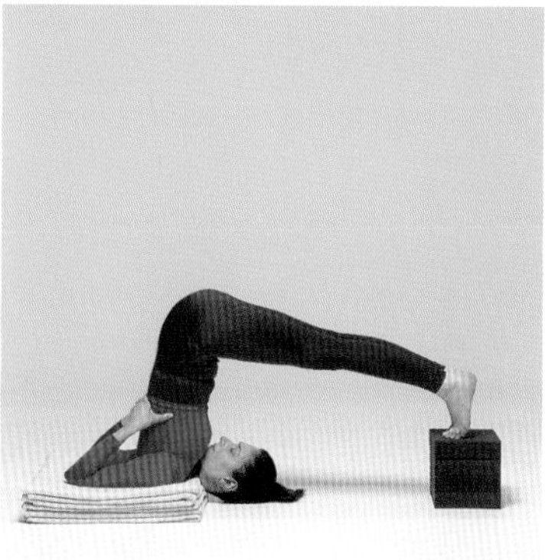

Do *Sarvāṅgāsana* (see Unit 5, page 93). Bend the legs and take the feet onto a support.

Straighten the knees and lift the hips and trunk. Breathe evenly.

Stay in the pose for 1 to 2 minutes. Bend the legs and gently slide down.

To Progress

Readjust the hands on the back to lift the trunk further. Bring the chest forward. Press the legs upward.

शवासन *Śavāsana*

Corpse Pose

The abdomen, which normally holds a lot of tension, relaxes when the legs are rested on a chair.

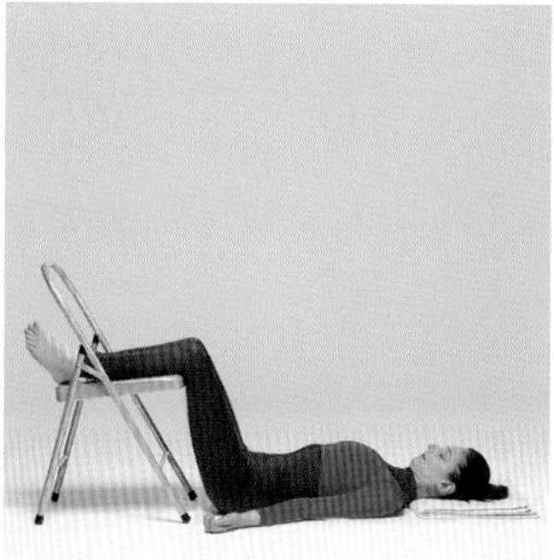

Sit in front of a chair. Lie down in a straight line, keeping the legs bent. Place the calves on the seat. Bring the chair closer, if necessary, so that it supports the entire length of the calves. Place a folded blanket under the head and neck. Press the shoulders down and move the shoulder blades in. Turn the upper arms outward so that the biceps face the ceiling. Stretch the arms and let them drop to the sides. Relax the hands, allowing the fingers to curl. Close the eyes and relax the face.

To Progress

Observe the relaxation of the abdomen and how this makes the whole body relax well, too.

The source of the world

KEY CONCEPT

Qualities of Matter This refers to three basic qualities inherent in Primordial Matter: illumination, activity, and inertia. In the broader sense it encompasses a wide range of attributes, such as colors; some authors take quality in this broad sense and build up a poetic image of Matter. Another meaning of this word is a "cord" or "rope." This sense contributes to the image of Matter as the binder of the soul.

Starting from the soul and its suffering, we traced the mind as the source of suffering. As release from a complex and deep-rooted disease is not possible unless the disease is thoroughly studied, we attempted to form an idea of the workings of the mind. Further search leads us to trace the source from which the mind emerges—Primordial Matter.

The Three Qualities of Matter

According to the *Sāṃkhya-Yoga* schools, the ultimate subtle, imperceptible source of the material world, *prakṛti*, has three qualities (*guṇas*): illumination (*sattva*), activity (*rajas*), and inertia, or darkness, (*tamas*). The world inherits these qualities from its cause, Primordial Matter. They account for the threefold response (knowledge, activity, and ignorance) every object in the world is capable of evoking. The *guṇas*, being the ultimate, basic attributes of the material world, can only be inferred.

Elaborating on the characteristics of the three qualities, it is stated that

1. the nature of *sattva* is bliss. Consequently it is associated with attitudes, such as contentment that result in happiness. It has illumination as its effect. It is light.

2. the nature of *rajas* is pain. Consequently it is associated with attitudes, such as hatred, that result in pain. It has activity as its effect. It is active.

3. the nature of *tamas* is confusion. Consequently it is associated with attitudes, such as fear, that result in confusion. Concealment and stagnation are its effects. It is heavy.

These qualities operate in three ways: in opposition, in mutual support, and by stimulating each other. They are complementary to each other in much the same way as oil, wick, and heat combine to produce a flame, or, to take another example, as the electron, neutron, and proton cooperate within an atom.

The Process of Evolution

As long as the qualities of Matter *(prakṛti)* are in equilibrium, the material world does not evolve and appear; however, its existence is assumed in a subtle form. As Matter evolves into the material world, it first gives rise to the principle of intelligence. From that evolves individuality. Without a sense of individual self, no further evolution is possible, for all creative activity first formulates in a "self-conscious" intelligence. I owe the coming into existence of the present writing to "my intellect," which comprises two elements: "my" and "intellect." Of these, "my" represents the "ego" element, and "intellect" represents the organization of the study I undertook during many decades. Because the sense of self depends on intelligence, this has to precede it.

From the sense of self, 16 faculties are produced. Eleven relate to sentient creation: five sense faculties (hearing, touch, sight, taste, and smell), five faculties of action (speech, hands, feet, anus, and generative organs), and the mind which partakes of both aspects, sensing and action.

The remaining principles that evolve from Matter relate to insentient creation. There are five essential properties of the elements (sound, touch, form-and-color, taste, and smell), from which arise the five gross elements themselves (space, air, fire, water, and earth).

The five sense faculties, five faculties of action, and five essential properties of the elements, together with the mind, intellect, and sense of self, constitute the subtle body. This is independent of the perishable physical body. It encases the soul, and by means of it the soul is incarnated. Liberation from the chain of birth, death and rebirth can be achieved only through the knowledge that the soul is distinct from Matter.

An endpaper from the undated *Bhagavad-Gītā* illustrated manuscript—held at the Bhandakar Oriental Research Institute in Pune, India.

The Emotional World

Apart from the material or elemental world, the *Sāṃkhya* school details an eightfold emotional world, which evolves from the principle of intelligence. It consists of four pairs of opposites: virtue and sin, knowledge and ignorance, detachment and attachment, power and weakness. (There is also another slightly different scheme.) Thus, there are two basic aspects to the world: (a) the actual machinery that entraps the soul (phenomenal world) and (b) the affective system that activates this machinery (emotional world). The twofold division is a logical necessity, as neither can operate without the other: In the absence of the subtle body (phenomenal world), no fate would come into existence; without a fate (emotional world), no subtle body would come into existence. As the two worlds are interdependent, it is again a logical necessity to regard their chain as having no beginning, as is the case with seed and tree. We cannot say which comes first.

Mind as Part of Matter

This theory of evolution presents mental faculties (intelligence, sense of individuality, and mind) as part of Matter, as distinct from the conscious principle, the soul (*puruṣa*), which is Spirit. That mind is part and parcel of

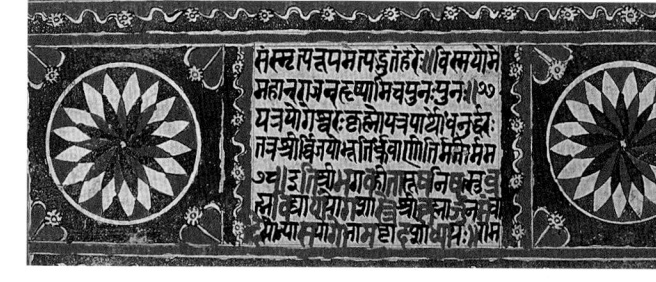

Matter can be understood by means of an analogy with the mechanical character of a computer, which is an instrument of "artificial" intelligence. It carries out a particular set of instructions until the user instructs it otherwise. In the philosophical way of thinking, the role of the soul is comparable to that of the user, whose distinct identity from the instrument and program is unquestionable. The soul, too, has a distinct identity, inasmuch as it can "change its mind." In other words, the identity of the soul is proved not so much by the continuation of mental function as by its change. The *Sāṃkhya-Yoga* argument that the soul and the mind are distinct by virtue of their roles as observer and observed may not be different from the argument that the computer user and the program are distinct.

Why Does Matter Act?

According to Yoga philosophy, the purpose of the activity of Matter (*prakṛti*) is the bondage and liberation of the soul (*puruṣa*). The soul is inactive and passive by nature; it is in itself uninvolved in the process of bondage and liberation. The sun remains unaffected as a cloud blocks the observer's vision and subsequently disperses; it is the cloud that comes and goes. The question is then raised as to what makes insentient Matter do what it does—first involving the soul in suffering and then effecting its release. This question is answered by saying that, although insentient, Matter acts for this twofold purpose by nature, in the same way that milk, which lacks conciousness, forms naturally for the nourishment of the calf. In other words, it is in the nature of Matter to subject the soul to suffering when it is ignorant of its real self, and to leave it alone when it comes to realize its pure nature. This reply implicitly admits the limitations of reasoning in defining reality and has given rise to counter-arguments from rival philosophical schools.

In Brief

The soul is different from the mind, since it observes the mind;
The insentient mind is stirred to act just by the presence of the soul.

The subtle body—comprising intelligence, individuality, faculties, and element properties—
Evolved from Matter; it is the cause of the soul's worldly life.

As long as the soul does not know itself to be different from that,
It suffers in life; knowing it, it attains liberation.

Unconscious Matter acts to bind and liberate the soul,
As insentient milk flows to nourish the calf.

For a wider perspective...

Variety in Life

The *Bhagavad-Gītā* explains how the "qualities" of Matter (*guṇas*) operate in life. The *sattva* quality is clean, enlightening, and healthy; it binds the soul through attachment to happiness and knowledge. The *rajas* quality is colored and gives rise to desire, attachment, avarice, and lack of peace; it binds the soul through attachment to action. The *tamas* quality emerges from ignorance and is deluding and averse to activity; it binds the soul through negligence, lethargy, and sleep.

In a *sattva*-oriented life, knowledge is of a kind that perceives an all-pervading single principle in all beings. Action is done without attachment to the outcome and is not prompted by love or hate. The performer is unattached, endowed with courage and drive, and unaffected by success or failure. Happiness is like poison initially but nectarlike finally.

In a *rajas*-oriented life, knowledge is of a kind that views diverse principles in all beings. Action is done with attachment to the outcome, and is ego-dominated and exerting. The performer is attached to benefits, is avaricious, violent, dirty, and is susceptible to joy and sorrow. Happiness is nectarlike initially but like poison at the end.

In a *tamas*-oriented life, knowledge is purposeless, narrow, and superficial. Action is done without consideration of its ill effects and is rooted in ignorance. The performer is discontented, uncultured, immodest, vengeful, lazy, depressive, and clumsy. Happiness is deluding, such as that obtained from sleep, laziness, and negligence.

The Eternality of the World

Unlike other systems of Indian philosophy, the *Sāṃkhya-Yoga* schools do not conceive of repeated creations and destruction of the world on a mass scale. The world evolved, once and for all, from Primordial Matter as the equilibrium of its three qualities (*sattva, rajas, tamas*) was disturbed by the sentient element, Spirit. However, cyclic processes of evolution and involution occur on an individual scale. The physical bodies of souls emerge from and merge into Primordial Matter in accordance with their fate. The only exception to this is liberated souls, for whom this process terminates, with the material stock belonging to them merging totally into their source. For unliberated souls the world goes on as before. It will cease to function only if all souls are liberated—an imaginary situation, considering the rarity of souls turning to the spiritual path and the even greater rarity of such souls reaching the stage of realization. Conclusion: the world will never stop.

Thus both Matter and Spirit, or soul, are eternal: the former, eternal as changing, and the latter, absolutely eternal—that is, unchanging. The eternality of Matter is supported by the fact that its identity continues despite change.

Unit 8

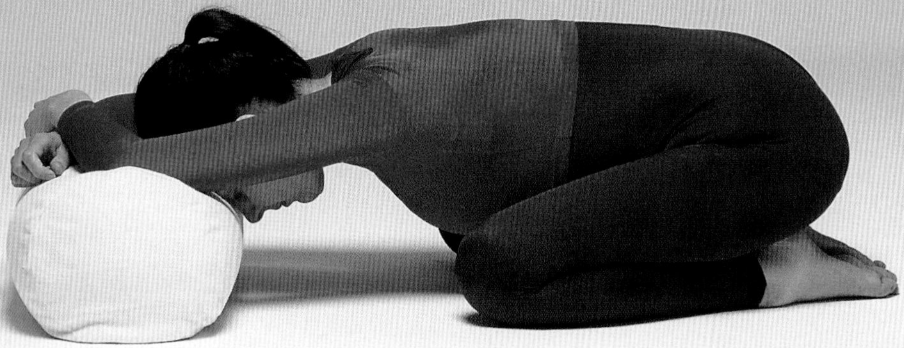

The immortal serpent, Ananta.

Yoga in life

TIME AND MIND

The chameleon Time
Alters
According to the context of the mind
Which gives it
Fleet or laggard markings.

The chameleon Mind
Modifies
The hue of words and deeds intended
To match
The setting of the present.

Why do we make time important in our lives? We position ourselves within it, use it as a reference point for our thoughts, emotions, and actions, try to bend it to our will, follow its dictates, and give it positive or negative associations. Yet the relationship of time with ourselves is a psychological construct, not a reality.

According to Yoga philosophy, time is an innate quality of objects, which contain in themselves their past, present, and future.[1] Development, existence, and decay, or completion, actuality, and potential constitute the reality of all material objects.

The tangible unit of existence is the moment, the fraction of time that is neither gone nor yet to come. It is only at the end of a succession of moments that the pattern of change in an object can be perceived.[2]

With this perspective of time as independent of the mind, the Yogin lives in the present and is not caught up in memories and hopes. For only the present is real, and only from the vantage point of the real comes clarity of mind.

---

[1] *Yoga Sūtra 4.12*

[2] *Yoga Sūtra 4.32*

Relaxing the head

If the body is the vehicle for life activities, it is also the vehicle for relaxation. The alleviation of physical pains and tensions contributes to mental well-being. However, the mind is subject to stresses of its own: anxieties, work pressures, emotional upsets, and so on. While these have repercussions on the body, their main location is the head, which houses the control center of sensory and mental activity, the brain. Overtaxing the senses and brain leads to fatigue; worrying and emoting lead to a state of mental restlessness.

When the senses and brain are tired, they need to be refreshed. Awash with emotion, the mind needs to be calmed and centered. However, it is difficult to control directly. In Yoga, access to mental states is gained through the body. The postures have psychological as well as physical effects. Thus by practicing certain sequences of poses, one can alter states of mind at will.

Whether mental tension has physical or psychological causes, the first step is to make the body relax in a simple supported pose. Shoulder-Balance Bridge (*Setu-Bandha-Sarvāṅgāsana*) acts like a restorative. As the body is lying down, tension eases away, but at the same time the intake of oxygen is encouraged by the bolster support for the chest. The altered spatial relationship between the head and the heart has a revitalizing effect on the brain. Other supported supine poses held for a length of time similarly revitalize the body and induce quietness.

Just as the body relaxes deeply when it is supported in various ways, so the head relaxes when it rests on a support. Most of the sense organs are located in the front half of the head. There is, therefore, a lot of tension in the face and the front of the brain. In everyday life, the face is held upright during the day and supine or sideways at night during sleep. Only rarely does it bend forward. Yet this position follows the direction of gravity and therefore instantly relieves strain. Even more benefit is felt when the head is supported.

In Intense Stretching Pose (*Uttānāsana*) and Dog Pose (*Adho-Mukha-Śvānāsana*), the head is inverted and supported. The spine is also inverted, and the resultant relief to the nerves increases the tranquilizing effect of these poses.

The prone position of the head in forward bends makes the neck relax, thereby easing tension on the brain. At the same time, the forehead presses gently onto the support. This gentle pressure produces a soothing sensation, which replaces agitation of mind.

Forward bends can be hard on the back, but the strain is relieved by rotating the spine in a simple twisting pose. The peaceful state of mind created by all these poses is continued and reinforced in a final inverted pose and Corpse Pose (*Śavāsāna*).

सेतुबन्ध-सर्वाङ्गासन

Setu-Bandha-Sarvāṅgāsana

Shoulder-Balance Bridge

Stretching out in a gentle arch allows tensions to be eased away from body and mind.

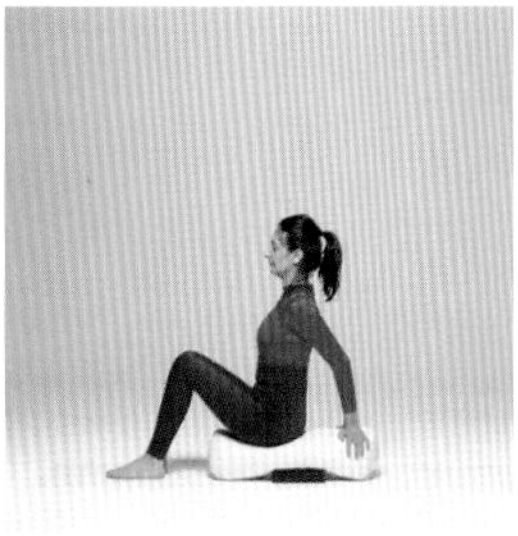

Place a bolster on top of a block or folded blanket so that the middle of the bolster is raised. Sit on the bolster and hold one end.

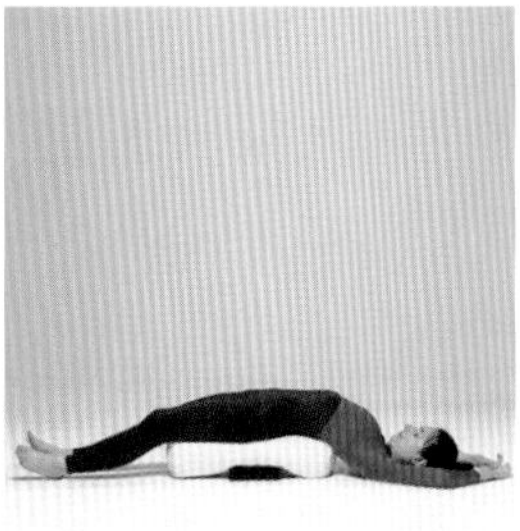

Move forward a little and lean back. Lie down so that the back and thighs are supported on the bolster and the head and shoulders are on the floor. Stretch out the legs. Take the arms over the head. Breathe evenly and relax. Stay in the pose for 2 to 5 minutes.

To come down, slide backward off the bolster.

Bend forward in simple cross-legs, resting the head on the bolster.

Help

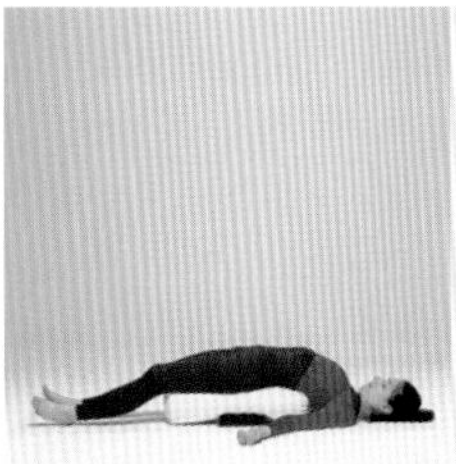

- **If the chest collapses, rest the arms beside the trunk.**

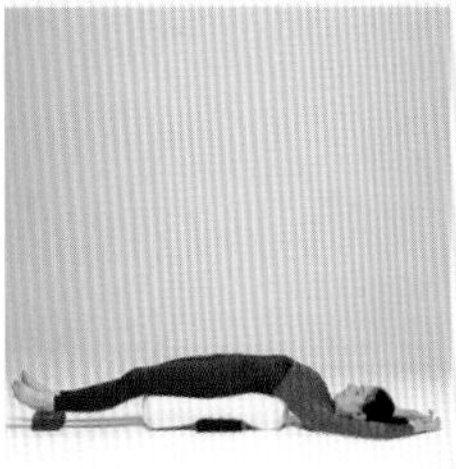

- **If the back feels strained, raise the feet on a support.**

To Progress

Increase the height of the center support—for example, by placing a second bolster crosswise under the top one.

मत्स्यासन *Matsyāsana*

Fish Pose

When the legs are crossed, the abdomen relaxes; this helps directly to calm the mind.

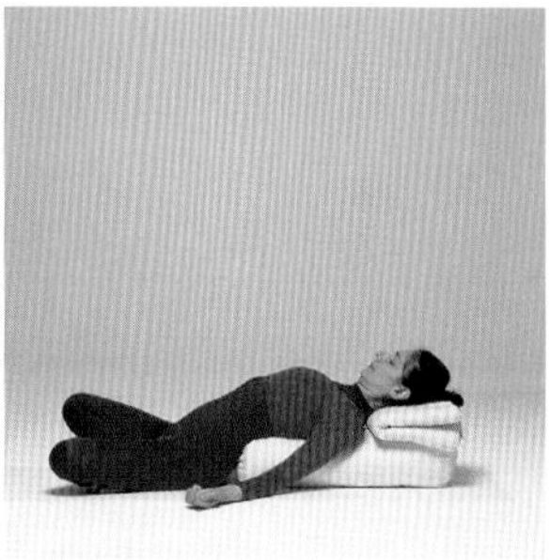

Follow the method given in Unit 4 (page 73).

To Progress

Make the back slightly concave, so that the rib cage lifts, but do not sink into the bolster.

सुप्त-बद्धकोणासन *Supta-Baddha-Koṇāsana*

Supine Bound-Angle Pose

Lying on a horizontal bolster extends the abdomen and inverts the chest, quickly inducing relaxation.

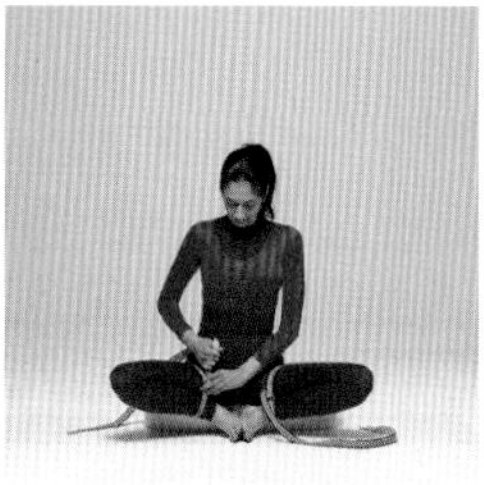

Sit on a bolster placed horizontally. Bend the knees out to the sides, and join the soles of the feet. Bring the heels toward the pubis. To allow the legs to relax, tie the thighs and shins together, using two belts. Pass each belt around the top of the thigh and bottom of the shin. Pull it tight, with the buckle between the thigh and calf.

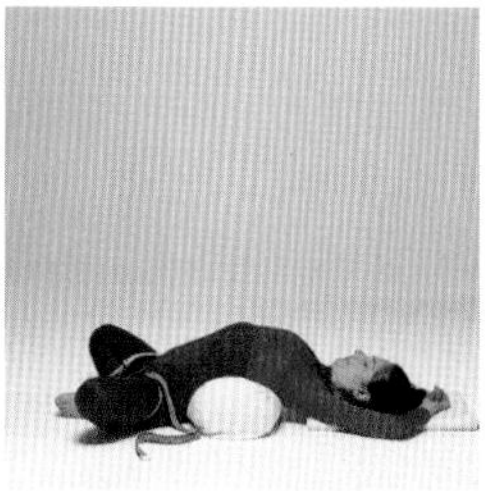

Slide down off the bolster and lie back over it. Place a folded blanket under the head and neck. Take the arms over the head. Breathe evenly and relax.

Stay in the pose for 2 to 5 minutes. Raise the knees and undo the belts. Turn to the side and come up.

To Progress

Pull the belt tighter.

Help

- **If the back feels strained, place the bolster lengthwise. Keep the arms beside the trunk.**
- **If the hip joints or groin feel strained, place supports under the thighs.**

उत्तानासन *Uttānāsana*

Intense Stretch

When the head presses lightly on a support, the buzz of thoughts is stopped.

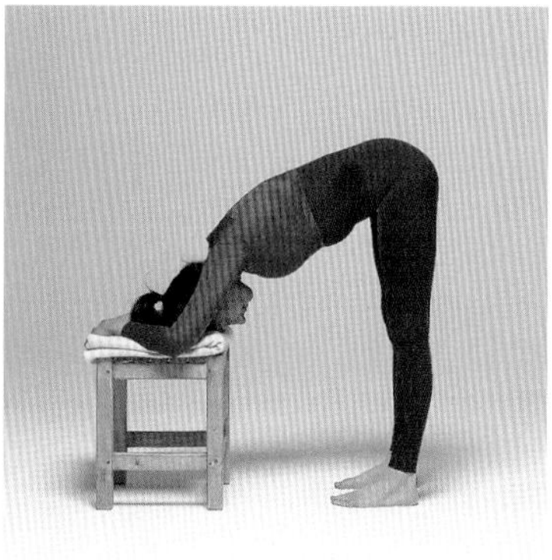

Follow the method given in Unit 4 (page 76).

To Progress

Actively maintain the stretch of the legs without disturbing the relaxation of trunk and head. Press the outer edges of the feet down, and lift the arches and inner ankles. Keep the knees tight, and pull up the thigh muscles. Relax the throat and ears.

अधोमुख-श्वानासन *Adho-Mukha-Śvānāsana*

Dog Pose, Head Down

The more the body takes the shape of this pose, the better the relaxation.

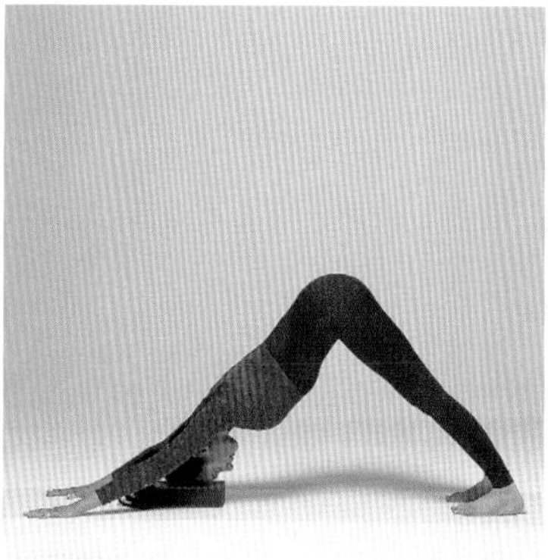

Follow the method given in Unit 4 (page 75).

To Progress

Press the legs strongly away from the trunk, and bring the trunk toward the legs. Lift the hips.

Help

- **Place the hands against the wall (see Unit 7, page 119).**

अधोमुख-वीरासन *Adho-Mukha-Vīrāsana*

Hero Pose, Head Down

With the forehead lightly pressed on a support, the brain feels relief from tension.

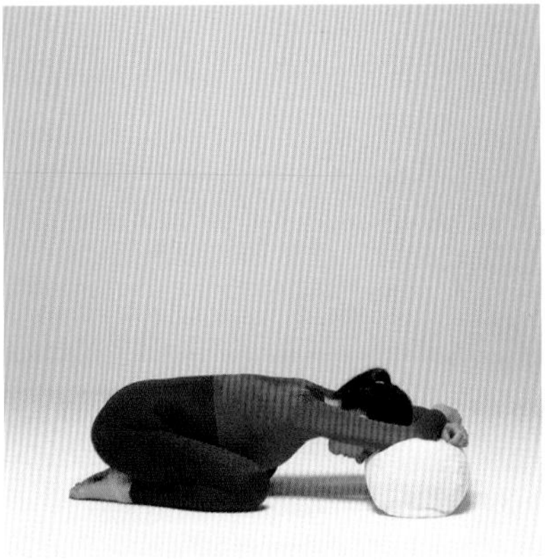

Kneel in front of a bolster. Bring the toes together, and take the knees apart to the width of the trunk.

Exhale and bend forward from the hips. Rest the head and arms on a bolster.

Stay in the pose for 20 to 30 seconds. Inhale and come up. Bring the legs forward.

To Progress

Lengthen the front of the body, and move the bolster forward.

Help

- **See "Help" in Unit 2, page 42.**

सुखासन *Sukhāsana*

Comfortable Pose

Staying quietly with the head resting on a support is wonderfully calming for the mind.

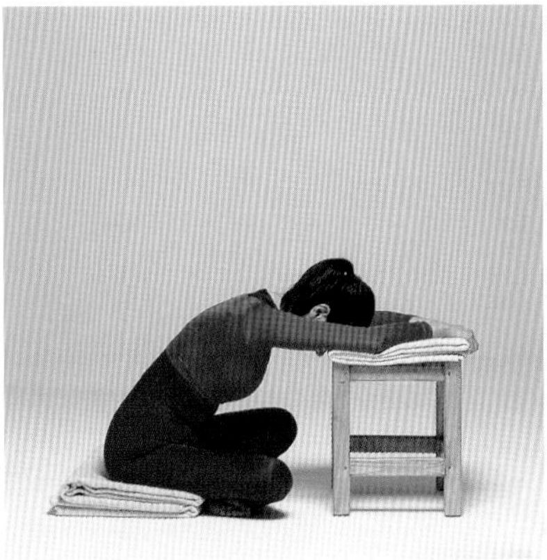

Follow the method given in Unit 4 (page 76).

To Progress

Lower the height of the support under the head.

जानुशीर्षासन *Jānuśirṣāsana*

Head-to-Knee Pose

One of the most restful of postures, this brings about a feeling of quiet peacefulness.

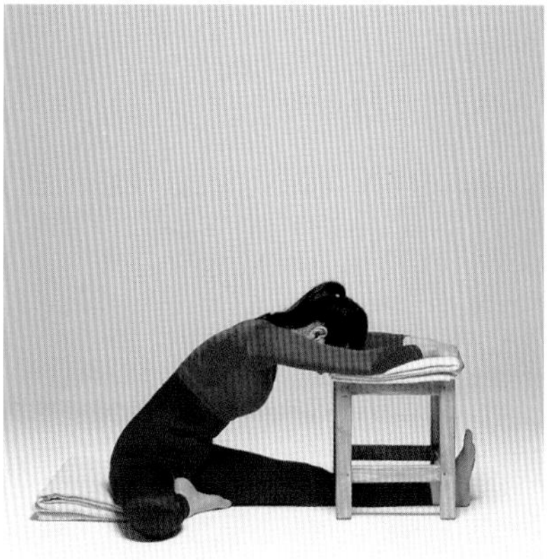

Sit on one or two folded blankets in front of a stool or chair with a blanket on the seat. Stretch the legs out under it. Bend the right leg to the side, bringing the heel to its own groin. Keep the left leg straight and the foot upright. Exhale and bend forward, resting the forehead and arms on the stool. Breathe evenly and relax.

Stay in the pose for 1 to 2 minutes. Inhale and come up. Repeat on the other side.

Help

- **If the back is stiff, sit higher.**

To Progress

As the back relaxes and the front of the body lengthens, move the stool a little forward, without raising the head.

एकपादवीर-पश्चिमोत्तानासन

Ekapādavīra-Paścimottānāsana

Posterior Intense Stretch with One Leg in Hero Pose

The continued resting of the forehead in this series of forward bends makes the feeling of calm unshakeable.

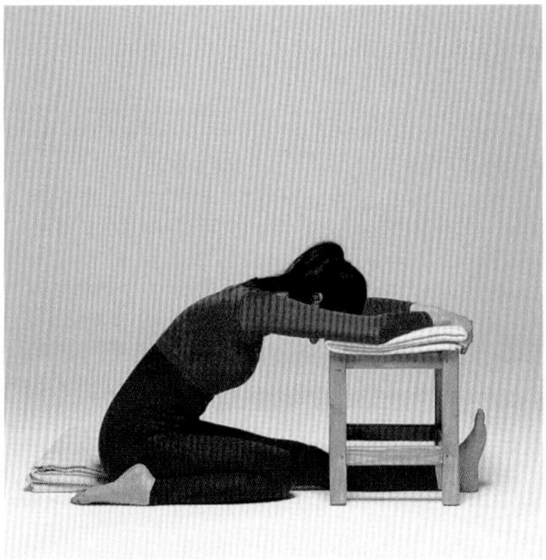

Sit on one or two folded blankets in front of a stool or chair with a blanket on top. Stretch the legs out under the stool. Move the blanket support so that it is under the left buttock. Bend the right leg back, keeping the knee facing forward. Keep the left leg straight and the foot upright. Exhale and bend forward, resting the forehead and arms on the stool. Breathe evenly and relax.

Stay in the pose for 1 to 2 minutes. Inhale and come up. Repeat on the other side.

Help

- **If the back is stiff or if it is difficult to balance, sit higher.**
- **If the ankles are stiff, place a rolled blanket under the lower shin (see Unit 2, page 42).**

To Progress

As the back relaxes and the front of the body lengthens, move the stool a little forward without raising the head.

पश्चिमोत्तानासन *Paścimottānāsana*

Posterior Intense Stretch

So cooling and soothing are these supported forward bends that they help to quell agitation of mind and lower blood pressure.

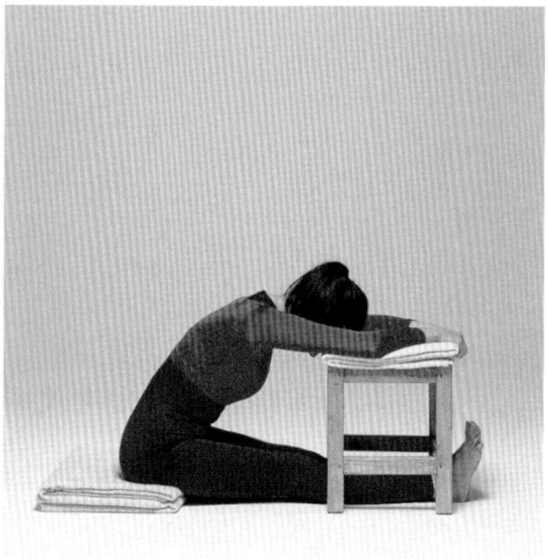

Sit on one or two folded blankets in front of a stool or chair with a blanket on the seat. Stretch the legs out under the stool. Straighten the knees and keep the feet upright. Exhale and bend forward, resting the forehead and arms on the stool. Breathe evenly and relax.

Stay in the pose for 2 to 3 minutes. Inhale and come up.

Help

- **If the back is stiff, sit higher.**
- **If the back aches after this series of forward bends, do *Parivṛtta-Sukhāsana* (see Unit 11, page 196).**

To Progress

As the back relaxes and the front of the body lengthens, move the stool a little forward without raising the head.

सेतुबन्ध-सर्वाङ्गासन

Setu-Bandha-Sarvāṅgāsana

Shoulder-Balance Bridge

Lying back after bending forward gives a taste of bliss. . . .

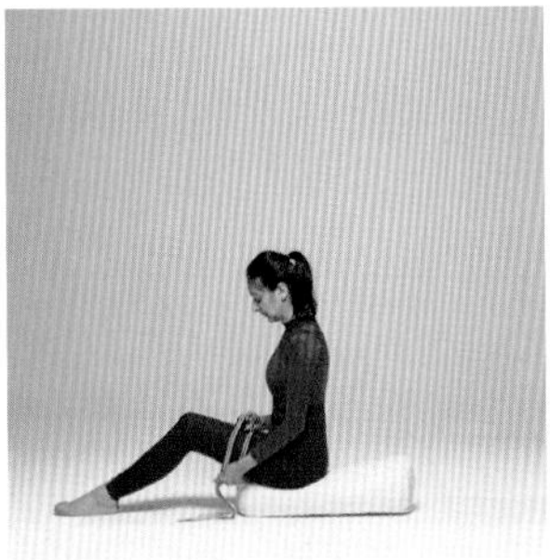

Sit at one end of a bolster. Tie the legs together at mid-thigh with a belt; this removes the effort of keeping the legs joined.

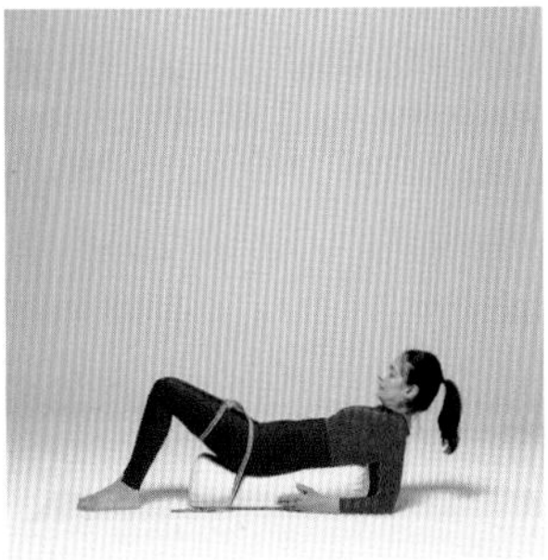

Move forward a little, and lean back so that the back and thighs are supported on the bolster.

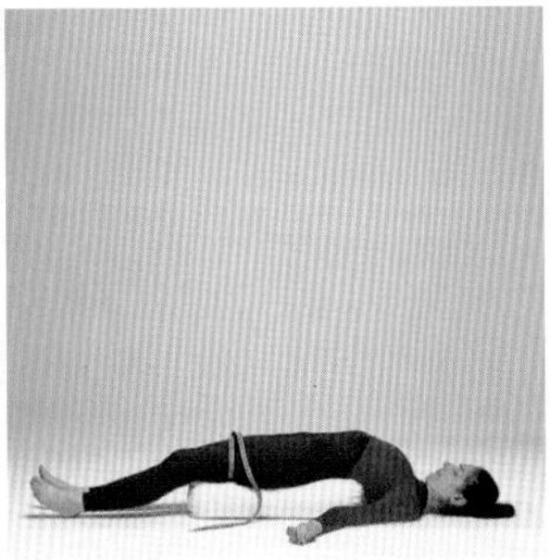

Lie down so that the head and shoulders are on the floor. Stretch out the legs. Rest the arms on the floor beside the trunk. Breathe evenly and relax. Stay in the pose for 2 to 5 minutes.

To come down, slide backward off the bolster.

Bend forward in simple cross-legs, resting the head on the bolster.

To Progress

Increase the height of the support—for example, by placing folded blankets on top of the bolster.

Help

- **If the back feels strain, raise the feet on a support.**

शवासन *Śavāsana*

Corpse Pose

After a session of restful poses, relaxation proper comes very well, with a feeling of inner space as well as lightness.

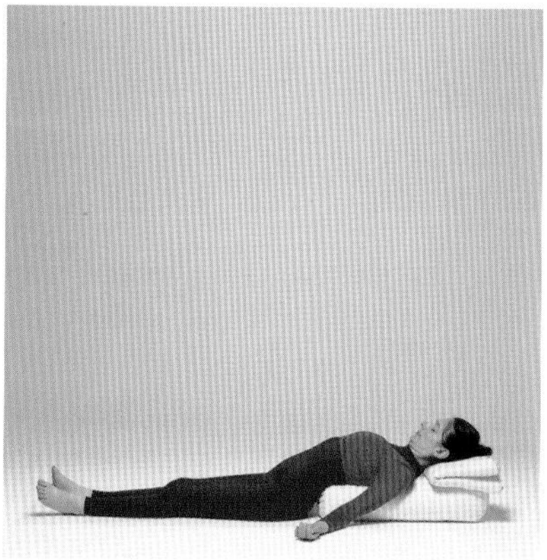

Follow the method given in Unit 4 (page 79).

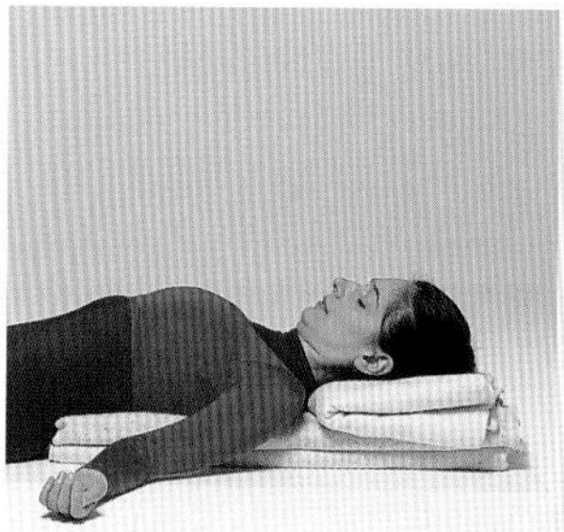

Help

- **If the bolster is too high for comfort, use one or two blankets folded into a narrow strip.**

To Progress

Feel the body opening out from the center of the chest. Do not let any part shrink back toward the center. Focus mental awareness uninterruptedly on this center.

Fate and reincarnation

We have seen how Primordial Matter (*prakṛti*) evolves into the body-mind complex which houses the soul, so that the soul can experience worldly life. The body-mind complex is mistaken by the soul as intrinsic to itself. As long as this mistaken notion persists, the soul is exposed to pleasure and pain. This experience ceases the moment the soul realizes that pleasure and pain belong not to itself but to the mind. This stage is known in Yoga as *kaivalya*, isolation or liberation of the soul from the elements that obscure it. The Yoga system analyzes the process that entangles the soul with material effects—chiefly, the mind.

KEY CONCEPT

Action (*karma*) In Indian philosophy the basic meaning of the word *karma*, "action," is extended to include its power to bring about consequences. These consequences may occur in lives other than the one in which the actions were performed. The actions of souls are analyzed into three categories:

1. Those whose powers have accumulated.
2. Those whose powers have come into effect so that their consequences are being experienced in the present life.
3. Those which are currently being performed and whose powers accumulate around the soul and await their turn to come into effect. The last category is known as "actions whose powers have begun;" only when their consequences have run their course are they considered to be finished.

The Operation of the Mind

The mind accesses objects through the sense organs, a process known as cognition. Cognition occurs when the mind is "colored" by the attributes of an object that is perceived through a sense organ. This explains why some objects within range of the sense organs remain unknown: they do not color the mind. Coloring is like registration. Insignificant objects, or objects in which the mind is not interested, are not registered, even though they pass in front of the senses. We are not aware of the objects within our sight when our mind is engrossed in thought. Otherwise, the mind is like a crystal; it reflects the object it faces.

The mind combines all the three factors of the process of knowledge—perceiver, means of perception, and object—when an object is perceived. At another level it reflects the perceiver, the soul.

The Accumulation of Fate

Memory imprints and instincts, as well as the root causes of suffering—ignorance, the sense of self and so on (see Unit 6)—prompt the actions that accumulate in a single life. Species type, length of life, and the nature of experiences are determined by past actions. This means that a human being in the present life may not have been one in past lives or may not be one in future lives. This chain of actions and lives shaped by them has no beginning; it can end only through the realization that the soul and mind are distinct. As the *Bhagavad-Gītā* observes, for one who is born, death is inevitable; for one who is dead, rebirth is inevitable. This basic doctrine of Indian philosophy is founded on the assumption that no action goes unpaid. It is this assumption that makes room for optimism in life: improve yourself and you will get a better next life; the present life is neither the first nor the last.

The theory of actions (*karma*) and their results assumes that no action is finished until its consequence is experienced by the performer. An invisible power is created by an action, which remains in existence after the action itself has ended. These powers or fates accumulate in a general stock, like the balance in a bank account. Reduced to a dormant form (like the image on a film, which emerges only after processing), they await their turn to bear consequences for the soul to experience. If they are very strong, they yield instant results. Barring this exception, the powers are said to become consolidated at the time of death. Their strength and priority are determined, and they come together to produce a single effect in the form of the next life. The length of the next life, as well as experiences during it, are determined by the dominant fate causing that life. Other fates either (a) lapse, (b) support another, major fate, (c) lie ineffective until a strong compatible fate provides the occasion for them to bear consequences, or (d) are destroyed by fates of an opposite nature (for example, good deeds cancel out bad ones). This is a theory proposed by Yoga; it rejects another view that actions accumulate in a queue as they are performed, and that their consequences emerge in the same order. If this theory is accepted, it is argued, the stock of actions or fates would never come to an end.

The Fate of the Enlightened

What happens to the fate of the enlightened? It is rendered infertile like burned seeds, which cannot yield a crop. It is only the fates of people trapped by the predispositions to suffering (ignorance, sense of self, and so on) that have the potential to cause life and consequently suffering. The *Bhagavad-Gītā* states that "the fire of knowledge reduces all fates to ashes." It further proclaims: "There is nothing in the whole world that is as purifying as knowledge."

The actions of an enlightened person *after* enlightenment are not treated as actions. Hence, they do not bear consequences. The logic is that the motivation of the performer gives an action its character as a binding force. For example, in the eyes of the law, a murderer is subject to punishment, for his act of killing is intentional. However, if a death is not motivated by self-interest, the action is not considered a crime. The judge's verdict results in the death of the murderer, but the judge is not a murderer because he is impartially carrying out his duty.

This logic leads further to the view that an enlightened man stays alive until the fate driving his current incarnation has run its course. This situation has given rise to the concept of the enlightened man being "liberated while alive," which is to be discussed in the next Unit.

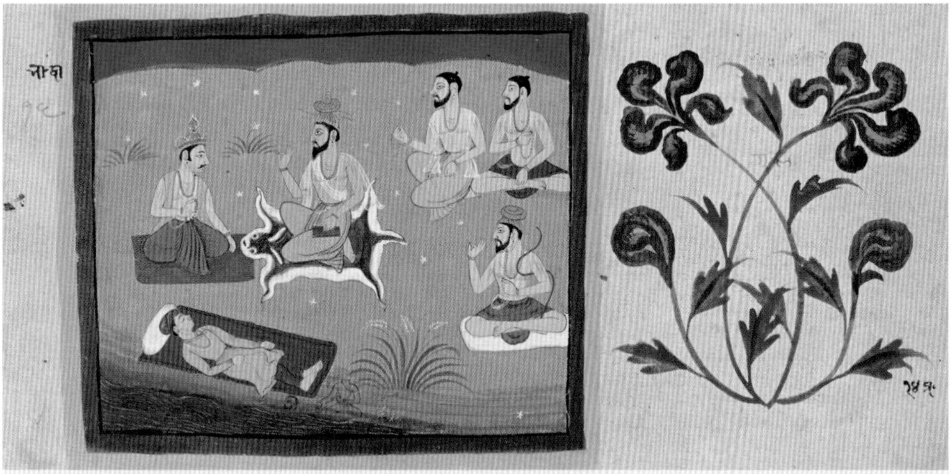

An illustration from the *Bhāgavata Purāṇa* manuscript dated A.D. 1648

In Brief

Rooted in ignorance, watered by the sense of self,
Fructifying in pleasure and pain, the tree called life ever torments the soul.

Life is the cause of fate; life is the result of fate.
Fate does not die unborne; it ends only through knowing that soul and mind are distinct.

Through fate, form and span of life after death are determined,
And appropriate instincts emerge from previous lives.

Burned by knowledge, fates do not fructify, even if numerous.
Burned by fire, do seeds in this world sprout again?

For a wider perspective ...

The Rationale behind Reincarnation

In an attempt to explain the otherwise inexplicable inequality and turns of events in life, the philosopher has proposed the hypothesis of actions, or *karmas*. He assigns these aspects of life to the good (meritorious) or bad (sinful) actions that souls have performed in their past incarnations. Actions have an invisible, potential, lasting form besides their physical one, which is visible and momentary. A physical action generates a power that clings to the subtle body of the soul and lasts till the soul experiences its consequences, unless it is countered by an action of an opposite nature. For instance, a good deed counters or cancels out a sin. It is because of the accumulation of actions and the waiting period before they bear consequences that the soul continuously moves in the cycle of births and deaths. The only exception to this rule is if the soul realizes its true nature. This realization liberates it, and it is never again caught in worldly sufferings. Liberation, once attained, is permanent. This theory of actions is shared generally by all Indian philosophical schools except the materialists.

Heaven, Hell, and Reincarnation

Indian tradition, shared by Yoga, views the organization of the universe from two aspects: location and status. The universe consists of seven "worlds," one above the other, with the earth at the center and the world of the Creator at the top. Heaven is separated from earth by the world called space. Souls in heaven and the worlds above it, generically termed gods, are considered successively higher in status. All the worlds above earth are sometimes referred to as heavens.

The lowest world is hell, which has six divisions where sinners suffer the consequences of their sins. Above hell are seven nether regions, arranged one above the other. Souls in these units are successively lower in status. All these, together with the earth, are counted as one world in the seven-world scheme of the universe.

This organization of the universe ties in with the concepts of actions and their consequences leading to transmigration. Meritorious souls go to heavenly abodes and enjoy the fruits of their good deeds till they are finished; sinners go to hell and suffer for their sinful deeds till these are finished. Heaven and hell are thus classed as places for experiencing the results of actions, while the earth is classed as the place for performing actions. At the expiry of their "visa" to heaven or hell, souls are reborn on earth in a species appropriate to their fate or accumulated actions. Their actions during the succeeding life are credited to their "account" and determine their future life. Depending on the nature of their actions, souls are also born directly in the next life in a species suited to their actions. Good deeds, as a general rule, lead the soul to a life in a superior species; bad deeds generally lead the soul to a life in an inferior species. Species on earth are classified into two categories, human beings and the rest, broadly on the basis of the vertical and horizontal construction of their bodies, no less than their ability to shape their future.

Unit 9

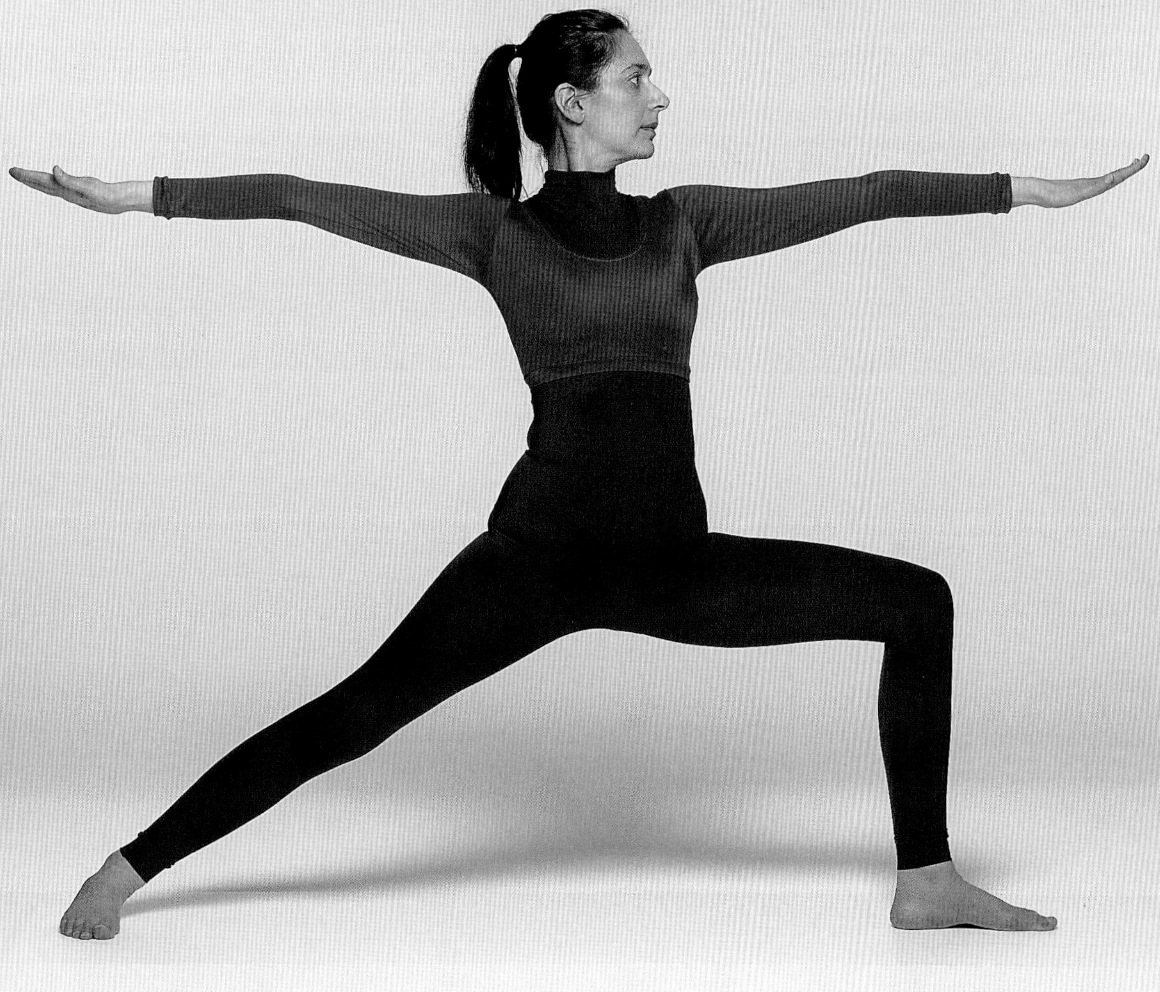

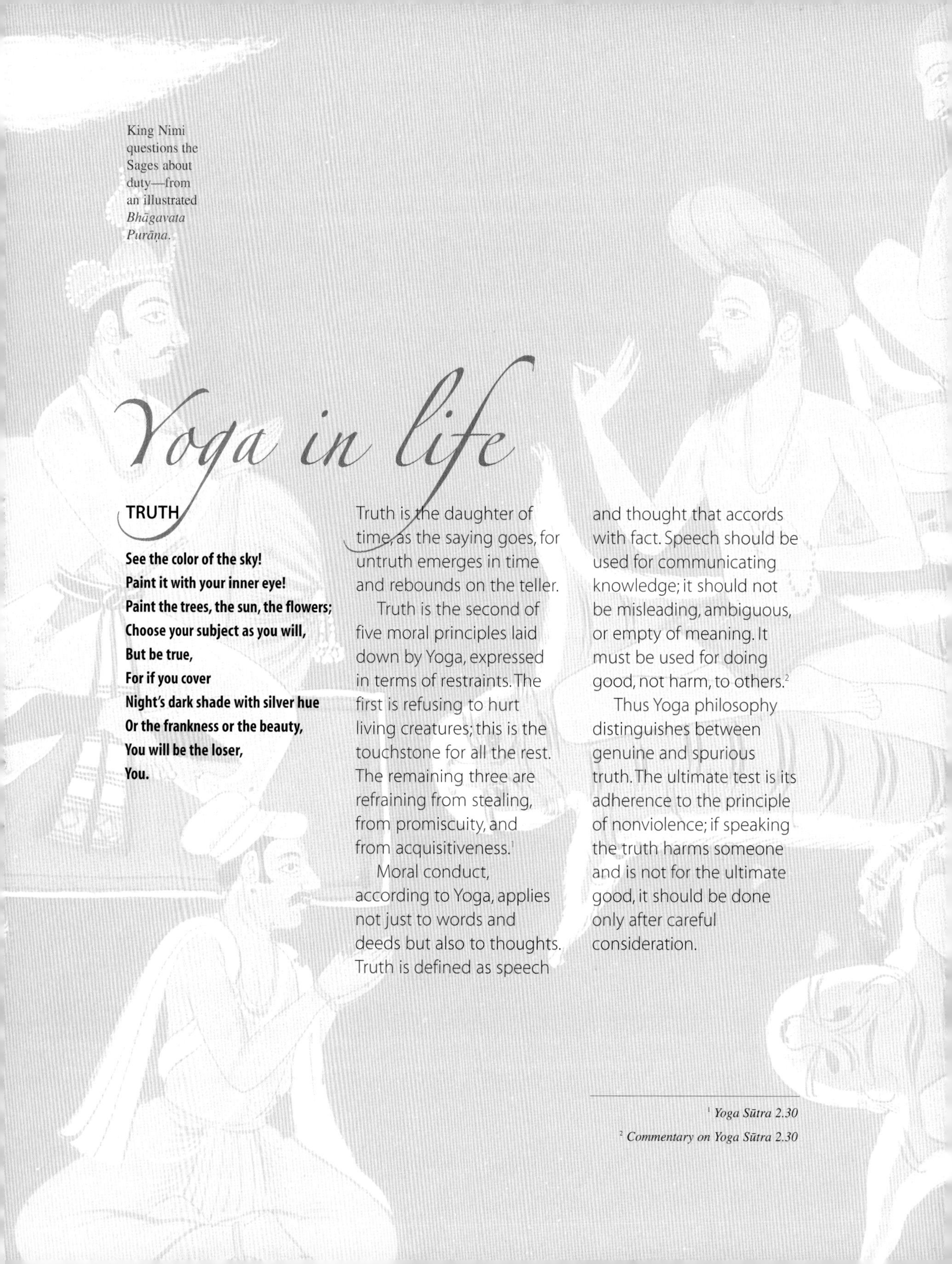

King Nimi questions the Sages about duty—from an illustrated *Bhāgavata Purāṇa*.

Yoga in life

TRUTH

See the color of the sky!
Paint it with your inner eye!
Paint the trees, the sun, the flowers;
Choose your subject as you will,
But be true,
For if you cover
Night's dark shade with silver hue
Or the frankness or the beauty,
You will be the loser,
You.

Truth is the daughter of time, as the saying goes, for untruth emerges in time and rebounds on the teller.

Truth is the second of five moral principles laid down by Yoga, expressed in terms of restraints. The first is refusing to hurt living creatures; this is the touchstone for all the rest. The remaining three are refraining from stealing, from promiscuity, and from acquisitiveness.[1]

Moral conduct, according to Yoga, applies not just to words and deeds but also to thoughts. Truth is defined as speech and thought that accords with fact. Speech should be used for communicating knowledge; it should not be misleading, ambiguous, or empty of meaning. It must be used for doing good, not harm, to others.[2]

Thus Yoga philosophy distinguishes between genuine and spurious truth. The ultimate test is its adherence to the principle of nonviolence; if speaking the truth harms someone and is not for the ultimate good, it should be done only after careful consideration.

[1] *Yoga Sūtra 2.30*

[2] *Commentary on Yoga Sūtra 2.30*

Stretching the legs

Strong, well-muscled and yet nimble legs are a boon in life. Strength and agility are complementary, but are not always found together. The former tends to be associated with rigidity and the latter with weakness. For example, bodybuilders develop thick, tight muscles, which limit joint movement, whereas ballet dancers have elongated muscles and supple joints, which are susceptible to injury. In general, men possess strength, while women enjoy flexibility. Both qualities are developed in Yoga.

As a result of the aging process and the action of gravity, muscles and joints become slack or stiff, or both. Tone and mobility are restored by stretching. This involves the lengthening of muscles and the tightening of joints. The procedure starts with the legs as the supporting struts of the body.

For many people, the burden of standing and walking is borne unevenly between the upper and lower legs. The shins become rigid and the calves powerful, whereas the thigh muscles tend to be lax. This is the opposite of what nature intended. No doubt a contributing factor to this is the loss of habitual movements of the haunches and thighs involved in sitting on the floor and squatting.

This unbalanced distribution of strength in the legs is rectified by standing poses. In these, the straight leg learns to stretch by several distinct actions: drawing the kneecap backward into the joint and extending the back of the knee, lifting the muscles at the front of the thigh (quadriceps) and stretching the hamstrings at the back. With repeated practice in a whole series of poses these actions transform weak legs, making them dynamic. The same actions can be performed while sitting, as in Seated-Angle Pose (*Upaviṣṭa-Koṇāsana*).

Stretching the legs continuously is strenuous; to relieve strain, these poses are followed by ones in which the legs are bent, as in Bound-Angle Pose (*Baddha-Koṇāsana*). Similarly, inverted poses relieve strain in the legs. In Unsupported Shoulder Balance (*Nirālamba-Sarvāṅgāsana*), so named because the back is not supported by the arms, the feet are rested against the wall. The relaxation of the legs is continued in Half-Plow Pose (*Ardha-Halāsana*) and in Corpse Pose (*Śavāsana*), using a chair.

Relaxing the legs is as important as stretching them. Relaxed muscles become soft and extend more. And with better extension comes better relaxation. The two aid each other.

In fact, the aim in Yoga practice is for extension to take place without tension. The key to achieving this is to keep the eyes, ears, throat, mouth, and brain passive. In this way energy is not diverted unknowingly to the mind and senses but is concentrated on the physical tasks at hand. Thus, the postures can be performed vigorously but at the same time with serenity, as indeed they should be.

अधोमुख-श्वानासन *Adho-Mukha-Śvānāsana*

Dog Pose, Head Down

The strength and direction of the leg stretch determine the shape of this pose.

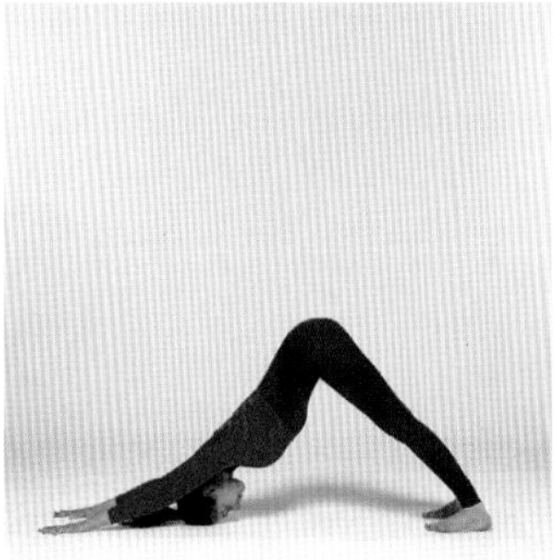

Follow the method given in Unit 3 (page 60).

To Progress

Press the shins toward the calves and the fronts of the thighs toward the backs of the thighs. Press the kneecaps in, and extend the backs of the knees. Increase the length of time in the pose.

ताडासन *Tāḍāsana*

Mountain or Palm Tree Pose

A rocklike firmness in the legs is the base for this pose.

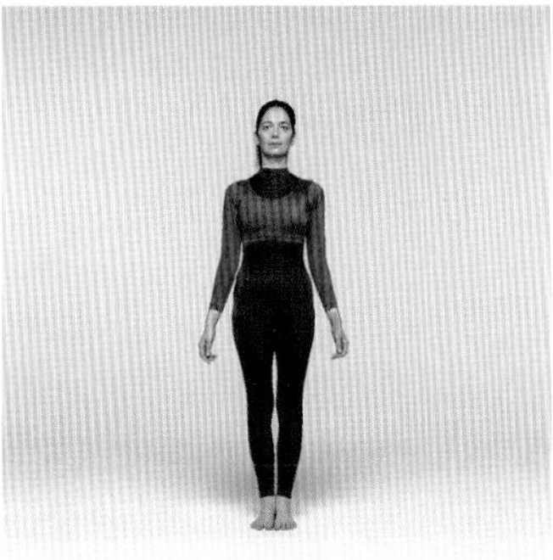

Follow the method given in Unit 1 (page 19).

Help

- **If the knees hyperextend, tighten them lightly and press the thighs strongly back.**

To Progress

Tighten the kneecaps at the bottom as well as at the top so that they engage actively with both shins and thighs. Lift the ankles and draw the shins up. Press the knees back, to extend the backs of the knees. Press the shins back, to extend the calves. Press the thighs back, to extend the backs of the thighs. Stretch the whole length of the leg up.

त्रिकोणासन *Trikoṇāsana*

Triangle Pose

Although standing diagonally, the legs have to stretch upward from base to top.

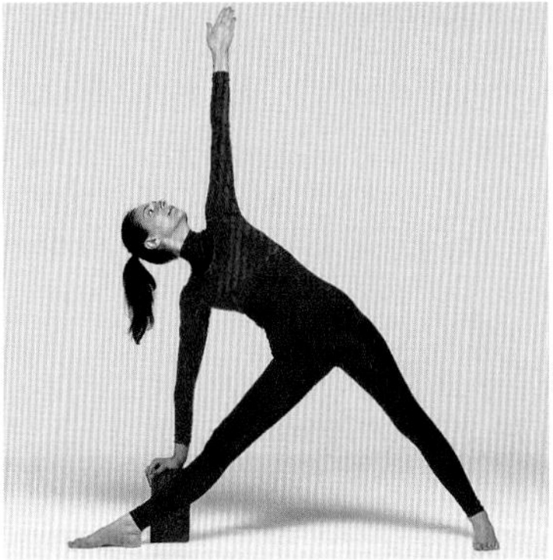

Follow the method given in Unit 2 (page 36).

To Progress

Revolve the whole length of each leg—ankle, shin, knee, and thigh—outward. When revolving the back leg, press the outer edge of the foot down and lift the arch and inner ankle. When revolving the front leg, press the inner edge of the foot and the big toe down. Maintaining their turn, stretch the legs up.

पार्श्वकोणासन *Pārśvakoṇāsana*

Side Angle Pose

To maintain the diagonal of the back leg, a strong upward lift from the inner to the outer leg is required.

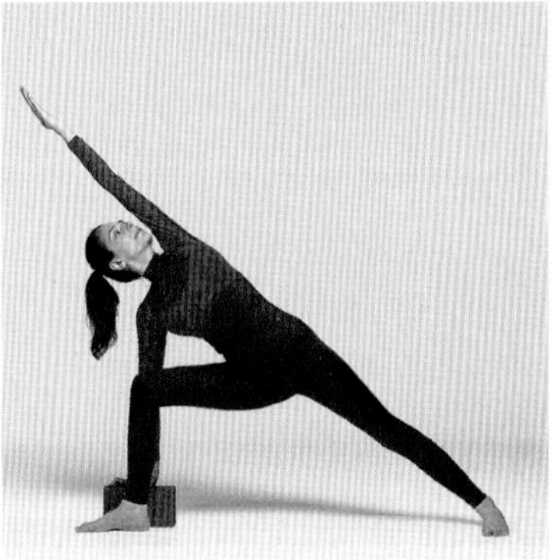

Follow the method given in Unit 2 (page 38).

To Progress

Stretch the inner edge of the back leg from ankle to groin. In particular, keep the inner edge of the knee firm. Press the inner leg toward the outer leg. Press the thigh back.

वीरभद्रासन १ *Vīrabhadrāsana 1*

Warrior Pose 1

A three-way stretch—the front leg forward, the back leg backward and the trunk and arms upward—makes this the most dynamic of standing poses.

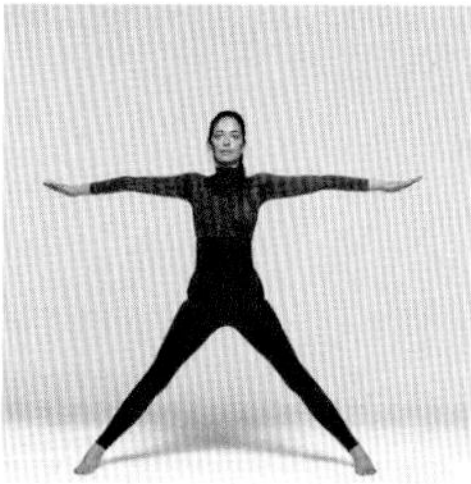

Stand in *Tāḍāsana* (see Unit 1, page 19). Take a deep inhalation and jump the feet 4–4½ feet apart, simultaneously extending the arms sideways to shoulder level with the palms facing down. Align the feet and make them parallel.

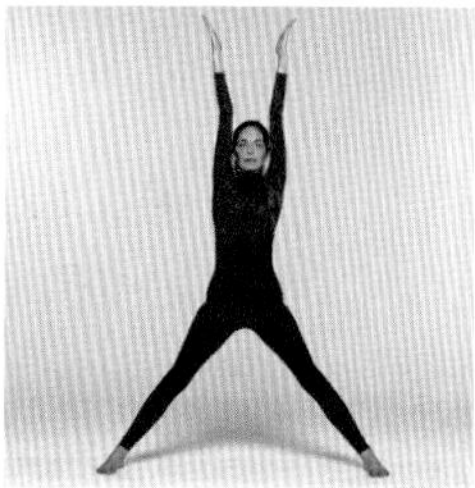

Turn the arms so that the palms face up. Keeping the elbows straight, raise the arms over the head, palms facing each other.

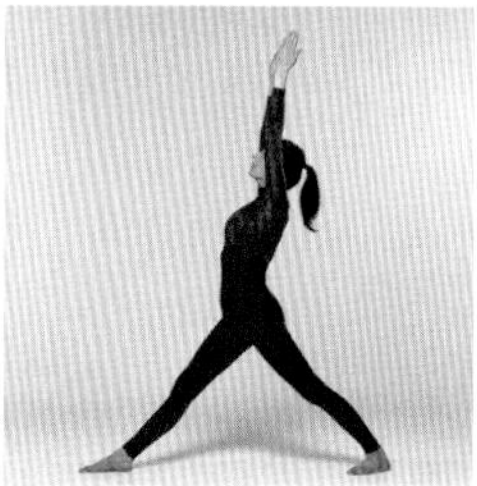

Turn the left foot 45–60 degrees in and the right foot 90 degrees out. At the same time, turn the trunk to the right. Align the centre of the right heel with the center of the left arch. Revolve the left leg inward, in the direction of the foot. Tighten the kneecaps and pull up the thigh muscles.

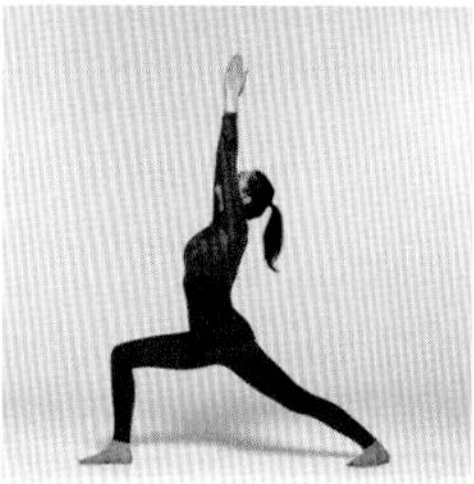

Exhale and bend the right leg to form a right angle, with the shin vertical and the thigh horizontal. Keep the trunk vertical. Take the head back and look up toward the ceiling. Breathe evenly and without strain. Stay in the pose for 20 to 30 seconds. Inhale and come up. Turn the feet to the front and rest the arms. Then repeat on the other side.

Inhale and come up. Bring the arms to horizontal. Exhale and jump the feet together, simultaneously bringing the arms down.

To Progress

Turn the pelvis farther to the right and lift it. Keep the inner edge of the back leg firm, and lift the knee and thigh. Simultaneously press the outer edge of the foot down.

उत्तानासन *Uttānāsana*

Intense Stretch

Activating different parts of the legs improves their ability to stretch and brings understanding of how they work.

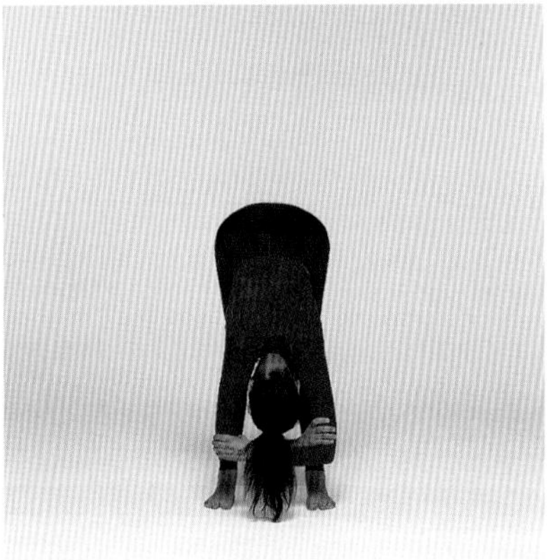

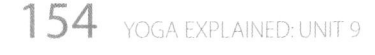

Follow the method given in Unit 5 (page 90).

To Progress

Press the outer edges of the feet down, and press the inner legs firmly toward the outer legs. Separate the buttock bones. Without lifting the heels, bring the body weight onto the front of the feet and stretch the backs of the legs.

वीरभद्रासन २ *Vīrabhadrāsana 2*

Warrior Pose 2

To maintain the equilibrium of this pose requires sturdiness of the back leg.

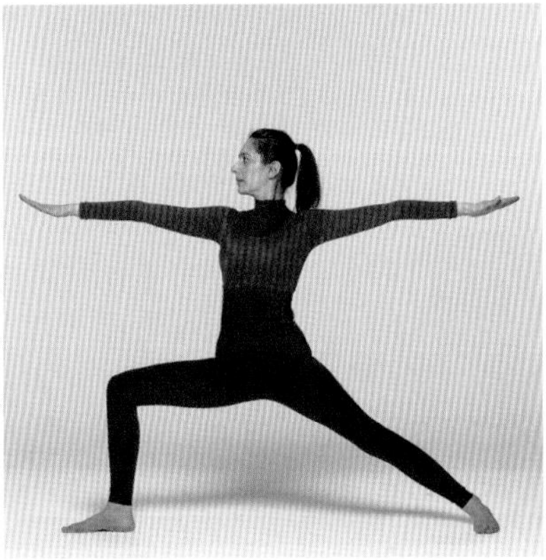

Follow the method given in Unit 2 (page 40).

To Progress

Press the outer edge of the left foot down, and bring weight onto the heel. Press the thigh back and stretch the back of the leg. Press the right knee back. Be aware of the back of the body.

वीरभद्रासन ३ *Vīrabhadrāsana 3*

Warrior Pose 3

Coordination and concentration are developed in this dynamic balancing pose.

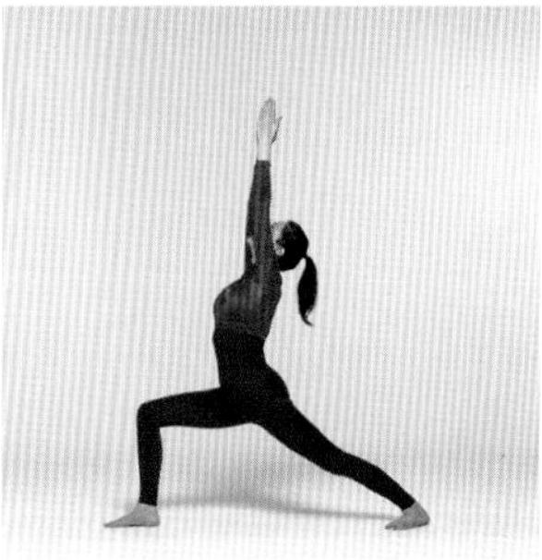

Follow the steps for *Vīrabhadrāsana 1* (see page 153).

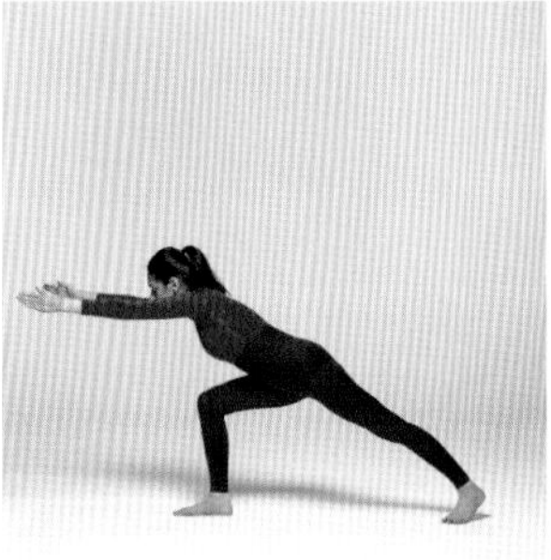

Exhale and bend forward over the right thigh, allowing the left heel to lift off the floor. Keep the arms straight and trunk extended.

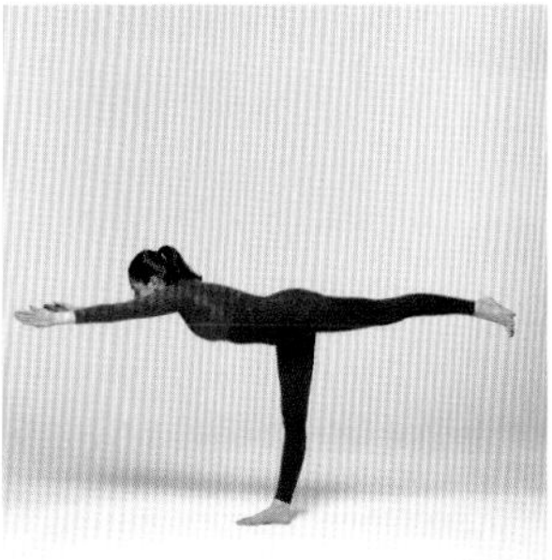

Inhale, straighten the right leg, and simultaneously raise the left leg up, parallel to the floor. Extend the trunk and arms forward.

Stay in the pose for 15 to 20 seconds. Go back into *Vīrabhadrāsana 1*. Inhale and come up. Turn the feet to the front and rest the arms. Then repeat on the other side.

Inhale and come up. Bring the arms to horizontal. Exhale and jump the feet together, simultaneously bringing the arms down.

To Progress

Keep both knees firm and stretch the legs strongly. Bring the hips a little forward, so that the right leg is vertical. Take the left buttock down so that the hips are level. Move the shoulder blades in, and raise the arms to keep the arms and trunk in line.

अर्ध-चन्द्रासन *Ardha-Candrāsana*

Half-Moon Pose

A crescent moon with the cusps facing downward is the inspiration for this pose.

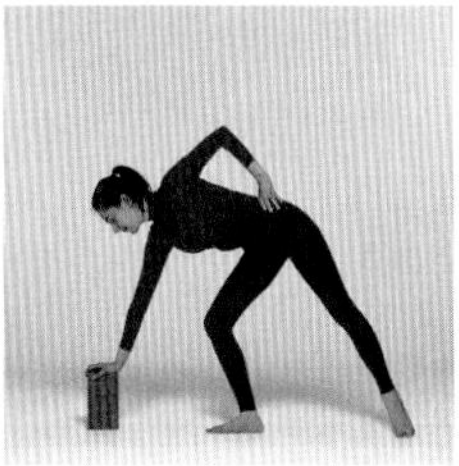

Do *Trikoṇāsana* (see Unit 2, page 36). Rest the right hand on the hip. Exhale, bend the right leg and bring the hand 1 foot forward, resting it on the brick. At the same time bring the left foot in a little.

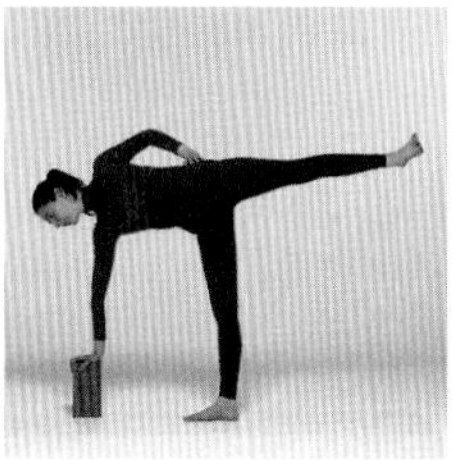

Straighten the right leg and raise the left leg up, foot facing forward. Revolve the trunk upward.

Raise the left arm up, palm facing forward. Turn the head to look up.

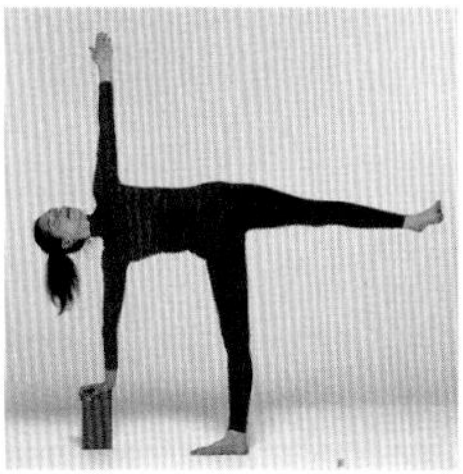

Stay in the pose for 20 to 30 seconds. Bend the right leg and lower the left foot to go back into *Trikoṇāsana*. Inhale and come up. Turn the feet to the front and rest the arms. Then repeat on the other side.

Inhale and come up. Exhale, jump the feet together, and bring the arms down.

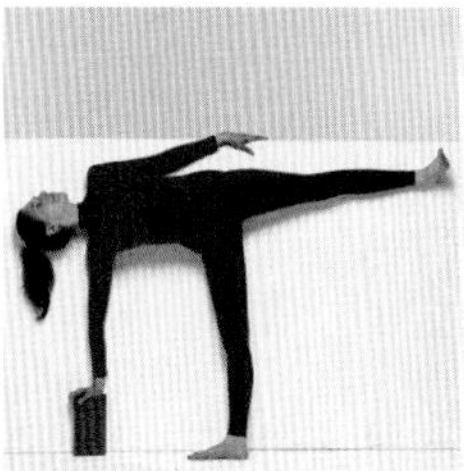

Help

- **If balance is difficult, do the pose with the back supported against a wall. If possible, hold on to a ledge in order to turn the trunk better.**

To Progress

Move the hips a little to the right to make the right leg perpendicular. Stretch the right leg up and the left leg away from the trunk. Lift the left hip.

पाश्र्वोत्तानासन *Pārśvottānāsana*

Sideways Intense Stretch

With the palms behind the back, the skill of balance is developed, in addition to strong stretches.

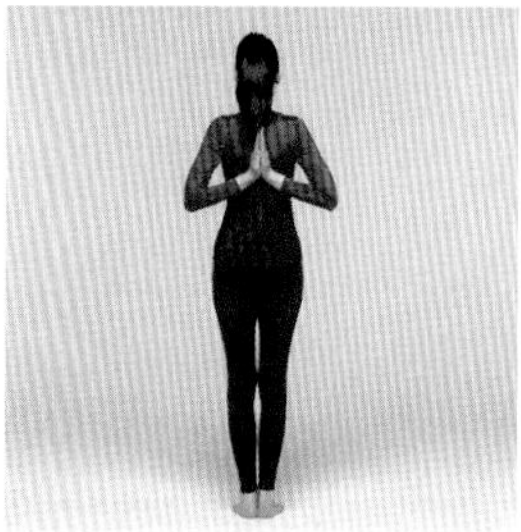

Stand in *Tāḍāsana* (see Unit 1, page 19). Join the palms behind the back, turn the hands inward and upward, and raise them as high as possible up the spine. Take the shoulders and elbows back.

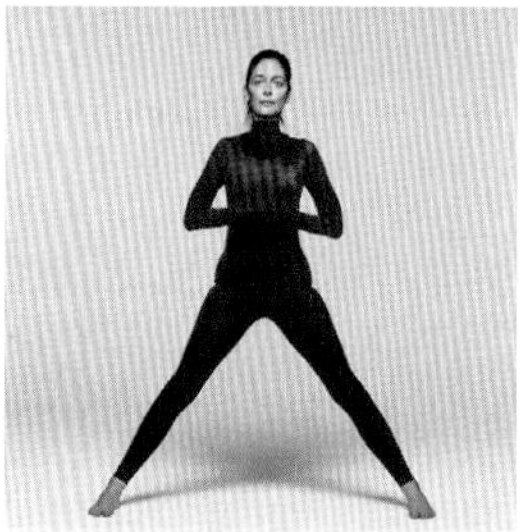

Exhale and jump the feet 3½–4 feet apart. Tighten the knees and pull the thigh muscles up.

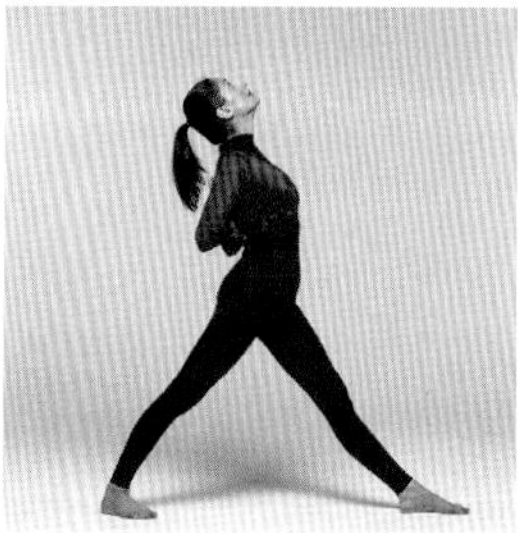

Turn the left foot 45–60 degrees in and the right foot 90 degrees out. Turn the hips so that the trunk faces to the right. Inhale and stretch up; take the head back.

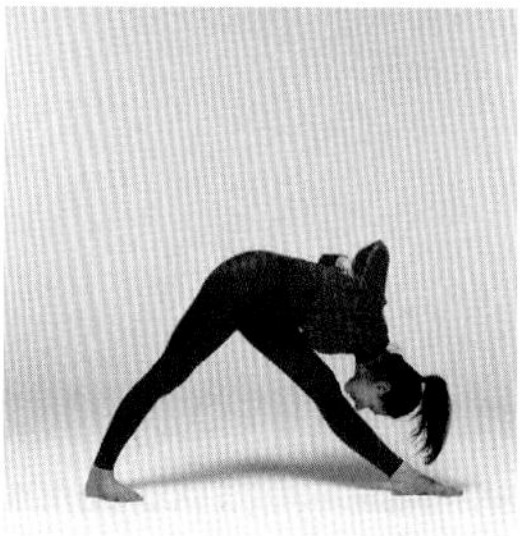

Exhale and bend forward from the hips, over the right leg. Keep the knees tight and stretch the legs up.

Stay in the pose for 20 to 30 seconds. Inhale and come up. Repeat on the other side.

Exhale, jump the feet together, and release the hands.

To Progress

In the forward bend, lengthen the front of the body and lift the arms away from the trunk. Make the back leg poker-stiff to counter-balance the weight of the trunk over the front leg.

पादाङ्गुष्ठासन *Pādāṅguṣṭhāsana*

Thumb-to-Toe Pose

With the hands connected to the feet, a circuit of energy flows in the body, allowing a powerful stretch of the legs and back.

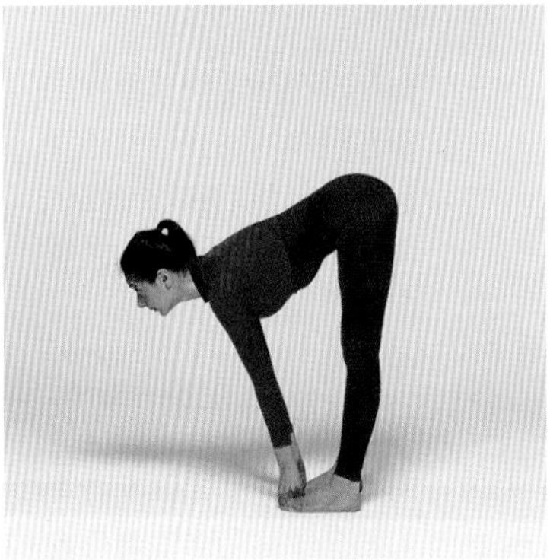

Stand in *Tāḍāsana* (see Unit 1, page 19). Take the feet hip-width apart. Tighten the knees and stretch the legs up. Exhale, bend down, and encircle the big toes with the thumb and first two fingers. Straighten the arms and extend the trunk forward. Make the back concave. Lengthen the front of the body and lift the chin.

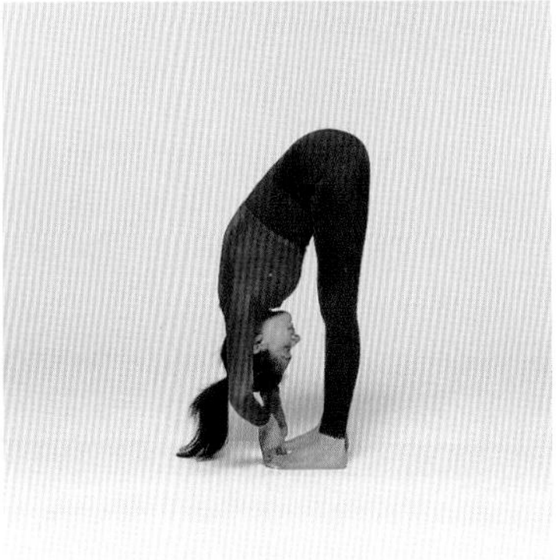

Exhale, bend the elbows outwards, and take the trunk toward the legs. Relax the head and neck.

Stay in the pose for 20 to 30 seconds. Inhale and raise the head and trunk. Release the toes and come up. Bring the feet together.

To Progress

Press the big toes down. In the concave position, press the sacrum (lower back) and thoracic spine down, and lengthen the waist. In the forward bend, pull the trunk down with the help of the arms and shoulders.

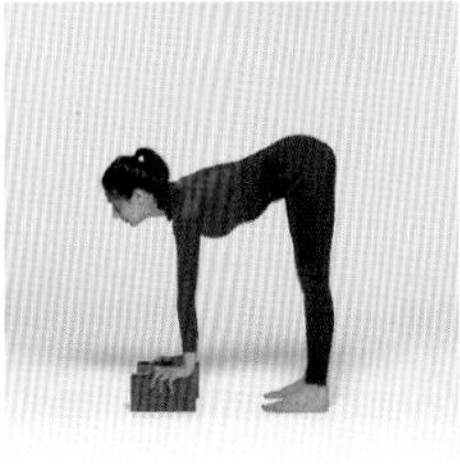

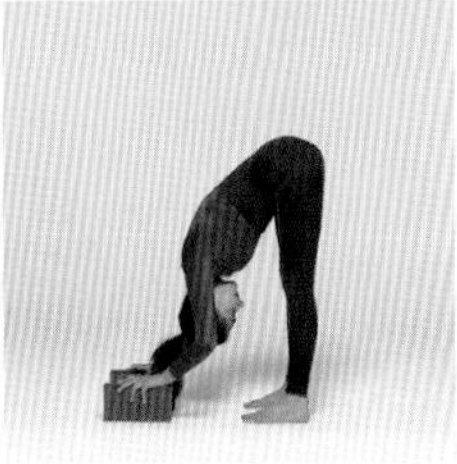

Help

- **If the back and legs are stiff, place the hands on bricks.**

प्रसारित-पादोत्तानासन
Prasārita-Pādottānāsana

Intense Stretch with Spread Legs

A feeling of spaciousness lightens the intensity of the extensions in this pose.

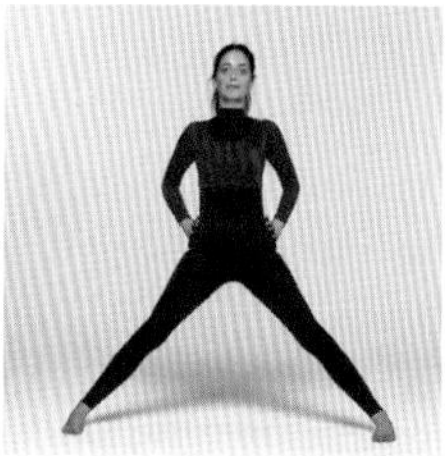

Stand in *Tāḍāsana* (see Unit 1, page 19). Inhale and jump the legs 5 feet apart. Place the hands on the hips. Turn the feet slightly in and press the outer edges down.

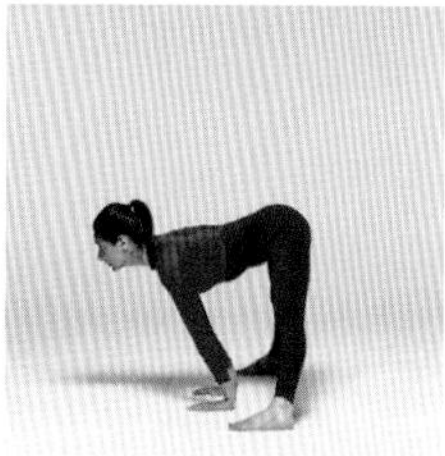

Exhale, bend forward, and place the hands (or fingertips) on the floor, shoulder-width apart. Keep the elbows straight. Make the back concave and lengthen the front of the body. Raise the chin.

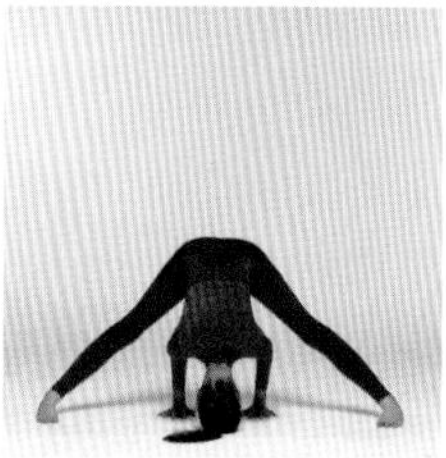

Exhale, bend the elbows back, lower the trunk, and rest the head on the floor. Take the hands back so that the forearms are vertical. Stay in the pose for 20 to 30 seconds. Inhale, straighten the arms, bring the feet in a little, and come up. Bring the feet together.

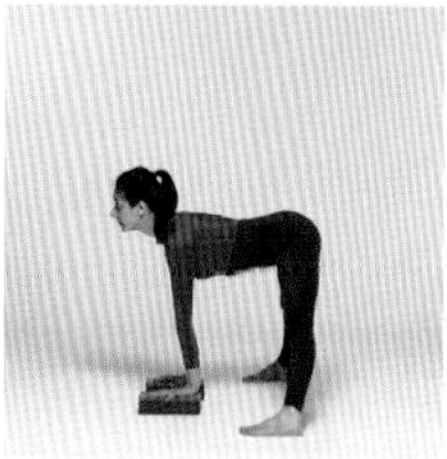

Help

If the back or legs are stiff:

- **Place the hands on blocks for the concave position.**

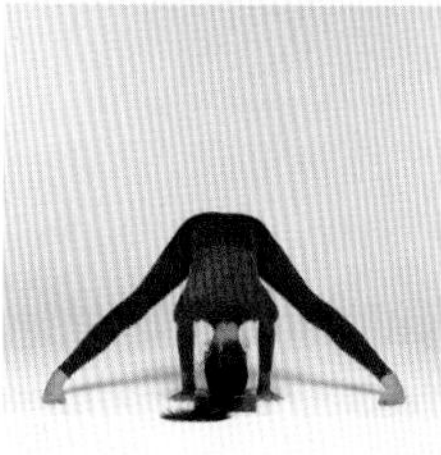

- **In the forward bend, rest the head on a support.**

To Progress

Make the inner legs firm and press them firmly toward the outer legs. Separate the buttock bones. In the concave position, press the sacrum and thoracic spine down and lengthen the waist. Lengthen the sides of the trunk. In the forward bend, lift the shoulders and keep the elbows in.

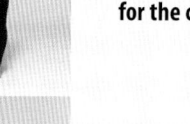

उपविष्ट-कोणासन *Upaviṣṭa-Koṇāsana*

Seated-Angle Pose

The widened groins, erect trunk, and stretched legs make this pose helpful during menstruation and for urinary complaints.

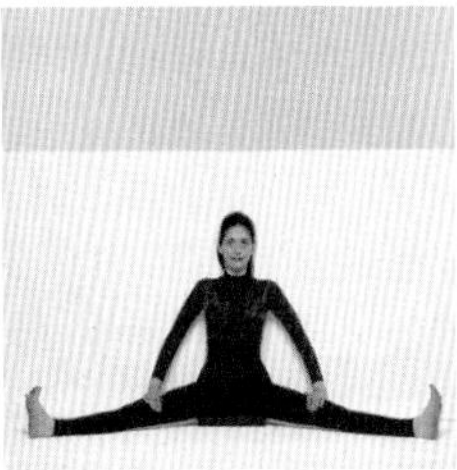

Sit against the wall on a support, such as one or two folded blankets or a block. Take the legs apart, as wide as possible. Keep the knees straight and feet upright. Rest the hands on the legs.

Stay in the pose for 30 seconds to 1 minute, or longer. Bend the legs and bring them forward.

To Progress

Tighten the thigh muscles and press the knees down. Stretch the inner legs from groin to heel. Lift the lower back and rib cage. Keep the shoulders pressed back against the wall.

बद्ध-कोणासन *Baddha-Koṇāsana*

Bound-Angle Pose

The better the legs stretch, the better they flex, and vice versa; here a neat fold at the knee brings the thighs and calves together along their whole length.

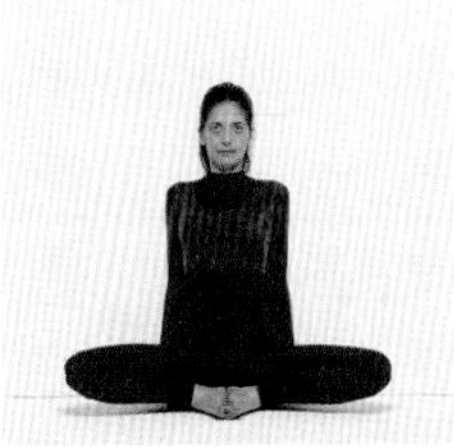

Sit against the wall on a support, such as one or two folded blankets or a block. Bend the knees outward, and bring the soles of the feet together. Bring the feet toward the pubis. Place the hands behind the hips and stretch the trunk up.

Stay in the pose for 30 seconds to 1 minute, or longer. Release the legs and bring them forward.

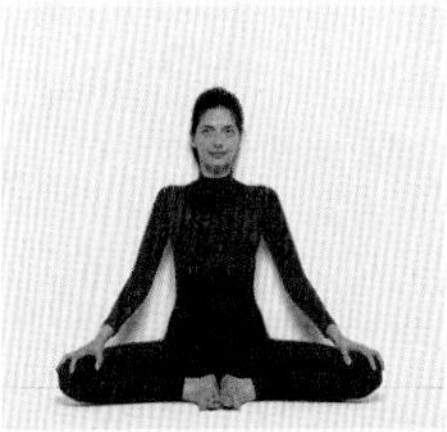

Help

- **To open the groins more, turn the soles of the feet upward with the help of the hands. Keep the outer edges of the feet together, and move the inner edges apart. Place the hands on the thighs and press them down.**

To Progress

Squeeze the hip sockets in so that the groins open more. Move the sacrum (lower back) forward and at the same time lift the pelvis. Roll the shoulders back towards the wall.

निरालम्ब-सर्वाङ्गासन

Nirālamba-Sarvāṅgāsana

Unsupported Shoulder-Balance

Initially this pose uses the wall as a support; ultimately it is performed independently, with no support from wall or arms.

Cautions

See Unit 3 (page 62).

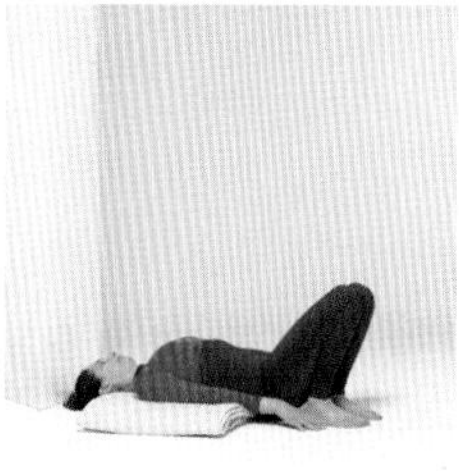

Fold a set of blankets (see Unit 5, page 94) and place them with the folded edges 1 foot away from a wall. Lie down with the shoulders on the folded edge of the sets of blankets and the head on the floor. Move the shoulders away from the neck and the shoulder blades in. Stretch the arms. Bend the legs, keeping the feet on the floor.

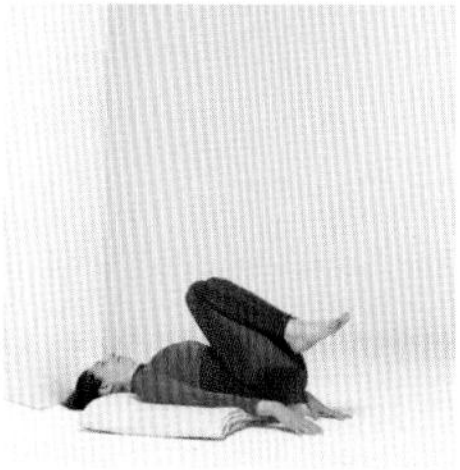

Bend the knees over the abdomen.

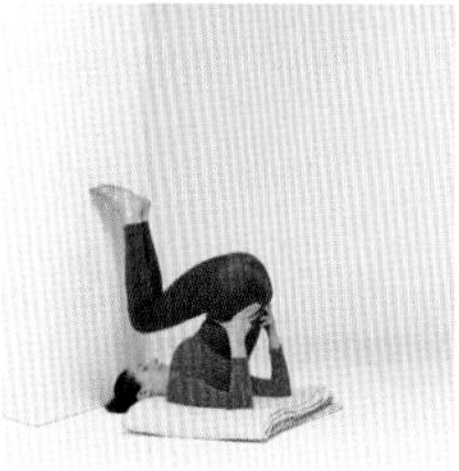

Lift the hips up, bring the feet to the wall, and support the back with the hands.

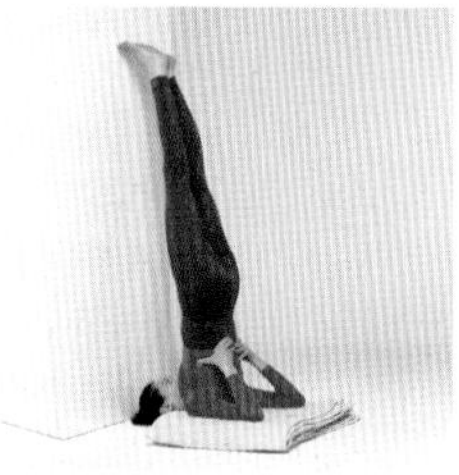

Take the feet higher up the wall and straighten the legs; at the same time bring the trunk forward. Take the hands lower down the back, and bring the elbows in to get a better support.

Stay in the pose for 1 to 5 minutes. Bend the legs, exhale, and slide gently down.

To Progress

Move the hips forward and stretch the whole body up. Keep the knees tight and stretch the legs.

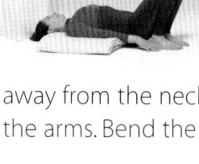

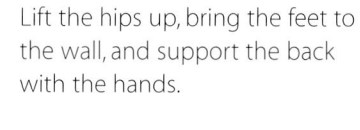

कर्णपीडासन *Karnapīḍāsana*

Ear-Pressing Pose

Contrary to the impression evoked by its name, this pose makes the ears and throat relax.

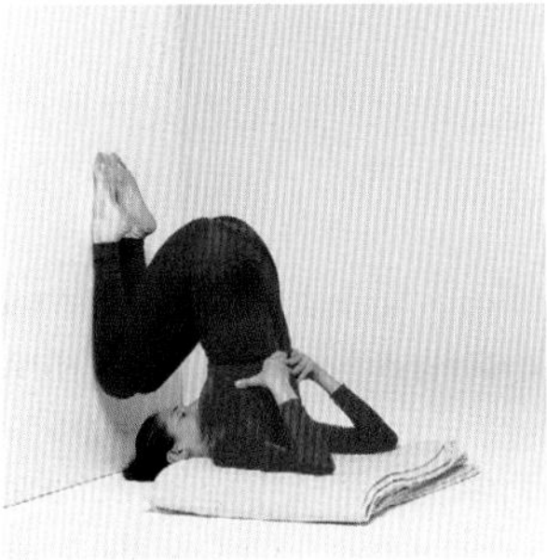

Do *Nirālamba-Sarvāṅgāsana* (see page 61). Bend the knees and rest the shins against the wall. Slide the shins down as far as is comfortable. Relax.

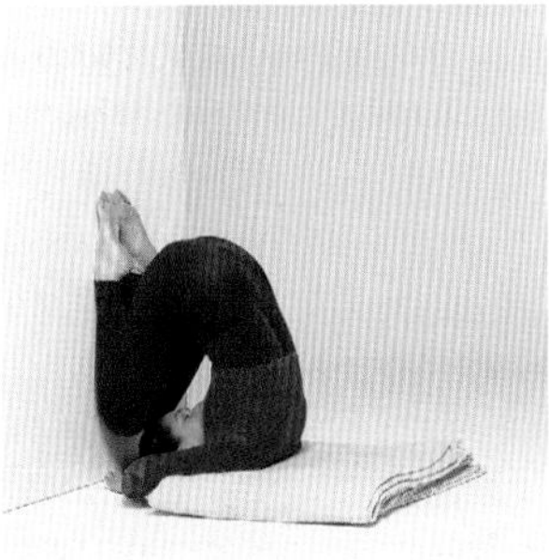

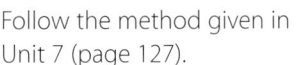

If possible, take the arms over the head. Relax.

Stay in the pose for 1 to 3 minutes. Exhale and slide gently down.

To Progress

Lift the trunk up.

Cautions

See Unit 3 (page 62).

शवासन *Śavāsana*

Corpse Pose

When the legs are rested on a chair they are both bent and inverted, giving a double-strength relaxation after exertion.

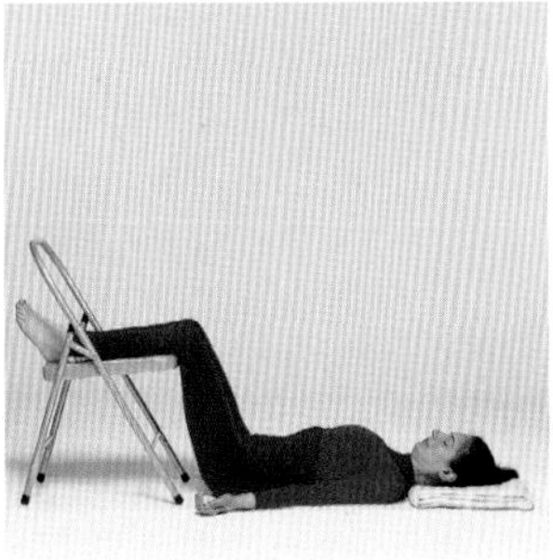

Follow the method given in Unit 7 (page 127).

To Progress

Observe how the body relaxes effortlessly and does not distract the mind. Quieten the sense organs more and more. Keep the eyes still and the ears passive, not straining to hear sounds. Relax the tongue, mouth, and throat. Let the skin become soft. Breathe softly.

Bondage and liberation

We saw earlier the framework of the Indian philosophical thought process. It starts with the concept of bondage and ends with that of liberation of the soul. Between the two is worldly life, characterized by the accumulation of fate (*karma*), by transmigration, and by suffering on the part of the soul through ignorance of its real nature. As in a dream, the soul assigns to itself what is in fact separate from it and experiences its effects—pleasure and pain. This is bondage. To be released from bondage, it is necessary first to understand it.

Release from Suffering

The soul and mind as viewed by Yoga are the observer and the observed. These terms are equivalent to the those previously used, subject and object, and conscious (sentient) and unconscious (insentient). Once the mistaken union of the observer (soul) and the observed (mind) is identified as the cause of suffering, it becomes clear that release from suffering would result from the breaking of this union. What does a doctor do except break the union of the patient with his ailment? Health, which already exists but is obscured, is restored only by the doctor's medicine. This fact makes the commentator on the *Yoga Sūtra* compare worldly life to a disease and a philosopher to a physician. This breaking of the painful

KEY CONCEPT

Discriminating knowledge The term "knowledge" conveys a range of meanings. It is generally understood as an intellectual phenomenon. In philosophical contexts, knowledge undoubtedly starts at the intellectual level, but does not end there. For the achievement of its goal, liberation, the knowledge that the soul is distinct from the mind needs to be translated into experience; and this requires persistent practice of Yoga. When the goal is achieved, even this discriminating knowledge ceases to exist. This is perfectly logical: how could there be liberation if the soul continues to be aware of its distinctness from the mind, when the mind, the principal instrument of knowledge, is itself eliminated?

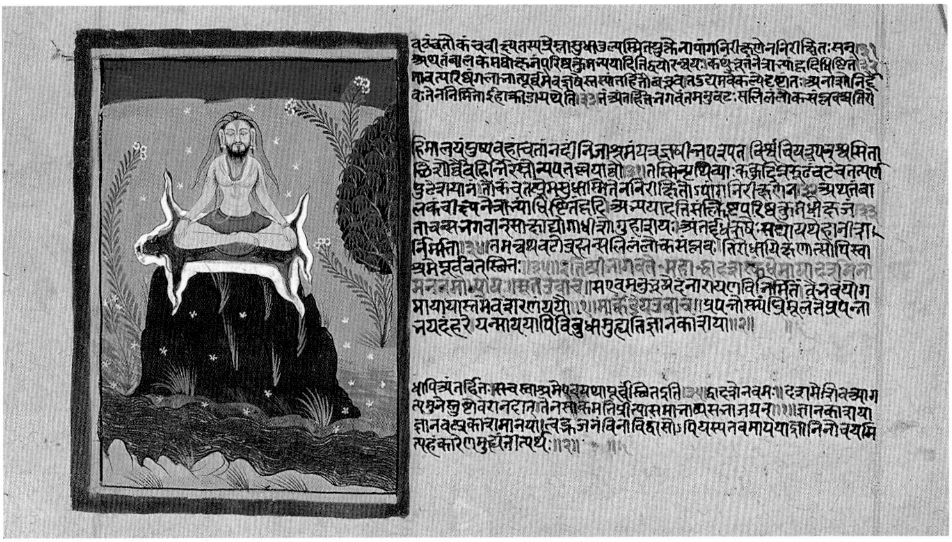

Sage Mārkaṇḍeya is liberated from the world.

union with the mind in worldly life is equivalent to the isolation or liberation (*kaivalya*) of the observer. In this state, the observer attains or regains its genuine nature—that is, pure consciousness untouched by the three qualities of Matter (*guṇas*) that permeate the world.

What is Liberation?

Liberation is defined as the dissolution of qualities of Matter (*guṇas*) in their cause, Primordial Matter (*prakṛti*), a situation that is equivalent to the repose of pure consciousness (the soul, *puruṣa*) in itself. This is the logical end of the three qualities, which can exist only for another entity, having no purpose to serve when the liberation of the soul has taken place. What happens to a mold when the cast is ready? It disintegrates in the heat, as it exists only for the sake of the cast. Yoga philosophy, therefore, says that Matter exists not for itself but for the soul, the entity that can utilize it, albeit under the influence of ignorance. When the three qualities cease to exist, the machinery of experience, which gives rise to pleasure and pain, also ceases to exist. Since the mind is the principal instrument of this experience, liberation is, in effect, the total and permanent annihilation of the mind, while meditation is a temporary suspension of it. In both cases, the soul attains its original pure character. The doctor gives painkillers as a temporary relief to the patient; the lasting cure is to remove the cause of the pain through appropriate treatment.

The Logical Necessity for the Soul

This raises the question of whether the soul exists as a permanent entity, distinct from the mind. *Patañjali* argues in favor of its existence on the following grounds:

1. The mind is continuously understood by the soul, the subject. (This is supported by everyone's personal experience: we are aware of what is going on in our mind.)

2. It is illogical to think of the mind as both the object and the subject, as the subject-object relationship cannot rest on a single entity (see Logic and Faulty Logic on page 167).

3. The hypothesis that the mind is understood by *another* mind, as a substitute explanation, involves similar logical defects, whether we assume only one more mind, or whether we assume a series of minds, each comprehending the previous one.

The first two points call for some discussion. When one person observes another, it is a case of one body-mind-soul complex observing another. The roles of subject and object can be reversed, with the observed becoming the observer. This goes against the hypothesis that subject and object are mutually exclusive. This argument is misleading because, in both alternatives, it is the sense organs that view their objects—that is, color, form, sound, and so on. That they can do this is due to the supporting presence of the mind and soul. An electrical device can work only when supported by electricity. The ultimate source of energy in all cognitive experiences is the soul, which is beyond the power of the sense organs to grasp.

What remains to be decided is the reason that forces us to regard the soul as a distinct entity from the mind. If we observe our cognitive process, we find that we are aware of the changes in our minds. Who is aware of it? Not the mind, which itself is the object. This situation leads us to suppose an entity other than the mind. That is the soul. In case this other entity is taken to be another mind, we are caught in illogicality, as shown in point 3 above.

The only logical explanation of worldly cognition has therefore to be based on the hypothesis that (a) the mind, being material, lacks consciousness and merely reflects the soul, as a mirror reflects light; and (b) as a result, the soul, as consciousness, appears to be the author of the cognitive process when an object is registered on the mind through the sense organs. This phenomenon is explained by the analogy that the victory or defeat of soldiers in battle is credited to their king. The corollary of the thesis is that bondage and liberation are in fact attributes of the mind. The recognition of a spiritual principle, the soul, as a distinct conscious entity is therefore a logical necessity.

Liberation in Life

The state of liberation has nothing to do with death; it can be experienced even while one is alive. The expression "liberated-while-alive" (*jīvan-mukta*) reflects this belief. This state of experience is thought to be nothing but liberation. Such a continuation of life after liberation is explained on the basis of remaining fate (*karma*). This concept has its root in the hypothesis that, even though the experience of Reality nullifies all fates, the specific fate causing the current incarnation of the liberated Yogin cannot stop bearing consequences in midstream.

Status of the World after Liberation

While the world ceases to be experienced by a particular liberated soul, it continues to exist for others. This is comparable to its existence for creatures in the waking state, and its nonexistence for one in deep sleep. Deep sleep isolates a person from others and is thus, to a limited extent, like liberation. Meditation also has points of similarity with liberation. Thus, liberation is individual in character. It has no social relevance. The deliverance of mankind by a prophet, as is often claimed, can mean only that the prophet shows his fellow beings the path to release. Treading the path and the progress on it depend on the will and effort on the part of the individual concerned.

The Means of Release

The direct means of release from suffering is "Discriminating Knowledge," that is, knowledge that discerns the difference between the soul and Matter. The causal relation between this knowledge and liberation is more metaphorical than real. The suffering of the soul is caused by its union with Matter, and this union is created by the mistaken identity of the soul. Discriminating knowledge corrects or annihilates this mistake. At its annihilation, liberation, which is in the very nature of the soul, manifests itself. It is like waking from the state of dream and rediscovering our normal identity. By the standard of worldly experience, what we find ourselves to be, in a dream, is false; it is corrected when we return to the waking state and recover our lost identity.

This knowledge that distinguishes the mind from the soul is attained through Yoga. The basic meaning of the word Yoga is "a means," and, in common usage, it stands for a chain of means and ends.

In Brief

Matter and Spirit are distinct. The mind is a product of Matter.
The Spirit is the perceiver; the mind the perceived. How can they be identical?

Thinking itself to be identical with the mind, the soul is afflicted by the latter's sufferings.
Separation from Matter is liberation for the soul, its own natural state.

Liberation is different from death; it can occur even during life.
The body survives as long as fate already unrolling remains.

Rare in the world is the man who has gained the knowledge of this distinctness;
The rest are ignorant and bound. Hence this world continues.

For a wider perspective...

Logic and Faulty Logic

The consistency of logic with fact and with itself is an essential condition for its acceptance. The purpose of logic is to help understand unseen aspects of reality by means of inference, and not to indulge in speculative explanations aimed at proving some doctrinal view. It is here that belief and rational thinking part.

In philosophical debate faults, in logic are considered to make an argument invalid. The faults in logic corresponding to defective suppositions recognized in the Sanskrit tradition and relevant in the present context are

1. Self-dependence. This occurs when the argument supposes that a single entity depends on itself. For instance, "The tree stands by itself."

2. Inter-dependence. This occurs when the argument supposes that two entities depend on each other. For instance, "The tree and the ground support each other."

3. Infinite regress. This occurs when the argument supposes an unending series in which each preceding entity depends on the successive entity—for instance, "Book A is based on book B, book B on book C, book C on book D," and so on. When such a chain arises in hypothetical reasoning, the argument is invalid. In the Yoga context, if the mind is supposed to be observed by another mind, it will lead to such a fault in logic, for the second or each successive mind is hypothetical, and not a matter of experience.

How to Recognize a Liberated Person

The *Bhagavad-Gītā* describes an enlightened, liberated man. He has transcended the qualities of Matter (see Unit 7), being unmoved by earthly phenomena. He is equal-minded in pleasure and pain, and always calm. A clod of earth, a stone, and a nugget of gold are the same to him. He is the same in praise or blame, honor or dishonor, and to friend or foe. His actions are unmotivated. Without desires, he is content within his soul. He is not disturbed by calamity or attracted to pleasures. He is free from passion, fear, and anger. He withdraws his senses from their stimuli as a tortoise draws in its limbs. He moves in the world without attachment or hate; this leads him to the peace that ends all woes. He sees the world but is unmoved by it, just as the ocean, though constantly filled, remains stable.

Unit 10

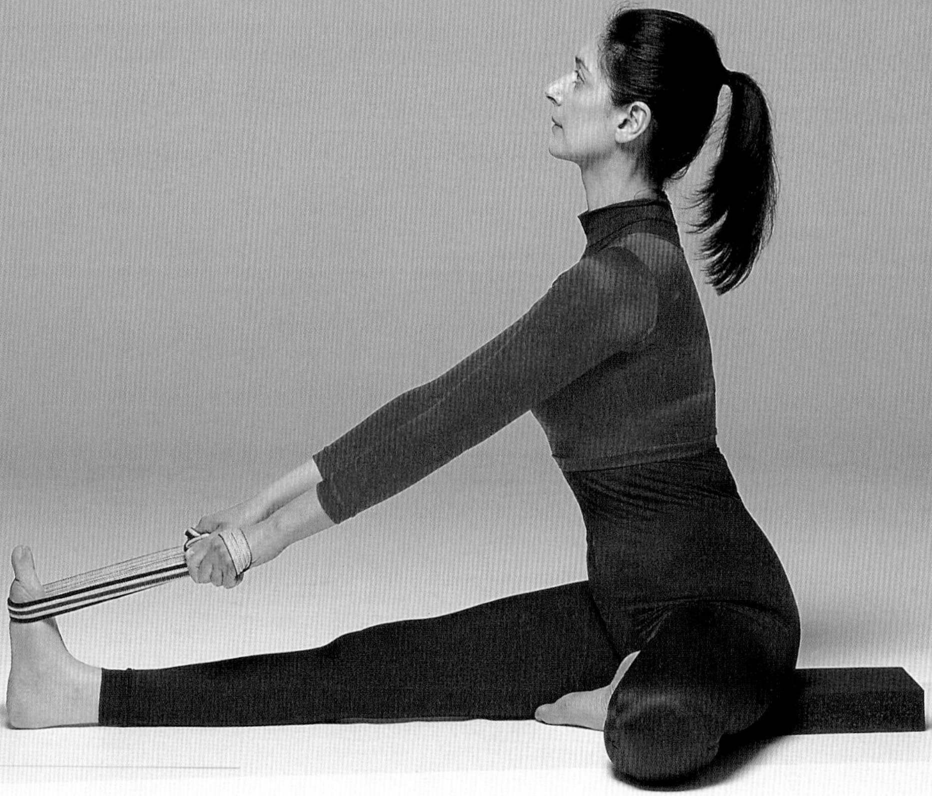

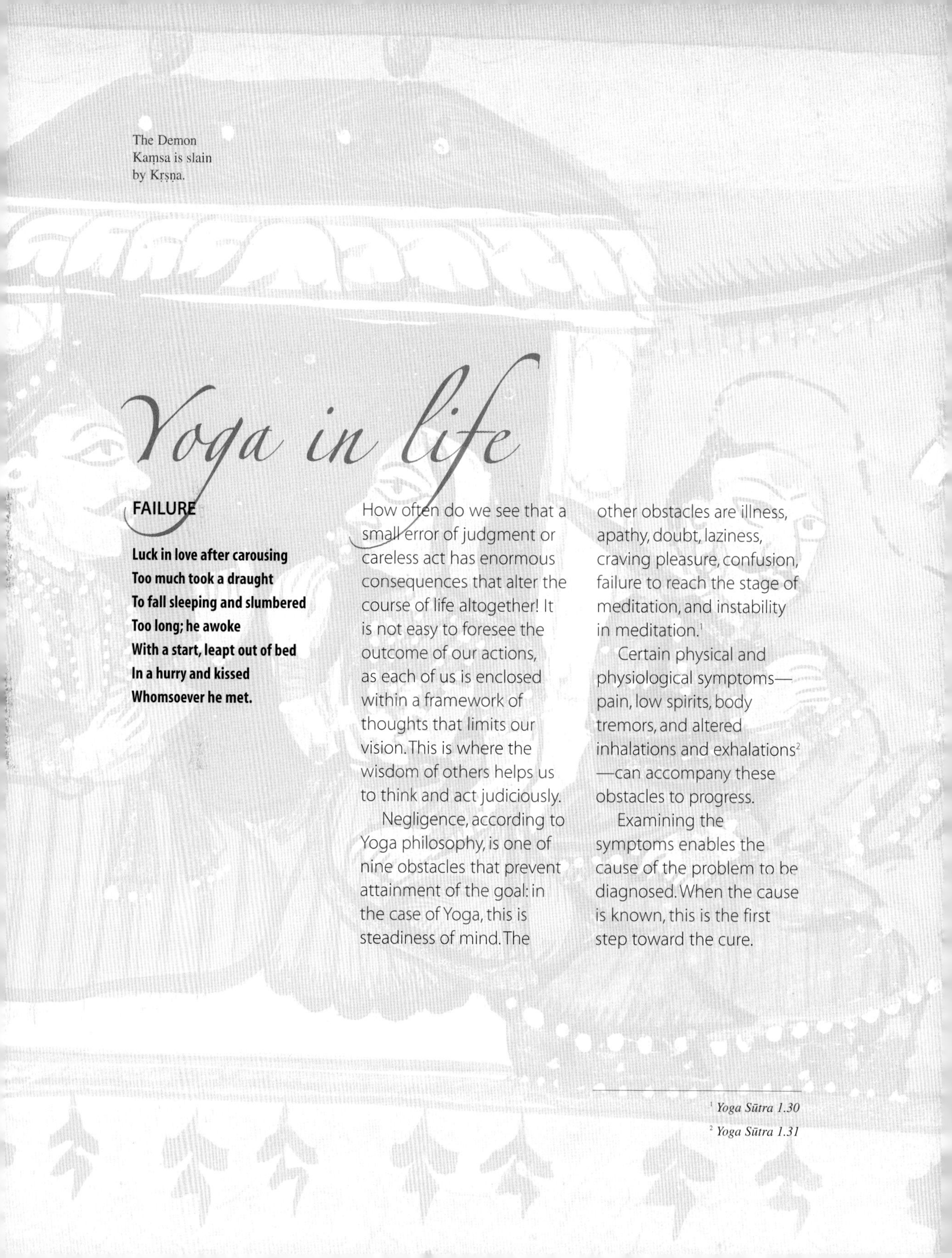

The Demon
Kaṃsa is slain
by Kṛṣṇa.

Yoga in life

FAILURE

Luck in love after carousing
Too much took a draught
To fall sleeping and slumbered
Too long; he awoke
With a start, leapt out of bed
In a hurry and kissed
Whomsoever he met.

How often do we see that a small error of judgment or careless act has enormous consequences that alter the course of life altogether! It is not easy to foresee the outcome of our actions, as each of us is enclosed within a framework of thoughts that limits our vision. This is where the wisdom of others helps us to think and act judiciously.

Negligence, according to Yoga philosophy, is one of nine obstacles that prevent attainment of the goal: in the case of Yoga, this is steadiness of mind. The other obstacles are illness, apathy, doubt, laziness, craving pleasure, confusion, failure to reach the stage of meditation, and instability in meditation.[1]

Certain physical and physiological symptoms—pain, low spirits, body tremors, and altered inhalations and exhalations[2]—can accompany these obstacles to progress.

Examining the symptoms enables the cause of the problem to be diagnosed. When the cause is known, this is the first step toward the cure.

[1] *Yoga Sūtra 1.30*

[2] *Yoga Sūtra 1.31*

More leg stretches

A helping hand is often needed in life to overcome a difficulty or to achieve something that is impossible through independent effort. It is the same with stretching. A little aid given in the right direction can bring enormous advances. The instrument of assistance is simple: a belt.

If the leg stretches when the foot is on the floor, as in standing poses, the downward pressure of the foot lends force to the upward extension. In poses where the foot is in the air, however, the extension tends to be weak. It is strengthened by making the foot push against the hands or a belt. There is then a circuit of energy that connects the arms and legs, empowering them both.

Upright Leg Raise (*Utthita-Hasta-Pādāṅguṣṭhāsana*) and Supine Leg Raise (*Supta-Pādāṅguṣṭhāsana*) are twin poses that involve stretching each leg upward and laterally. In the final, advanced pose the fingers grip the big toe, making a very intense stretch. A realistic beginning is to place a belt around the foot, in this way extending the reach of the arms.

This method is also used for Upward Leg Extension (*Ūrdhva-Prasārita-Pādāsana*) where the lower back has to remain flat on the floor with the legs perpendicular to it. Empowered by the hands holding the belt, the legs can stretch up while the hips press down.

Forward bends, which involve extending one or both legs along the floor, are similarly facilitated by using a belt. In addition to the leg stretch, these poses involve bending the elbows to give the arms strength to pull the trunk forward. The belt makes this action possible for people who cannot catch their feet.

In all the above poses the primary line of extension is along the inner leg from the groin to the inner heel. To maintain this line, the inner edge of the knee has to be held firm. This applies also to inverted poses. The stretch of the inner leg gives a feeling of lightness and spaciousness in the legs.

The poses so far have involved hands clasping legs. In others, the hands link to each other. Interlocking the fingers, pressing the palms together, catching hands: these various hand connections give strength to the arm stretches and flexions involved. Here, too, a belt can be used if the hands do not reach, for example, in Cow Head Pose (*Gomukhāsana*).

A belt is also used to link the arms in Shoulder Balance (*Sarvāṅgāsana*). The arms have a tendency to slip outward, making it difficult for them to support the back. When they are held together by a belt, two purposes are served. First, they stay in line with the shoulders, so that they can function effectively as supports. Secondly, their individual strengths are combined in a solid support. For this reason it is helpful always to use a belt in this pose and in Plow Pose (*Halāsana*).

उत्थित-हस्त-पादाङ्गुष्ठासन

Utthita-Hasta-Pādāṅguṣṭhāsana

Upright Leg Raise

The separated legs stretch in different directions to achieve the same end: straightness.

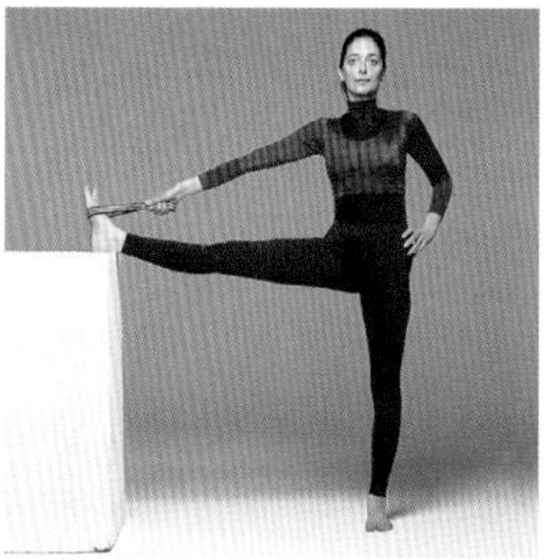

(a) Sideways

Stand in *Tāḍāsana* (see Unit 1, page 19) with the right side 2½–3 feet away from a ledge. Bend the right leg and turn it outward. Raise the leg and place the heel on the ledge, in line with the hip. Loop a belt around the foot, and hold it with the right hand; place the left hand on the left hip. Straighten both the legs. Lift the trunk and take the shoulders back. Keep the head level. Breathe evenly.

Stay in the pose for 30 seconds to 1 minute. Repeat on the other side.

To Progress

Keep the knees firm. Press the left thigh back and bring weight onto the heel. Stretch the leg up. Revolve the right leg outward, keeping the foot upright. Press the thigh down and stretch the leg toward the heel.

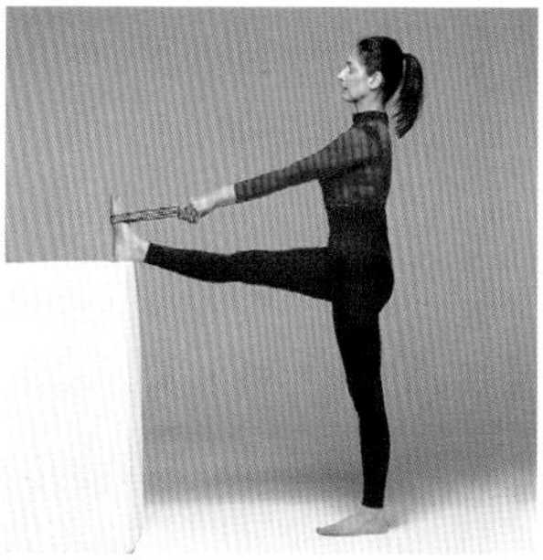

(b) Forward

Stand in *Tāḍāsana* (see Unit 1, page 19) 2½–3 feet away from a ledge and facing it. Bend the right leg, raise it, and place the heel on the ledge in line with the hip. Loop a belt around the foot and hold it with the left hand; place the right hand on the right hip. Straighten both the legs. Lift the trunk and take the shoulders back. Keep the head level. Breathe evenly.

Stay in the pose for 30 seconds to 1 minute. Repeat on the other side.

To Progress

Keep the knees firm. Keep the left foot facing forward. Press the left thigh back and bring weight onto the heel. Stretch the leg up. Press the right thigh down and stretch the leg toward the heel.

सुप्त-पादाङ्गुष्ठासन

Supta-Pādāṅguṣṭhāsana

Supine Leg Raise

The stable leg controls the movement of the mobile leg and therefore the degree of stretch.

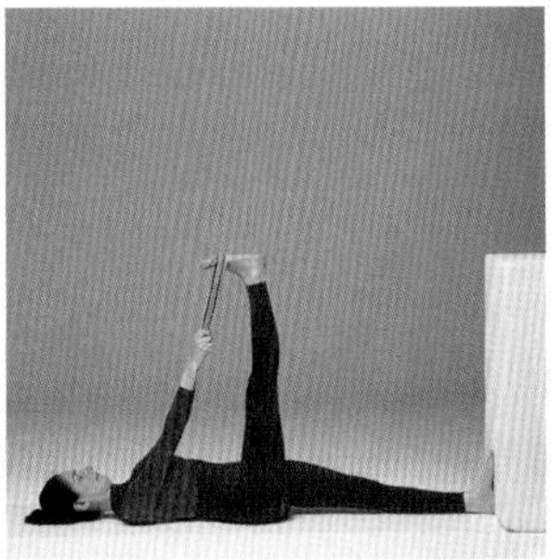

(a) Upward

Lie with the feet pressed against the wall. Bend the right leg over the abdomen, loop a belt around the foot, and hold each end of it separately. Straighten both the legs. Keep the chest expanded and the shoulders down.

Stay in the pose for 30 seconds to 1 minute. Bend the right leg and bring it down. Repeat on the other side.

To Progress

Keep the knees tight. Press the left thigh down, extend the back of the leg, and press the heel into the wall. Press the right thigh back. Keeping the right hip down, stretch the leg up toward the heel.

Help

- **If the back or legs are stiff, support the raised leg against a column.**

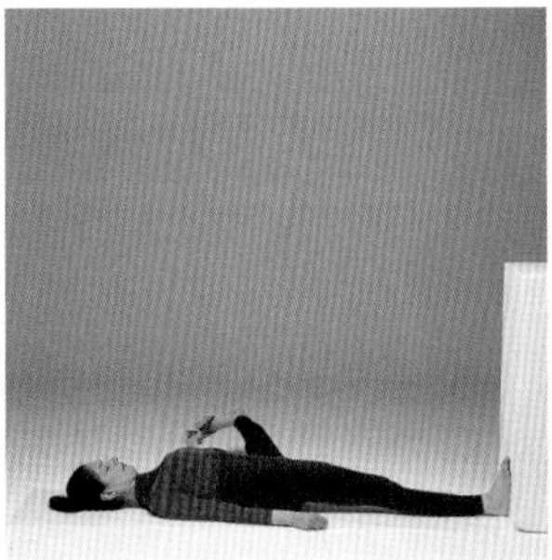

(b) Sideways

Lie with the feet pressed against the wall. Bend the right leg over the abdomen, loop a belt around the foot, and hold it with the right hand. Revolve the leg outward and take it out to the side. Straighten both the legs. Keep the chest expanded and the shoulders down.

Stay in the pose for 30 seconds to 1 minute. Bring the right leg up, bend it and take it down beside the left leg. Repeat on the other side.

To Progress

Keep the knees tight. Press the left thigh down, extend the back of the leg, and press the heel into the wall. Press the right thigh back and stretch the leg toward the heel.

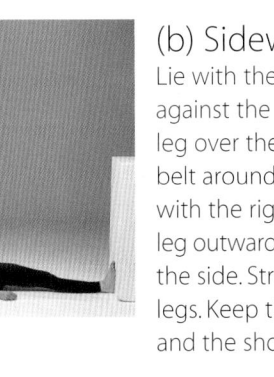

ऊर्ध्व-प्रसारित-पादासन *Ūrdhva-Prasārita-Pādāsana*

Upward Leg Extension

To form a sharp right angle between the legs and trunk, opposite forces come into play: downward for the hips and upward for the legs.

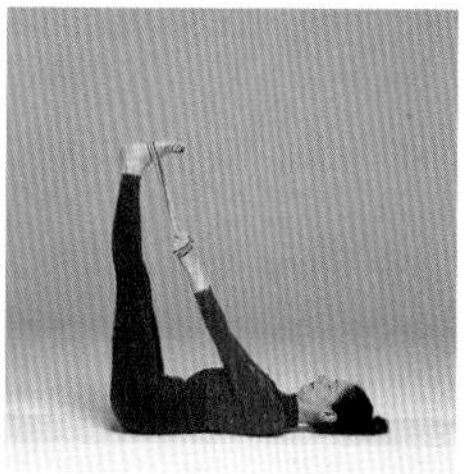

Lie in a straight line. Bend the knees over the abdomen and loop a belt around the feet. Straighten the legs up to a vertical position. Keep the arms straight. Extend the trunk and press the shoulders down.

Stay in the pose for 30 seconds to 1 minute. Bend the legs and come down.

To Progress

Press the hips down. Press the thighs back, extend the backs of the legs, and press the feet against the belt.

जानुशीर्षासन *Jānuśīrṣāsana*

Head-to-Knee Pose

When the trunk bends forward over the legs they get an intense extension; one leg at a time is the way to begin.

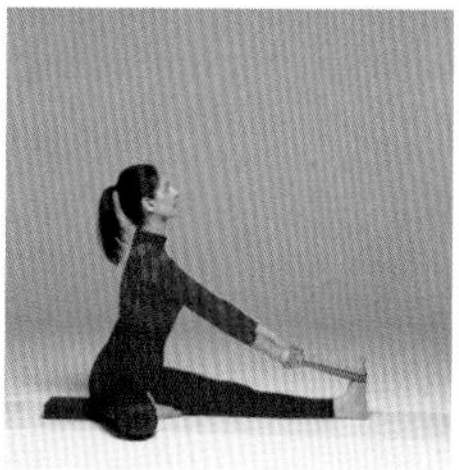

Sit on one or two folded blankets with the legs stretched out in front. Bend the right leg to the side, bringing the heel to the groin. Keep the left leg straight and the foot upright. Loop a belt around the left foot and catch the two ends separately. Inhale, straighten the arms, and stretch the trunk up. Make the back concave and lengthen the front of the body. Look up. Breathe evenly.

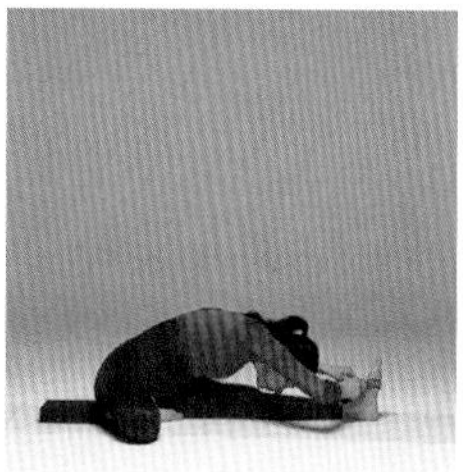

Exhale, bend the elbows outward, and take the trunk down over the left leg.

Stay in the pose for 20 to 30 seconds. Inhale and come up. Repeat on the other side.

To Progress

Keep the left knee tight and the thigh muscle pulled up. Move the trunk forward from the lower back. Keep the right knee relaxed.

Help

- **If the back is stiff, sit higher.**

एकपादवीर-पश्चिमोत्तानासन

Ekapādavīra-Paścimottānāsana

Posterior Intense Stretch with One Leg in Hero Pose

There are pluses and minuses in this pose: with one leg bent back, the trunk bends more freely over the legs but is less balanced.

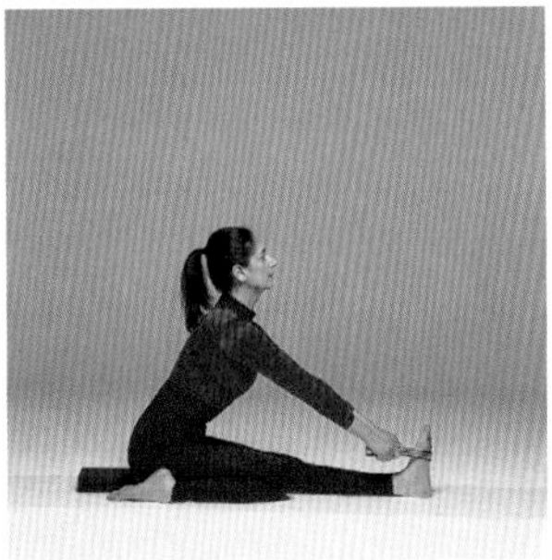

Sit on one or two folded blankets with the legs stretched out in front. Move the blanket support so that it is under the left buttock. Bend the right leg back, keeping the knee facing forward. Keep the left leg straight and the foot upright. Loop a belt around the left foot, and catch the two ends separately. Inhale, straighten the arms, and stretch the trunk up. Make the back concave and lengthen the front of the body. Look up. Breathe evenly.

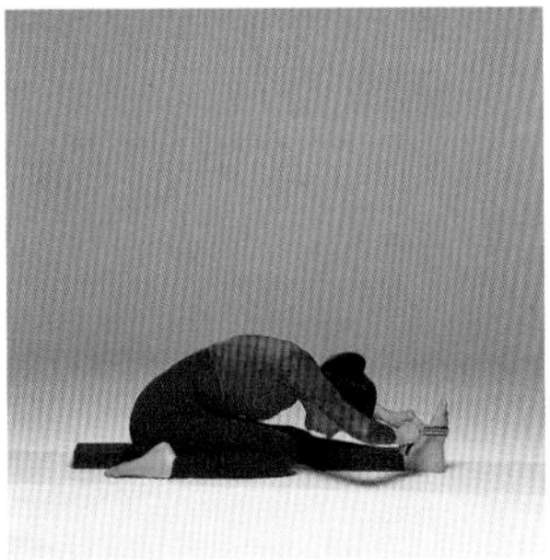

Exhale, bend the elbows outward and take the trunk down over the left leg.

Stay in the pose for 20 to 30 seconds. Inhale and come up. Repeat on the other side.

Help

- **If the back is stiff or if it is difficult to balance, sit higher.**
- **If the ankles are stiff, place a rolled blanket under the lower shins (see Unit 2, page 42).**

To Progress

Keep the left knee tight and the thigh muscle pulled up. Move the trunk forward from the hips. Roll the right thigh outward and press the shin down.

मरीच्यासन १ *Marīcyāsana 1*

Marici's Pose 1

When one leg is bent upward the lower back tends to collapse; the strong forward thrust required to counter this develops lower back strength.

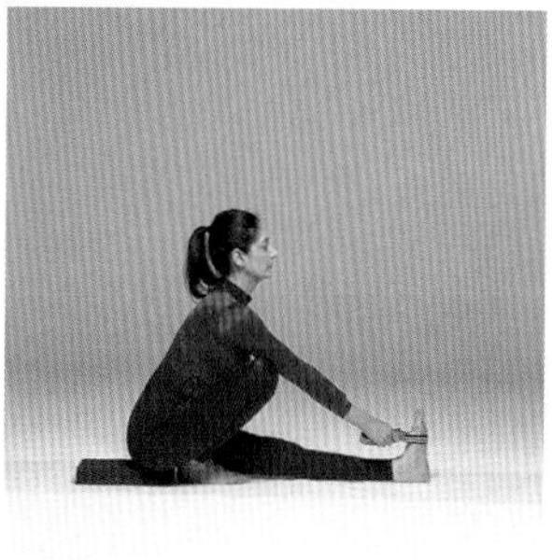

Sit on one or two folded blankets, with the legs stretched out in front. Bend the right leg up, taking the foot against the left inner thigh and the heel against the right thigh. Keep the left leg straight and the foot upright. Loop a belt around the left foot, and catch the two ends separately. Inhale, straighten the arms, and stretch the trunk up. Make the back concave and lengthen the front of the body. Look up. Breathe evenly.

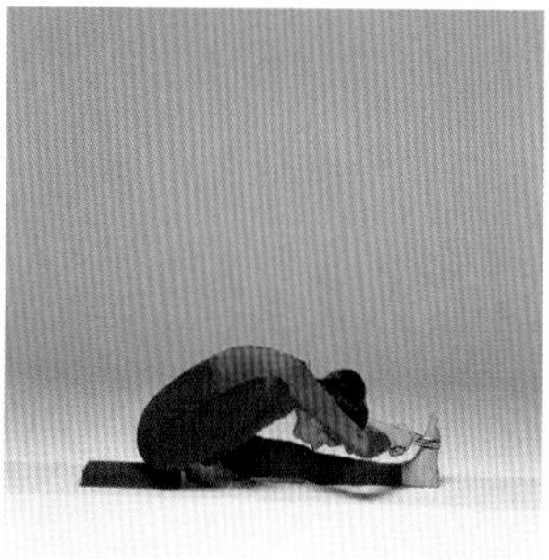

Exhale, bend the elbows outward, and take the trunk down over the left leg.

Stay in the pose for 20 to 30 seconds. Inhale and come up. Repeat on the other side.

Help

- **If the back is stiff, sit higher.**

To Progress

Keep the left knee tight and the thigh muscle pulled up. Move the trunk forward from the lower back. Keep the right leg upright.

पश्चिमोत्तानासन *Paścimottānāsana*

Posterior Intense Stretch

This forward bend is said, in ancient works on Yoga, to stimulate digestion, make the abdomen flat, and remove diseases.

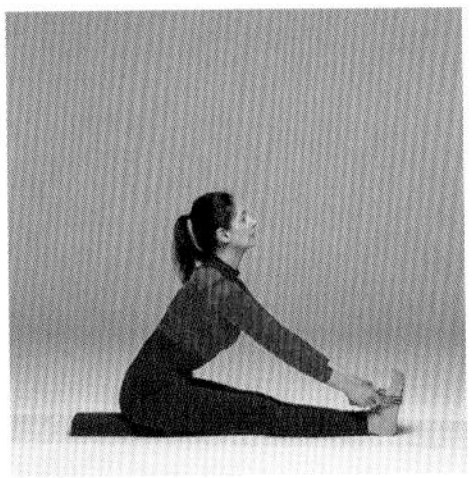

Sit on one or two folded blankets with the legs stretched out in front. Straighten the knees and keep the feet upright. Loop a belt around the feet, and catch the two ends separately. Inhale, straighten the arms, and stretch the trunk up. Make the back concave and lengthen the front of the body. Look up. Breathe evenly.

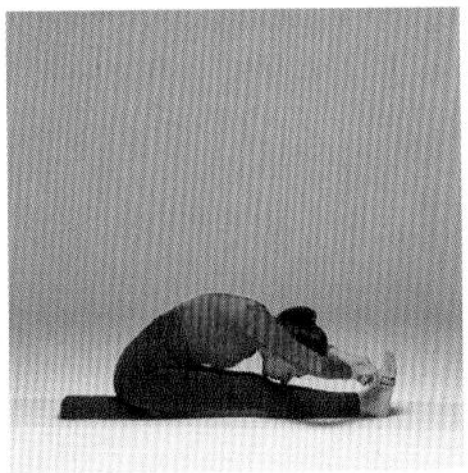

Exhale, bend the elbows outward and take the trunk down over the legs.

Stay in the pose for 20 to 30 seconds. Inhale and come up.

Help

- **If the back is stiff, sit higher.**

To Progress

Keep the knees tight and the thigh muscles pulled up. Move the trunk forward from the lower back. Pull on the belt to extend the sides of the trunk.

पर्वतासन *Parvatāsana*

Mountain Pose

After having been stretched, the legs remain elongated, even in a flexed position.

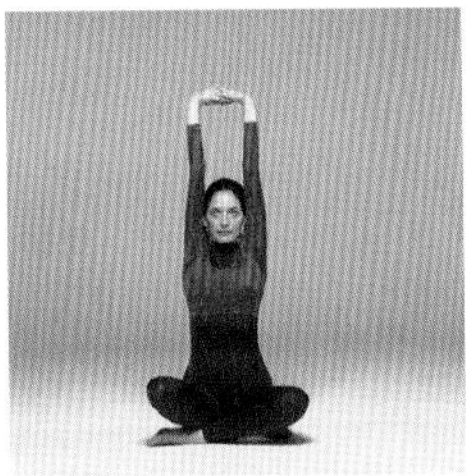

Follow the method given in Unit 2 (page 43).

To Progress

Observe the effect of prior stretching on the position of the legs and their ability to relax.

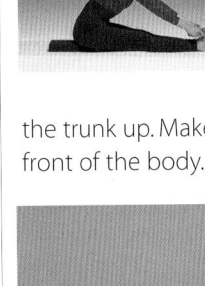

सपर्वतासन वीरासन
Vīrāsana with Parvatāsana

Hero Pose with Mountain Pose

The nature of a stretch alters according to the configuration of limbs; in this pose the lower back moves freely, facilitating extension from the base of the trunk.

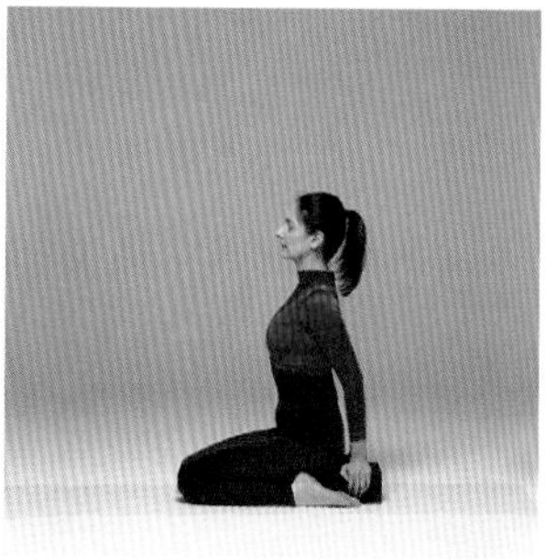

Sit in *Vīrāsana* (see Unit 6, page 107).

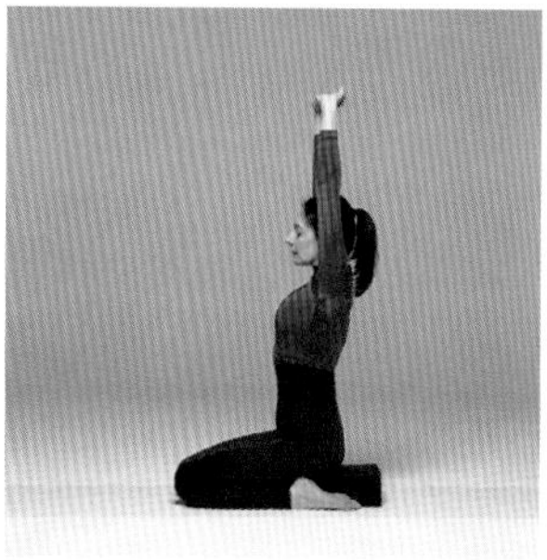

Interlock the fingers. Turn the palms outward and stretch the arms up. Tighten the elbows. Keep the face and neck relaxed.

Stay in the pose for 20 to 30 seconds. Bring the arms down, change the interlock of the fingers, and repeat. Bring the legs forward.

To Progress

Move the shoulder blades in. Press the wrists upward and lift the arms higher. Take the arms back till they are vertical, and extend the armpits.

नमस्ते *Namaste*

Salutation

The lift of the chest produced by this arm position brings a corresponding lift of spirits.

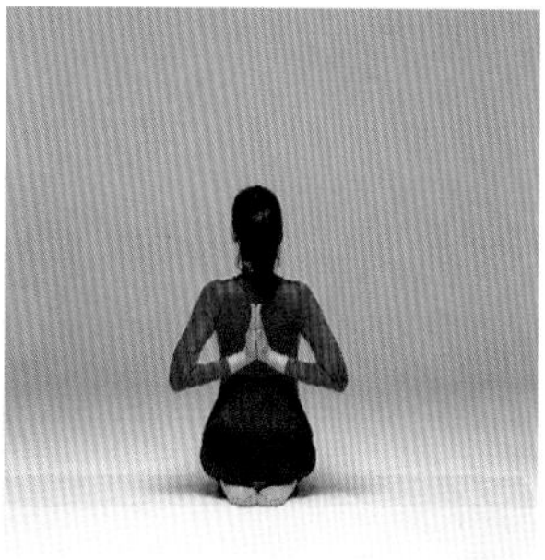

Follow the method given in Unit 6 (page 106).

To Progress

Press the fingers and thumbs evenly against each other. Press the wrists together.

गोमुखासन *Gomukhāsana*

Cow-Head Pose (a) Arms Only

Holding the arms in different positions greatly increases the mobility of the shoulder girdle, neck, and upper back.

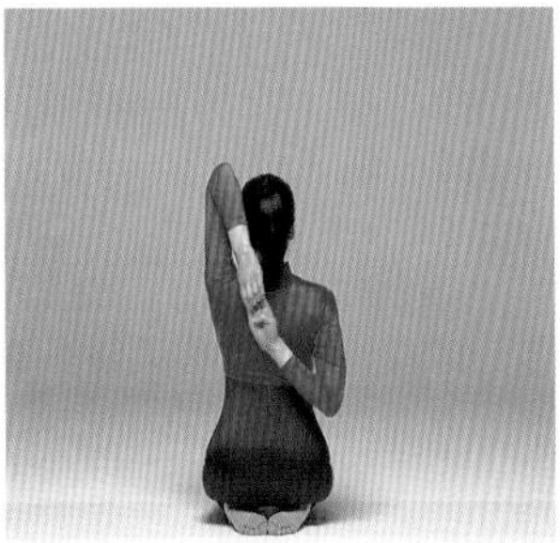

Follow the method given in Unit 6 (page 106).

To Progress

Grip the fingers strongly and pull equally with the right and left hand.

गोमुखासन *Gomukhāsana*

Cow-Head Pose (b) Legs Only

Moving the legs into different positions brings flexibility to the hips and lower back.

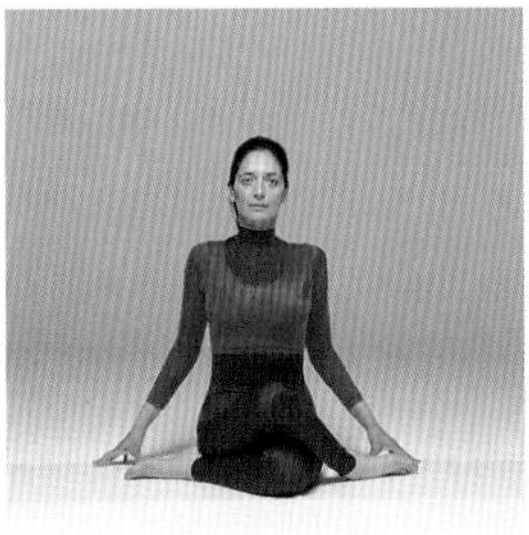

Sit with the legs stretched out in front. Bend the right leg and place the foot beside the left outer thigh. Bend the left leg and place the foot beside the right outer thigh. Place the hands beside the hips, making a cup shape with the fingers. Stretch the trunk up. Breathe evenly.

Stay in the pose for 30 seconds to 1 minute. Repeat on the other side. Bring the legs forward.

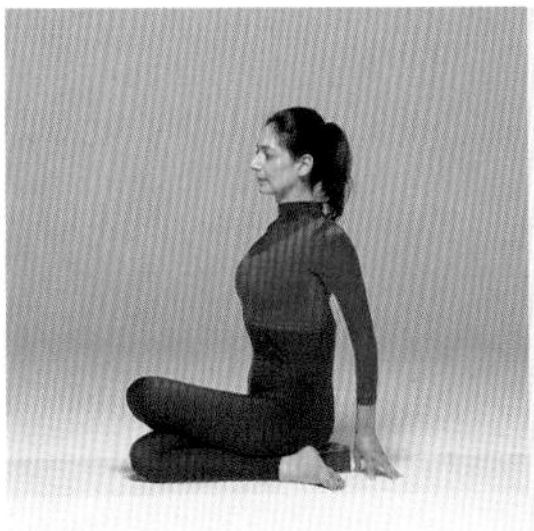

Help

- **Sit on a height, such as a block, bolster or folded blanket.**

To Progress

Open the groin of the top leg so that the knee goes down. Lift the lower back.

सर्वाङ्गासन *Sarvāṅgāsana*

Shoulder Balance

Lightness and lift are the essence of this pose: the body feels as if it is flying upward.

A belt is tied around the upper arms. This stops the elbows from slipping outward and helps the arms support the trunk strongly.

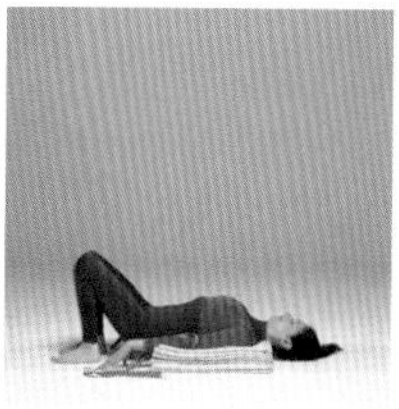

Fold three or four blankets and place them above one another with the folded edges neatly on one side. When folded they should be broader than the shoulders and longer than the upper arms. The blanket support prevents compression of the neck and throat. Take a belt and make a loop the width of the shoulders. Put the belt loosely around the right upper arm just above the elbow. Lie down with the shoulders on the folded edge of the sets of blankets and the head on the floor. Move the shoulders away from the neck and the shoulder blades in. Stretch the arms. Bend the legs, keeping the feet on the floor.

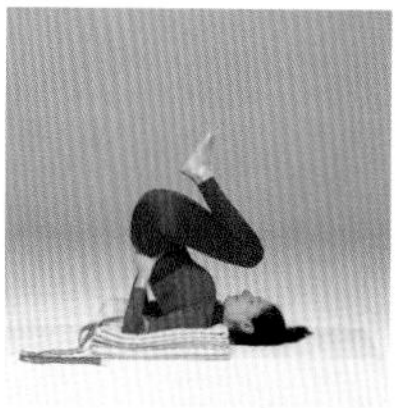

Bend the knees over the abdomen. Lift the hips up and support the back with the hands.

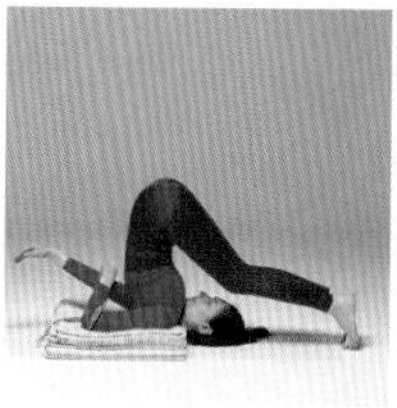

Take the feet over the head to the floor. Slip the loop of the belt over the left upper arm just above the elbow. Move the shoulders away from the neck, and stretch the upper arms back.

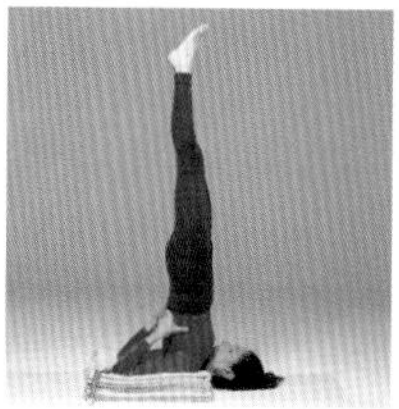

Lift the legs up and straighten them. Adjust the hands on the back, and bring the whole body as much as possible towards the vertical.

Stay in the pose for 1 to 5 minutes. Bend the legs, remove the belt, exhale, and slide gently down.

To Progress

Use the hands strongly to lift the upper trunk. Use the thumbs to lift the sides of the trunk. Move the sacrum (lower back) forward and tighten the buttocks. Keep the knees tight and stretch the backs of the legs.

Cautions

See Unit 3 (page 62).

हलासन *Halāsana*

Plow Pose

While the legs stretch, the back is soothed by being inverted and the mind is peaceful.

Cautions

See Unit 3 (page 62).

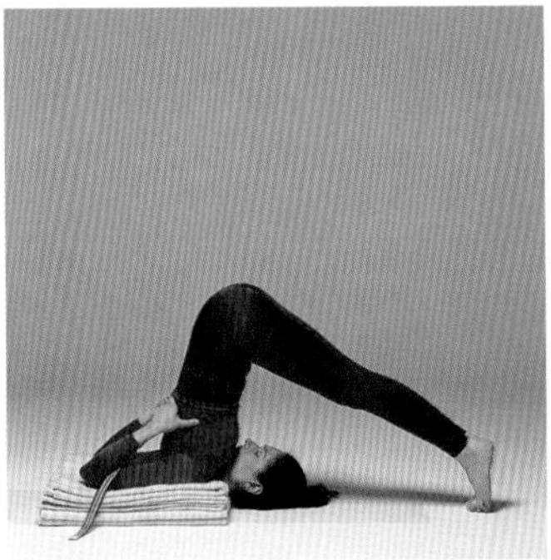

Do *Sarvāṅgāsana* (see page 179). Bend the legs and take the feet to the floor. Straighten the knees and lift the hips and trunk. Breathe evenly.

Stay in the pose for 30 seconds to 1 minute. Bend the legs, remove the belt, and gently slide down.

To Progress

Use the hands strongly to lift the upper trunk and move the sternum (breastbone) forward. Keep the knees tight and stretch the backs of the legs. Lift the shins, knees, thighs, and hips.

शवासन *Śavāsana*

Corpse Pose

When tension is deep-seated, pervading the whole body, it is eased by relaxing from the extremities inward.

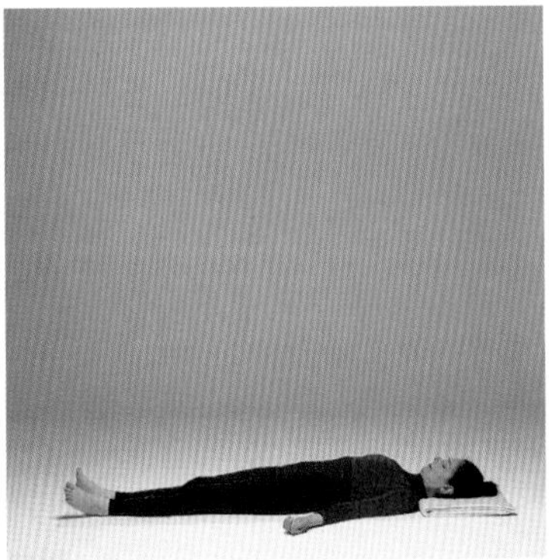

Follow the method given in Unit 1 (page 26).

To Progress

Relax the legs along their whole length. Let the thighs, knees, and lower legs roll out farther. Let the feet drop farther to the sides, and relax the arches. Similarly relax the arms along their whole length. Relax the palms. Relax the abdomen.

The constitution of the mind

KEY CONCEPT

Modes of the mind The entire process of knowledge and its preservation is an act of the mind. In Yoga philosophy the mental modes of correct knowledge and error are separate. The moment the process of knowledge stops, the mind is no longer active but is reduced to a potential form. This is the mode of deep sleep. This implies that the other states of consciousness, namely waking and dreaming, are the major realm of the mind. The mental mode of memory includes dreaming, as this reflects the experiences of the waking state, albeit in a distorted form. The final mode is conceptualization, the unique factual or fictional knowledge based on language.

We now know the Yoga view that (a) life is full of suffering, (b) the mistaken identification of the soul with the mind is the cause of suffering, and (c) the knowledge that the soul is distinct from the mind is the means to end this suffering—in other words, to be liberated. To attain liberation, implying disjunction from the mind, it is necessary to know thoroughly what the mind is and how it works. This alone equips us to control the mind and progressively sever all ties with it, thus paving the way to its elimination in the sense of its regression into its cause, Primordial Matter. Mind control is Yoga; severance from the mind is liberation.

The Modes of the Mind

The most obvious role of the mind is as coordinator of information received by the sense organs. The mind is, as it were, colored by this information. The study of the mind does not end here. A thorough analysis leads Patañjali to view it as having the following five modes: (1) valid cognition or knowledge, (2) erroneous cognition or knowledge, (3) conceptualization, (4) deep sleep, and (5) memory. The states of valid cognition and erroneous cognition relate to the waking condition. The mode of dream is included in memory.

According to Yoga, there are three means of valid cognition: perception, inference, and authority.

1(a). Perception is the means by which cognition is obtained, broadly, of the *special* characteristics of external objects, which possess both general and special characteristics. We identify a cow as a cow by the characteristics it shares with other cows; we distinguish it from other cows by its special characteristics, such as its color, size, and so on. The characteristics it shares with other cows become special when it comes to distinguishing the cow from a horse.

(b). Inference is the means by which cognition is obtained, broadly, of the *general* characteristics of objects; this is on the basis of characteristics that are present in similar objects and absent in dissimilar ones. Footprints on mud lead us to deduce what animal has visited the farm; they do not tell us about its special characteristics, such as color and age.

(c). Authority is the knowledge obtained through the words of a trustworthy person (or a similar source such as a text) who obtains it by perception or inference.

2. Erroneous cognition can be briefly described as follows: When a rope in a poor light is mistaken for a snake, it is erroneous knowledge—the cognition of an object as something it is not.

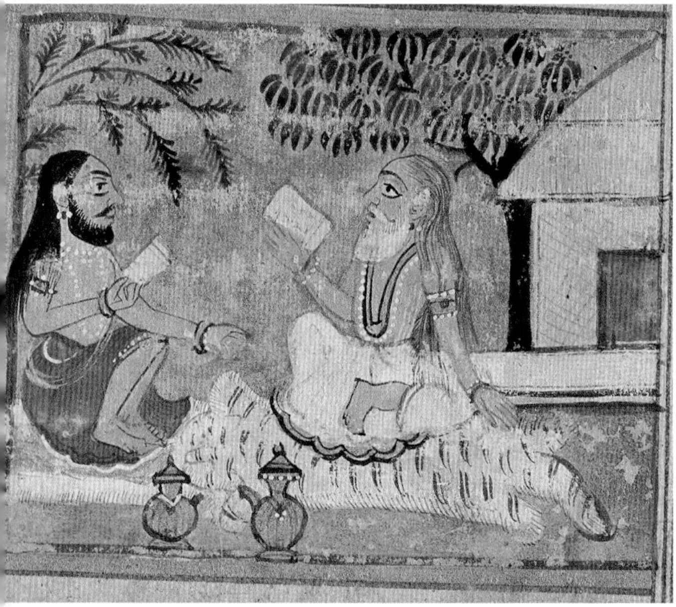

A sage teaching a disciple, from a collection of ancient illustrated manuscripts held at the Bhandarkar Research Institute in Pune, India.

3. Cognition through conceptualization. Words in a language create mental images or concepts that may or may not correspond to reality. Take, for example, the expression "Consciousness is the nature of the soul." In actual fact, the soul itself is consciousness; and yet the statement implies a distinction between the soul and consciousness by giving them a relationship of subject and predicate. "The tip of the tongue" is another instance; the tip is part of the tongue. The part as distinct from the whole is a construct of imagination and a matter of convenience, not of fact. Words are symbols of realities. Language works on the basis of an imagined equation of the symbols and the symbolized. As an ancient Indian philosopher of language observes, language is the means of seeking reality on the basis of unreality.

4. Deep sleep is the mode in which the daytime activities of the body and the sense organs cease temporarily, in contrast to the waking state, in which they are active. Deep sleep gives us an experience similar to that of liberation and is, hence, akin to meditation and liberation. The distinction between these may be briefly noted as follows:

Liberation: the experience of the soul is total and permanent.

Deep meditation in its advanced stage: the experience of the soul is total, controlled, and impermanent.

Deep sleep: the experience of the soul is total but uncontrolled and impermanent.

5. Memory is the recall of mental

imprints (*saṃskāras*) of experiences. The memory of experience in deep sleep proves that sleep is not the absence of experience. It is a positive state.

All the five modes of the mind, including memory, are capable of creating memories as they leave imprints of themselves on the mind. These imprints are mental images of experiences that lie dormant in the deep layers of the psyche, unless and until they are revived by stimulating conditions. The content of memory can be equal to or less than the experience that causes it.

Instincts

Instincts are deep-seated memory records carried through many incarnations in different life forms; they are aroused in appropriate situations in a relevant life form. For example, a cat pounces on a mouse by instinct. The instinct inherited from an earlier life as a cat remains latent and manifests itself only when the soul is reborn as a cat. It is like the image on a photographic plate, which remains invisible until it is developed with the help of appropriate chemicals.

The Limitation of Valid Cognition

Control of the mind implies the suspension of all its states. In other words, the mind as an instrument for knowing the world is suspended during meditation. Further, what is valid cognition for worldly dealings is not relevant to the cognition of the highest Realities through Yoga. Even in practical life, the human body is viewed differently by a medical man than by a layman. It is the outlook of the viewer that changes the perspective. When the mind is thus suspended in meditation, the soul emerges in its real nature—that is, pure consciousness. During active states of the mind, the soul becomes erroneously identified with it and ascribes the experiences of the mind to itself. In experiencing the emotions of Hamlet while reading or watching the play, we temporarily identify ourselves with Hamlet. This is aesthetic identification, a deliberate act of will that has a limited duration. In the experience of the "play" called life, the identification of the soul (the spectator) with the mind (Hamlet) is not a deliberate act of will; hence it is unlimited in duration.

The Soul Enables the Mind

What is the role of the soul in the operations of the mind analyzed above? It is true that the soul does not take an active part in these operations; but its mere presence enables the mind to act. This phenomenon is conventionally explained on the analogy of a magnet, which activates iron filings although it is itself inactive. This is true of many an energy source. The sun's mere presence in the sky enables us to work, even to live, on the earth. Air and fire are additional instances. All basic supports are of this nature. The point that is lacking in these analogies is the element of suffering in the soul. This is the limitation of analogies: they illustrate, but do not give exact parallels.

Mind and Soul Reflect Each Other

The mind appears to be sentient because it reflects the sentient soul; the soul reflects the mind in that it considers pleasures and pains of the latter (mind) as if they relate to it (soul). Like a crystal or a mirror, each shows as its own the attributes that belong in fact to the reflected object. The soul is able to reflect the mind with its attributes because of its nature as pure consciousness (cognition, knowledge), which displays as its own the character of whatever object is close to it. The mind is able to reflect the soul because it consists primarily of the quality of illumination (*sattva*; see Unit 7). In other words, the cause of the soul's suffering is rooted in the ability of both, the mind and the soul, to show as their own what actually belongs to the other.

The Way to Transcend the Mind

Yoga teaches that the states of mind can be suspended by means of persistence and detachment. Detachment starts from indifference to worldly pleasures and matures into total indifference to the entire domain of nature. Following this logic to the limit, Patañjali asserts that, in the final analysis, the domain of nature or the material world includes the knowledge that discriminates between the soul and mind, as all knowledge belongs to the mind. Therefore transcendence of knowledge implies liberation of the soul.

In Brief

The soul in this life is overlaid by pleasures and pains and moves in suffering,
Imagining that it is identical with the mind, which is influenced by sense organs and their objects.

Living beings in this world have five modes of mind:
Valid knowledge, false knowledge, conceptualization, deep sleep, and memory.

All these, surviving as imprints, generate memory
When awakened at the right time, even though interrupted by other lives.

The mind engages in its affairs merely by the presence of the soul,
But the soul considers its activity as its own.

The mind is inoperative in deep sleep, meditation, and liberation of the soul.
In the first two it re-emerges; liberation is deemed to be permanent.

For a wider perspective...

Means of Knowledge

There are three major means of valid knowledge accepted by **Patañjali**: perception, inference, and authority. However, other schools of philosophy accept additional means of knowledge, depending on their emphasis on or ignoring minute distinctions in the process of knowledge. Accordingly, knowledge by comparison (ice is like glass), circumstantial conclusion (Mr. X is fat, but never eats during the day—therefore he must be eating at night), and knowledge of absence (there is no one on the street, since no one is seen) are three more means. With slight variations, the number reaches twelve.

How We Understand Language

Words or a series of audible sounds, conventionally related to meanings, create mental images, which, when integrated, create knowledge in the mind of the listener. It is similar for the process of reading. The images thus formed may or may not correspond to actual objects or facts. Linguistic theorists in the Sanskrit tradition conceive a permanent mental image of a word to account for the receiving of knowledge from the impermanent serial sounds of words. The gist of the theory is that as a word is uttered, the sounds create mental impressions. When the last sound is uttered, the permanent image is aroused, yielding the meaning in a flash.

Unit 11

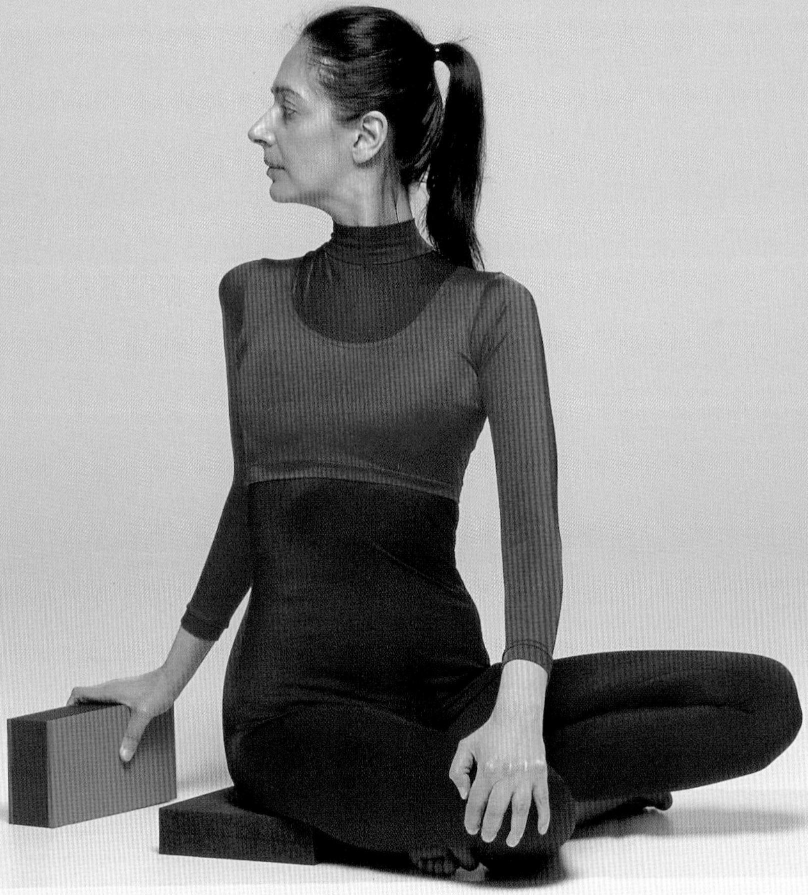

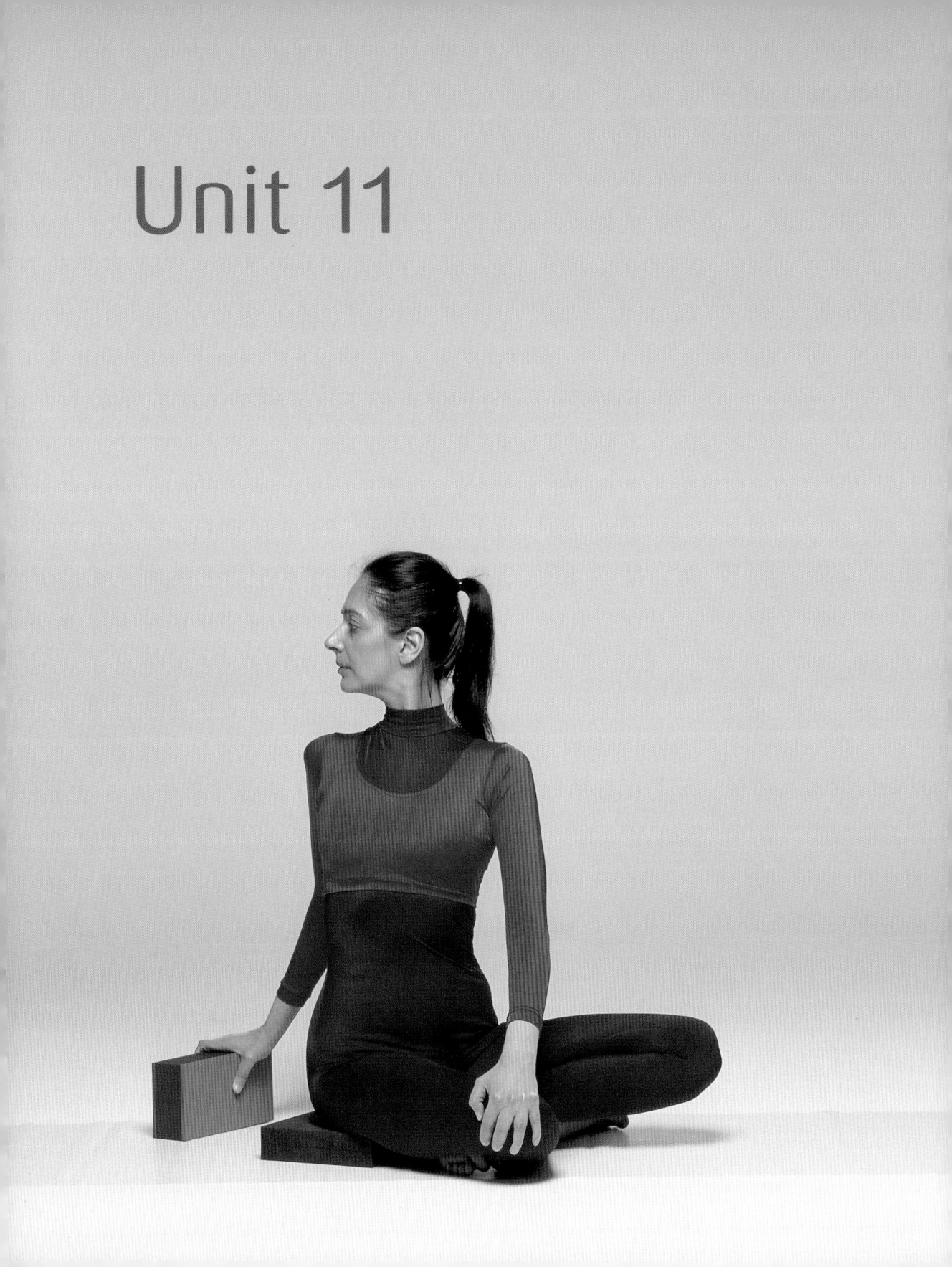

Kṛṣṇa navigates the Pāndava brothers to success—from the illustrated *Bhagavad-Gītā.*

Yoga in life

SUCCESS

Sometimes Wisdom for the
way ahead
Needs a lamp to see by
And a stick to lean on
To help it find its path,
Lest it falter, not through fear,
But from a taxed, taxed dry
endurance,
At the stark straitness of the pass.

Let it remember then
A mother's loving arms and care
And endlessly supporting strength.

Success in any endeavor may be due to many factors, luck and talent among them, but surely one of the most important is perseverance in the face of obstacles.

Yoga philosophy recognizes that mental and physical discipline are necessary for succeeding, particularly persistence in practice and dispassion.[1] The former refers to making repeated, vigorous efforts toward the goal. In this way, over time, steadiness is achieved.[2]

"Dispassion" refers to being unmoved by the desire to gain benefits.[3] A detached stand allows us to continue making efforts without being disheartened, and prevents pride, through which all can be lost. Such an attitude makes us master of our exertions rather than the victim of circumstance.

These disciplines are essential for achieving the aim of Yoga, control of the mind, if success is to be sustained and not ephemeral.

---

[1] *Yoga Sūtra 1.12*

[2] *Yoga Sūtra, and Commentary 1.13—14*

[3] *Yoga Sūtra, and Commentary 1.15*

Spinal rotation

Throughout nature, plants and animals are gifted with the ability to turn in different directions. The human being is no exception. Axial rotation is designed into the spine, and its gift is versatility of movement.

Certain Yoga postures exploit this ability to rotate, using it both to restore and to increase the spine's robustness and flexibility. Revolving movements are always done after stretching, so that space is created between the vertebrae, allowing room for the turn.

The different areas of the back—sacral, lumbar, thoracic, and cervical—have different degrees of lateral movement. The tendency is for the stiffer parts, sacrum and thorax, to become immobile and for the supple parts to do all the moving. This pattern of underuse and overuse causes strain, which can culminate in injury.

Twisting poses help to rebalance the uneven kinetic energy of the spine. This is because they involve the whole length of the spine from tailbone to neck. The turning action starts at the hips and proceeds upward like a spiral.

At the same time, the sacrum, thoracic spine, back ribs, and shoulder blades are made concave. These areas usually collapse outward and downward, giving rise to a hunched upper back and tilted lower back, shapes that characteristically accompany back pain. Thus the poses involving spinal rotation are supremely effective in revitalizing the back and relieving pain.

They also stimulate the digestive system by massaging the intestines.

Revolving the spine is done in both standing and sitting poses. The very simplest use a chair support, and for this reason they can be attempted even when the back is aching.

Standing poses performed in series give the training in stretching that is a prerequisite to revolving the spine. Revolved Triangle Pose (*Parivṛtta-Trikoṇāsana*) then builds on this preparation and makes the body turn 180 degrees over the legs, so that it faces literally back to front.

For seated twists, a number of leg positions can be assumed. Each gives a different action by facilitating access to a different region of the trunk. For example, when sitting cross-legged, it is easier to turn the hips and lower back than when kneeling; but when kneeling, it is easier to rotate the rib cage. In Bharadvaja's Pose (*Bharadvājāsana*) the shoulders and shoulder blades can be turned strongly.

Sometimes after Shoulder-Balance (*Sarvāṅgāsana*), the back feels strained. This strain is removed by the supine Abdomen-Revolving Pose (*Jaṭhara-Parivartanāsana*). Instead of the back twisting in relation to the stationary legs, as in standing and sitting poses, the legs are turned against the back, which is stable on the floor. This pose is also effective in alleviating backache from other causes.

भरद्वाजासन *Bharadvājāsana*

Bharadvaja's Pose

The name of this pose commemorates one of the seven great seers of Indian legend who passed on the timeless knowledge of the *Vedas*.

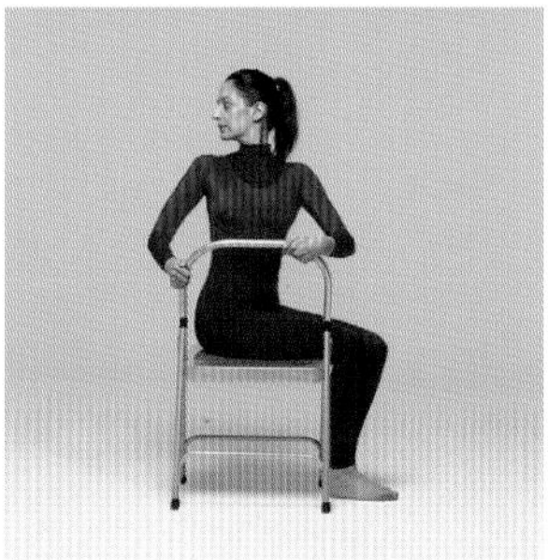

Sit sideways on a chair, with the right side toward the back of the chair. Keep the feet together. Stretch the trunk up and take the shoulders back.

Exhale, turn to the right, and hold the back of the chair. Turn the head and neck to the right. Breathe evenly.

Stay in the pose for 30 seconds to 1 minute. Release the hands and come to the center. Repeat on the other side.

To Progress

Keep the trunk upright, so that the spine revolves on its axis. Turn the hips, waist, rib cage, and shoulders. Move the thoracic spine and shoulder blades in. Lift the front of the body.

मरीच्यासन १ *Marīchyāsana 1*

Marici's Pose 1

This pose commemorates another of the seven great seers who bequeathed the sacred lore enshrined in the *Vedas*.

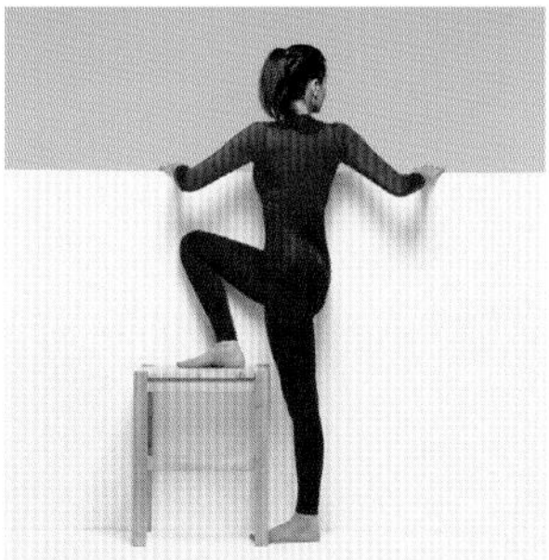

Place a high stool or chair against a wall or ledge. Stand in *Tāḍāsana* (see Unit 1, page 19) with the right side against the wall, facing the stool and close to it. Place the right foot on the stool, with the hip touching the wall. Exhale, turn the trunk toward the wall, and hold the ledge (or place the hands on the wall). Stretch the left leg up and keep it vertical. If necessary, step closer to the stool.

Stay in the pose for 30 seconds to 1 minute. Come to the center and bring the leg down. Repeat on the other side.

To Progress

Press the left hip toward the wall and the left thigh back. Keep the trunk upright, so that the spine revolves on its axis. Turn the hips, waist, rib cage, and shoulders. Move the thoracic spine and shoulder blades in. Lift the front of the body.

उत्थित-हस्त-पादाङ्गुष्ठासन *Utthita-Hasta-Padāṅguṣṭhāsana*

Upright Hand-to-Big-Toe Pose 3

Nothing relieves an aching back as fast as Yoga "twists."

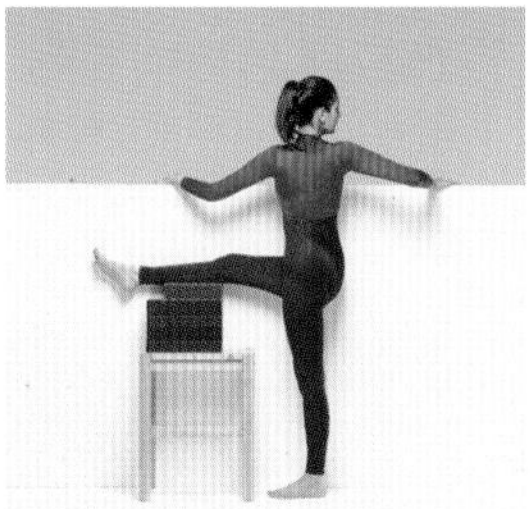

Place a high stool or chair against a wall or ledge, and place blocks on top to hip-height. Stand in *Tāḍāsana* (see Unit 1, page 19) with the right side against the wall, facing the stool and close to it. Place the right calf on the stool, with the hip touching the wall. Exhale, turn the trunk toward the wall, and hold the ledge (or place the hands on the wall). Stretch the left leg up and keep it vertical. If necessary, step closer to the stool.

Stay in the pose for 30 seconds to 1 minute. Come to the center and bring the leg down. Repeat on the other side.

To Progress

Press the left hip toward the wall and the left thigh back. Keep the trunk upright, so that the spine revolves on its axis. Turn the hips, waist, rib cage, and shoulders. Move the thoracic spine and shoulder blades in. Lift the front of the body.

त्रिकोणासन *Trikoṇāsana*

Triangle Pose

As postures are repeated, they imprint the physical memory necessary for the body to internalize their shape; ultimately physical and mental involvement should coincide.

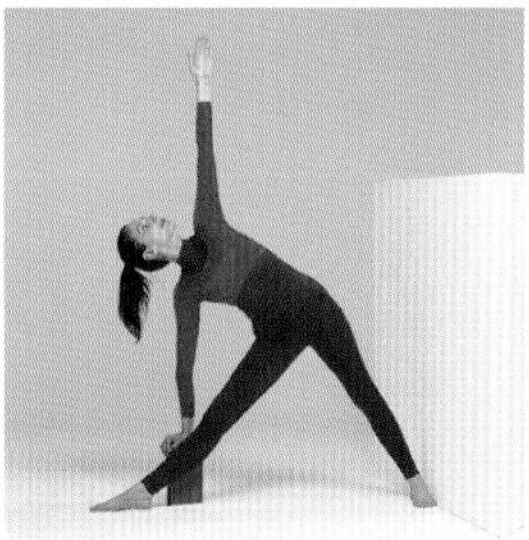

Follow the method given in Unit 7 (page 120).

To Progress

Uniformly revolve the whole of each leg outward, including thigh, knee, and lower leg. Uniformly revolve the whole trunk, both pelvis and rib cage. The support of the wall for the back foot and the brick for the hand aid these rotations. Move the thoracic spine in to turn the neck and head.

पार्श्वकोणासन *Pārśvakoṇāsana*

Side Angle Pose

Drawing strength from the wall and brick supports, body parts move forward, press back, stretch, or turn to bring alignment with the vertical plane.

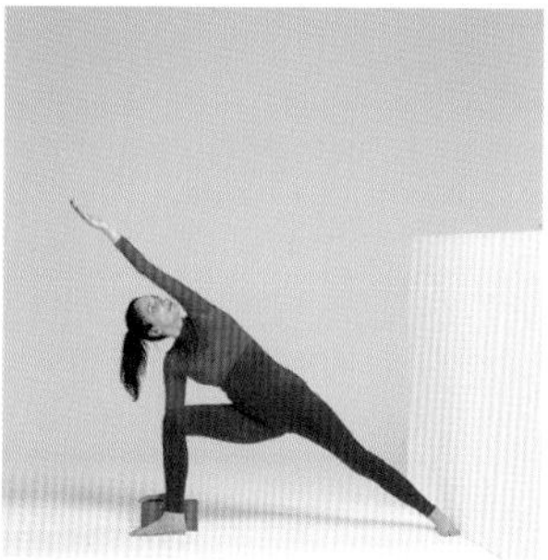

Follow the method given in Unit 7 (page 121).

To Progress

Uniformly revolve the whole of the left leg outward, including thigh, knee, and lower leg. Maintain the outward turn of the right thigh while bending it. Uniformly revolve the whole trunk, both pelvis and rib cage. Rotate the left arm from the shoulder, so that the palm faces down. Move the thoracic spine in to turn the neck and head.

वीरभद्रासन १ *Virabhadrāsana 1*

Warrior Pose 1

The wall support gives strength to the turn of the hips essential for this pose.

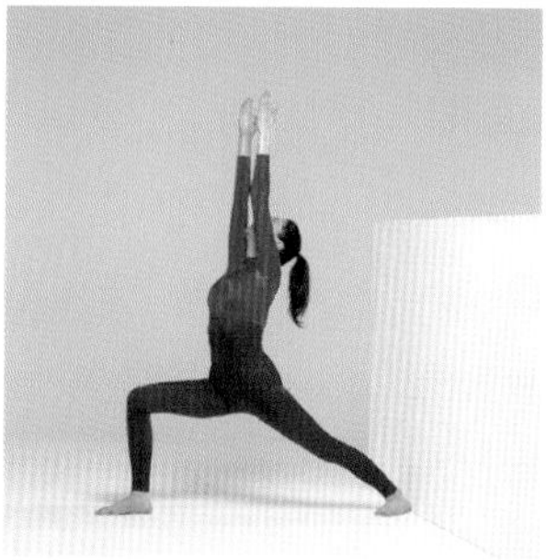

Follow the method given in Unit 7 (page 122).

To Progress

Uniformly revolve the whole of the left leg inward, including thigh, knee, and shank. Maintain the outward turn of the right thigh while bending it. Move the left buttock away from the right and turn the hips more. Uniformly turn the pelvis and rib cage. Rotate the outer arms inward and stretch them up from the shoulders. Press the thoracic spine in when taking the head back.

Lift the rib cage away from the waist.

उत्तानासन *Uttānāsana*

Intense Stretch

When the legs are slanting—a position made possible by resting against the wall—the trunk releases farther downward, and strain from exertion is speedily relieved.

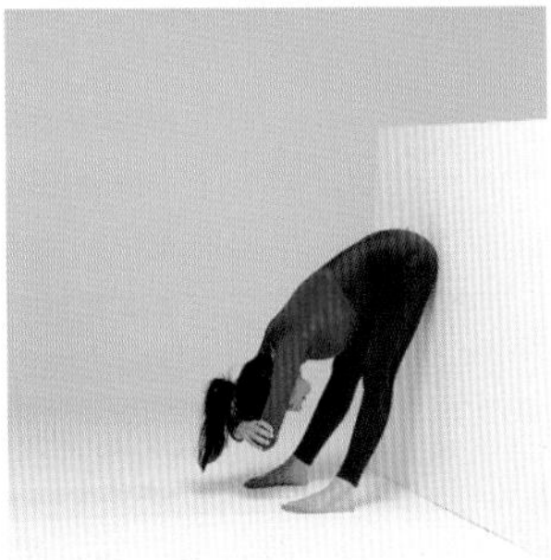

Stand in *Tāḍāsana* (see Unit 1, page 19) 1–1½ feet (30–45cm) away from a wall. Take the feet hip-width apart. Placing the fingertips on the wall for support, lean back and rest the buttocks against it. Manually move the flesh of the buttocks upward so that the bones are against the wall. Bend forward from the hips, and catch the elbows. Breathe evenly and relax.

Help

- **If the back is stiff, place the feet wider or do *Ardha-Uttānāsana* (Unit 2, page 41).**

To Progress

Keep the knees tight and stretch the whole of the legs upwards from the shins. Pull the trunk down from the shoulders, with the help of the arms. Move the base of the skull away from the neck to relax the head.

वीरभद्रासन २ *Virabhadrāsana 2*

Warrior Pose 2

Though this pose is popularly known as the Warrior, it is in fact named after a manifestation of the Indian god, Śiva, the fearsome embodiment of his wrath.

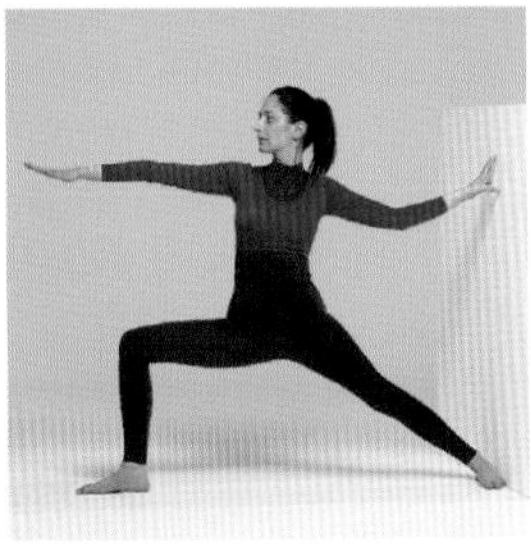

Follow the method given in Unit 7 (page 124).

To Progress

Uniformly revolve the whole of the left leg outward, including thigh, knee, and shank. Maintain the outward turn of the right thigh while bending it. Turn the trunk slightly from right to left so that it remains facing forward. Move the thoracic spine in to turn the neck and head.

परिवृत्त-त्रिकोणासन *Parivṛtta-Trikoṇāsana*

Revolved Triangle Pose

The trunk turns 180 degrees to fold backward over the legs, both necessitating and developing a powerful rotation of the spine.

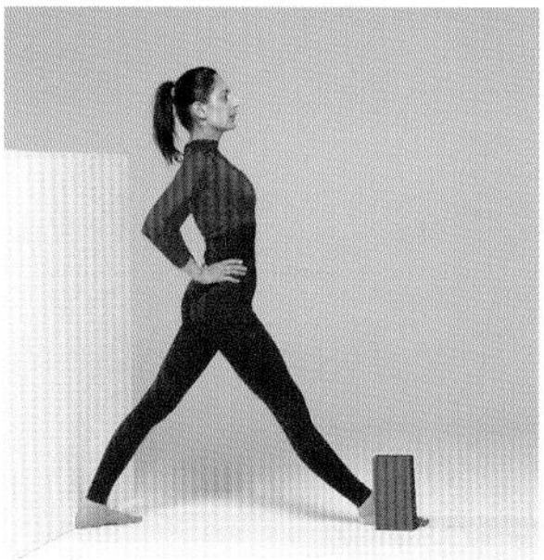

Stand in *Tāḍāsana* (see Unit 1, page 19) about 2 feet away from a wall, with the left side facing the wall. Take the left foot to the wall, placing the outer edge of the foot against it. Spread the legs $3\frac{1}{2}$–4 feet apart. Turn the right foot 90 degrees out and revolve the leg outward. Place a brick upright beside the outer edge of the right foot. Turn the left foot deep in (60 degrees), so that only the heel is against the wall. Revolve the left leg in at the same time. Align the center of the right heel with the center of the left arch. Place the hands on the hips, and turn the trunk to the right. Tighten the kneecaps and pull up the thigh muscles.

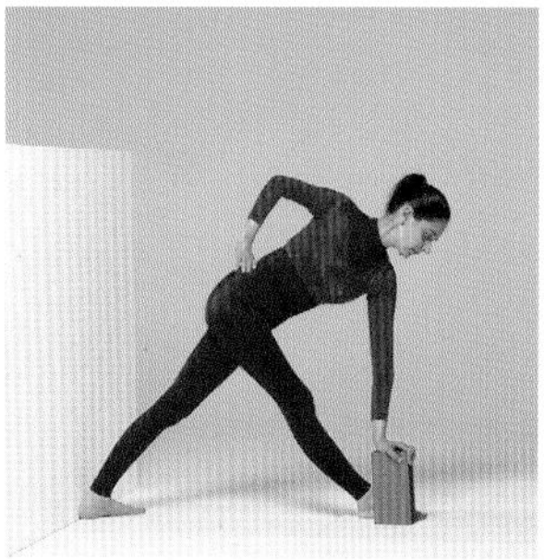

Bend forward from the hips, simultaneously turning the trunk to the right; place the left hand on the brick. Straighten the left arm. Lengthen the front of the body and take the right shoulder back.

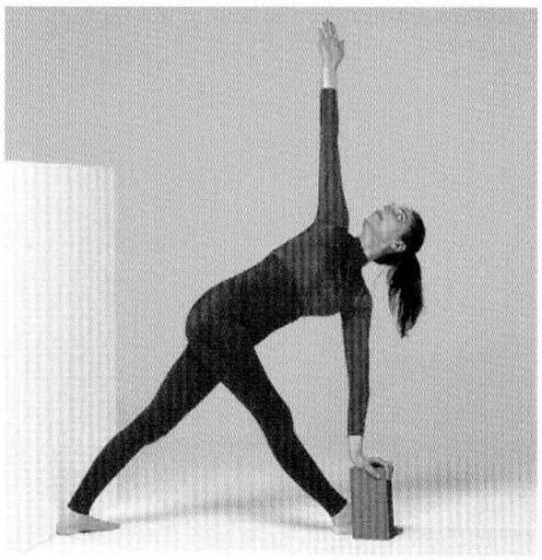

Raise the right arm vertically up, palm facing forward. Revolve the trunk farther. Turn the neck and head and look up. Breathe evenly.

Stay in the pose for 20 to 30 seconds. Inhale and come up. Repeat on the other side.

To Progress

Turn the hips, waist, ribcage and shoulders. Move the thoracic spine and shoulder blades in. Lift and expand the chest.

Help

- **If balancing and turning the trunk are difficult, place the brick on the inner edge of the right foot.**

अधो-मुख-वीरासन *Adho-Mukha-Vīrāsana*

Hero Pose, Head Down

After stretching the legs strongly, it is a relief to bend them; the actions, though contrasting, aid understanding of each other.

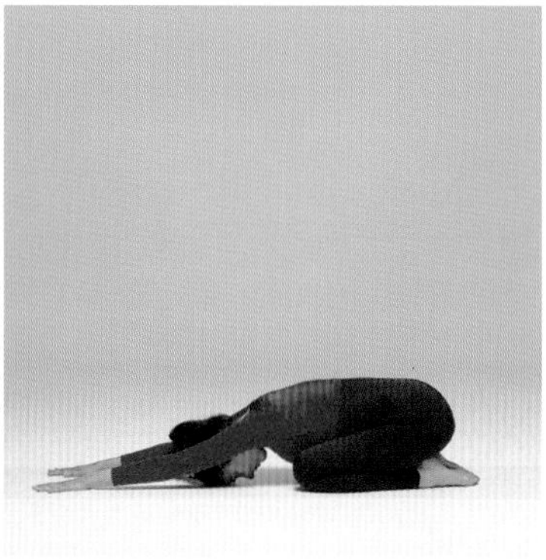

Follow the method given in Unit 2 (page 42).

To Progress

With the fingers, gently press in the flesh at the back of the knees, to tuck it into the joint. Whereas in stretching the backs of the knees project backward, in flexing they go deep in, so that the joint can fold comfortably. Bend evenly at the inner and outer knees.

पार्श्वोत्तानासन *Pārśvottānāsana*

Sideways Intense Stretch

The back stretches in tandem with the limbs; the more the arms and legs stretch, the better the back extends.

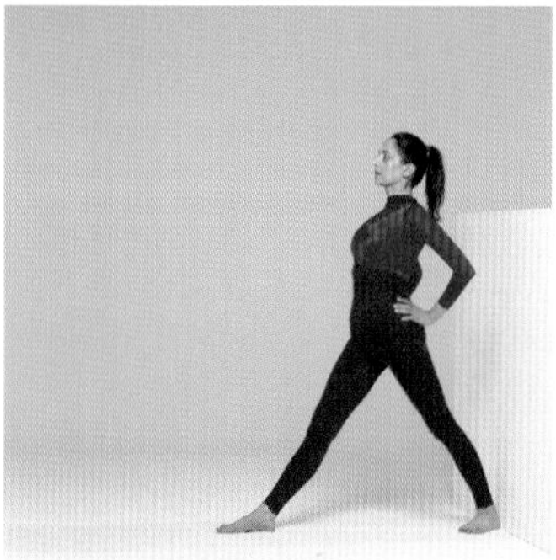

Stand in *Tāḍāsana* (see Unit 1, page 19) about 2 feet away from a wall, with the left side facing the wall. Take the left foot to the wall, placing the outer edge of the foot against it. Spread the legs 3½–4 feet apart. Turn the right foot 90 degrees out, and revolve the leg outward. Turn the left foot deep in (60 degrees), so that only the heel is against the wall. Revolve the left leg in at the same time. Align the center of the right heel with the center of the left arch. Place the hands on the hips and turn the trunk to the right. Tighten the kneecaps and pull up the thigh muscles.

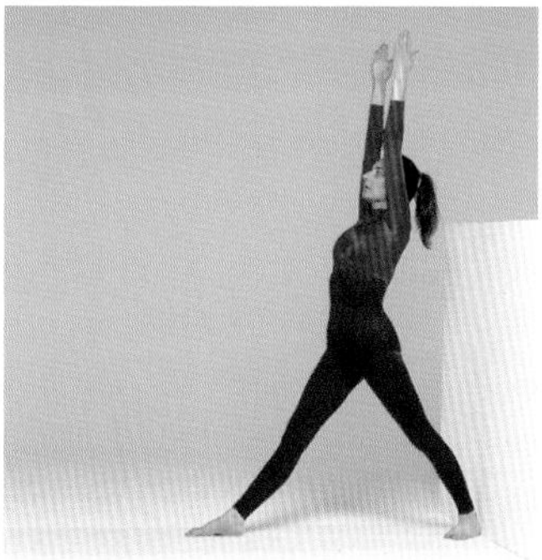

Inhale and raise the arms over the head, palms facing each other. Tighten the elbows and stretch the arms and trunk up.

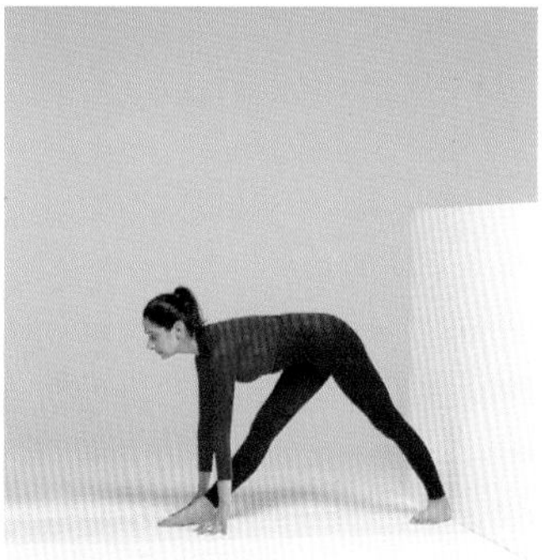

Bend forward from the hips and place the fingertips on the floor. Lengthen the front of the body and press the sacrum (lower back) and thoracic spine down to make them concave. Lift the head.

Help

- **If the hands do not reach the floor, place them on bricks.**

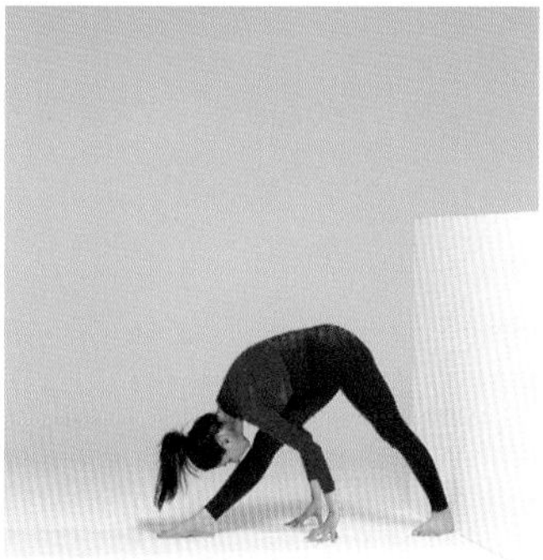

Bend the elbows, move the hands back, and take the trunk and head toward the right leg. Breathe evenly.

Stay in the pose for 20 to 30 seconds. Inhale and come up. Repeat on the other side.

If the legs are strained after this series of standing poses, kneel and bend forward in *Adho-Mukha-Vīrāsana* (see Unit 2, page 42).

To Progress

Draw the legs strongly up and make the hips level. Take the trunk toward the right leg, the right leg towards the left leg, and the left leg toward the wall.

परिवृत्त-सुखासन *Parivṛtta-Sukhāsana*

Comfortable Pose Twist

Simple yet effective, this spinal twist quickly relieves an aching back.

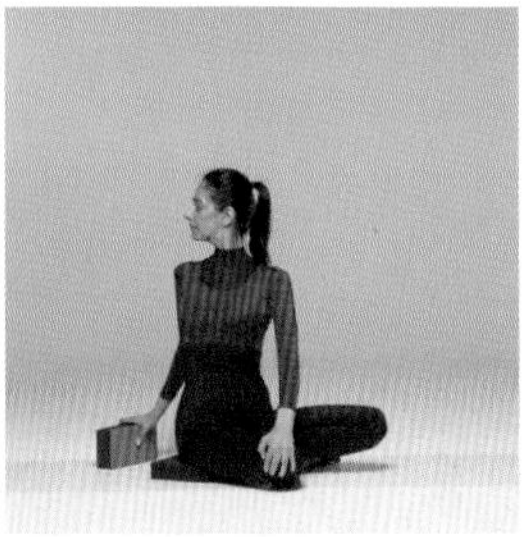

Sit on one or two folded blankets or a block and cross the legs simply. Place a brick or other support behind the back. Lift the lower back and stretch the trunk up. Take the shoulders back. Exhale and turn the trunk to the right, placing the left hand on the right knee and the right hand on the brick. Turn the neck and head to the right. Breathe evenly.

Stay in the pose for 20 to 30 seconds. Come to the center. Repeat on the other side. Then cross the legs the other way, and repeat on both sides.

To Progress

Turn the hips, waist, rib cage, and shoulders in succession. Move the back ribs and shoulder blades in. Take the shoulders back and down, and lift the chest.

Help

- **If the back or hips are stiff, sit on a higher support.**

परिवृत्त-वीरासन *Parivṛtta-Vīrāsana*

Hero Pose Twist

Different leg positions for the base alter the accent of the spinal twist; here the lower back moves relatively freely.

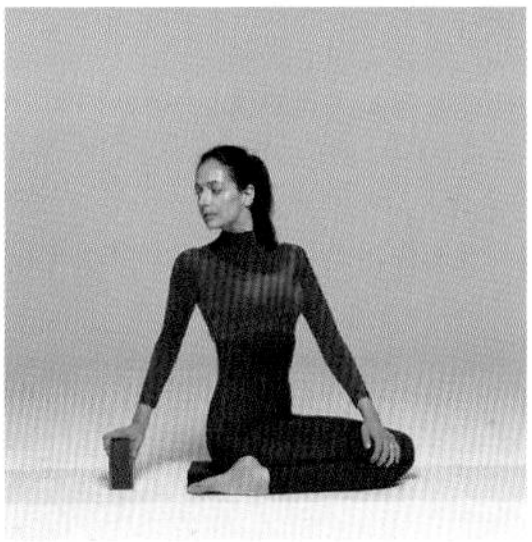

Sit between the legs in *Vīrāsana* (see Unit 6, page 107) with a support under the buttocks. Place a brick behind the back. Lift the lower back and stretch the trunk up. Take the shoulders back. Exhale and turn the trunk to the right, placing the left hand on the right knee and the right hand on the brick. Turn the neck and head to the right. Breathe evenly. Stay in the pose for 20 to 30 seconds. Come to the center. Repeat on the other side.

To Progress

Stretch the sides of the trunk upward with the help of the arms.

Help

- **If the back or hips are stiff, sit on a higher support.**

परिवृत्त-दण्डासन *Parivṛtta-Daṇḍāsana*

Staff Pose Twist

Like a spiral, the spinal rotation starts minimally and increases as it proceeds upward.

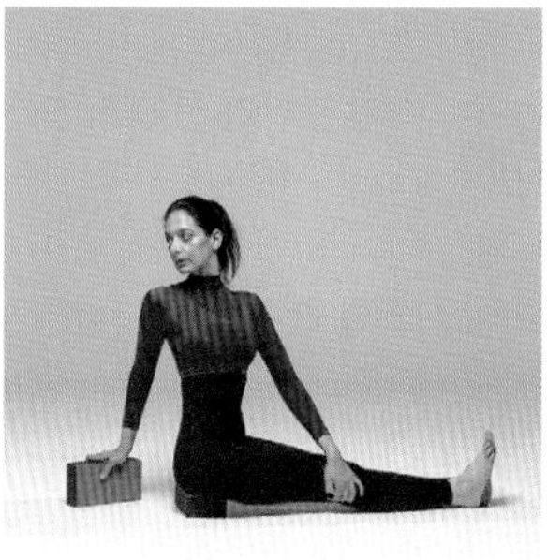

Sit on a support with the legs stretched out in front. Place a brick behind the back. Lift the lower back and stretch the trunk up. Take the shoulders back. Exhale and turn the trunk to the right, placing the left hand on the right knee or outer calf and the right hand on the brick. Turn the neck and head to the right. Breathe evenly.

Stay in the pose for 20 to 30 seconds. Come to the center. Repeat on the other side.

To Progress

Turn the hips, waist, rib cage, and shoulders in succession. Move the back ribs and shoulder blades in. Take the shoulders back and down, and lift the chest.

Help

- **If the back or hips are stiff, sit on a higher support.**

परिवृत्त-बद्धकोणासन *Parivṛtta-Baddha-Koṇāsana*

Bound-Angle Pose Twist

The knees actively press down to stabilize the base of this twist; otherwise the lower back cannot turn.

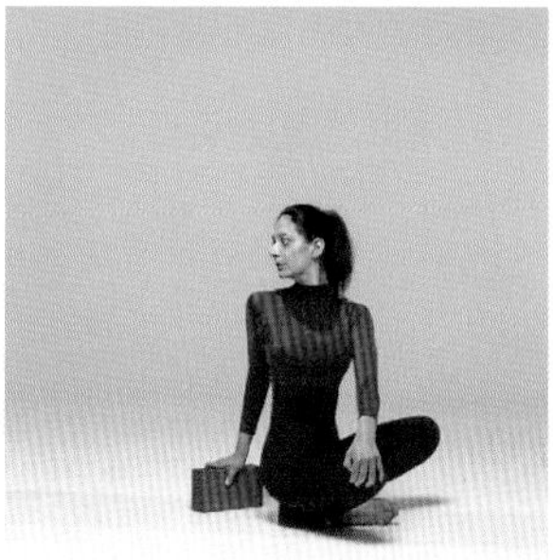

Sit on a support with the legs stretched out in front. Place a brick behind the back. Bend the legs outward into *Baddha-Koṇāsana* (see Unit 9, page 160). Lift the lower back and stretch the trunk up. Take the shoulders back. Exhale and turn the trunk to the right, placing the left hand on the right knee and the right hand on the brick. Turn the neck and head to the right. Breathe evenly. Stay in the pose for 20 to 30 seconds. Come to the center. Repeat on the other side.

To Progress

Stretch the sides of the trunk upward with the help of the arms.

Help

- **If the back or hips are stiff, sit on a higher support.**

भरद्वाजासन १ *Bharadvājāsana 1*

Bharad-vaja's Pose 1

The base of this pose is asymmetrical; this intensifies the effect of the spinal rotation.

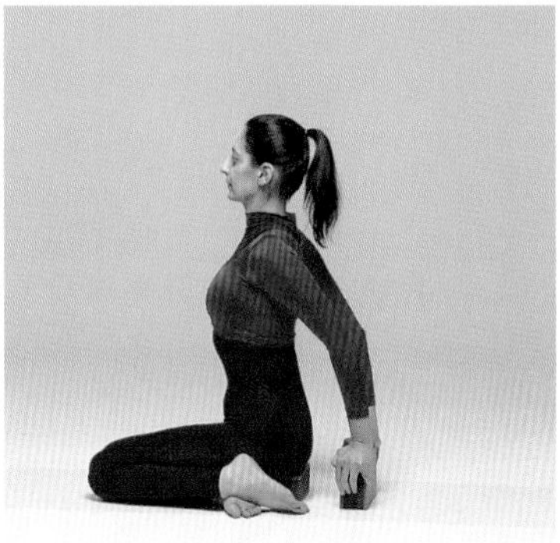

Sit on one or two folded blankets or a block, with the legs stretched out in front. Place a brick behind the back. Bend the legs to the left, and place the feet beside the left hip, with the left foot on the right instep and the left toes pointing back. Move the support so that it is under only the right buttock. Take the hands back and hold the brick. Lift the lower back and stretch the trunk up. Lift the chest and take the shoulders back.

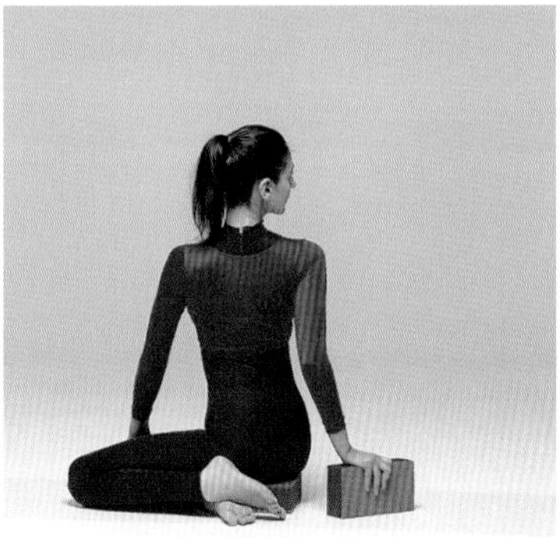

Exhale and turn the trunk to the right, placing the left hand on the right knee or thigh and the right hand on the brick behind the back. Turn the neck and head to the right. Breathe evenly.

Stay in the pose for 20 to 30 seconds. Come to the center. Repeat on the other side.

To Progress

Turn the hips, waist, rib cage, and shoulders in succession. Move the back ribs and shoulder blades in. Take the shoulders back and down, and lift the chest.

Help

- **If the back or hips are stiff, sit on a higher support.**

सर्वाङ्गासन *Sarvāṅgāsana*

Shoulder Balance

Each type of pose and series of poses affects subsequent ones; spinal rotation increases ease and freedom of the neck and back in inverted poses.

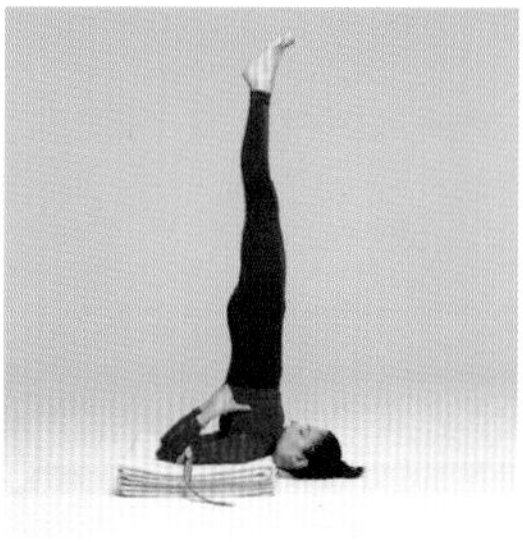

Follow the method given in Unit 10 (page 179).

To Progress

Press the elbows down so that the weight of the body does not fall onto the neck. Lift the upper trunk from the base near the shoulders. Move the coccyx (tailbone) in and tighten the buttocks. Lift the hips. Tighten the kneecaps and extend the backs of the knees. Stretch the legs up, keeping the feet relaxed.

Cautions **See Unit 3, page 62.**

हलासन *Halāsana*

Plow Pose

Some poses have natural links to others; Shoulder Balance does not feel complete without Plow Pose.

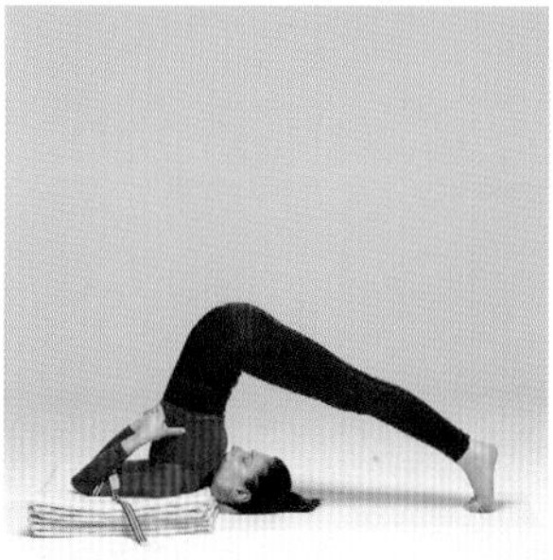

From *Sarvāṅgāsana* (above), bend the legs and take the feet to the floor. Straighten the legs.

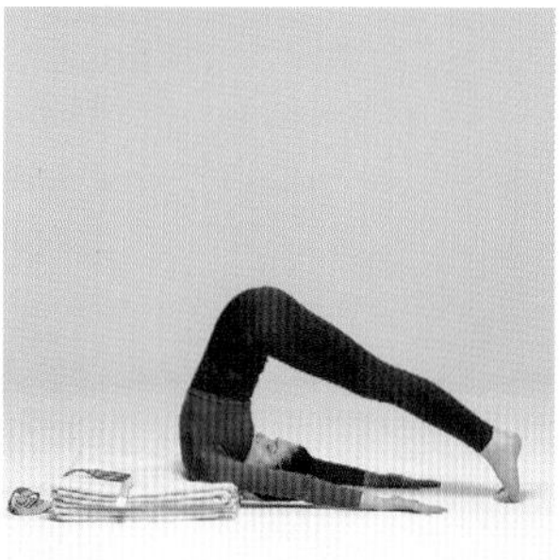

Remove the belt and take the arms over the head. Relax.

Stay in the pose for 2 to 5 minutes. Exhale and slide down.

To Progress

Be on the tips of the toes. Keep the knees firm and press the legs upward. Lift the trunk and hips.

Cautions **See Unit 3, page 62.**

जठर-परिवर्तनासन
Jaṭhara-Parivartanāsana

Abdomen-Revolving Pose

Quick relief from backache is often obtained by doing this pose.

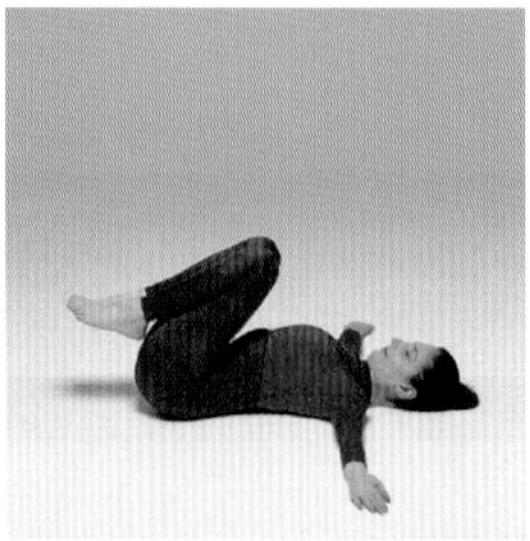

Lie down in a straight line. Take the arms out to the sides in line with the shoulders. Bend the knees over the abdomen.

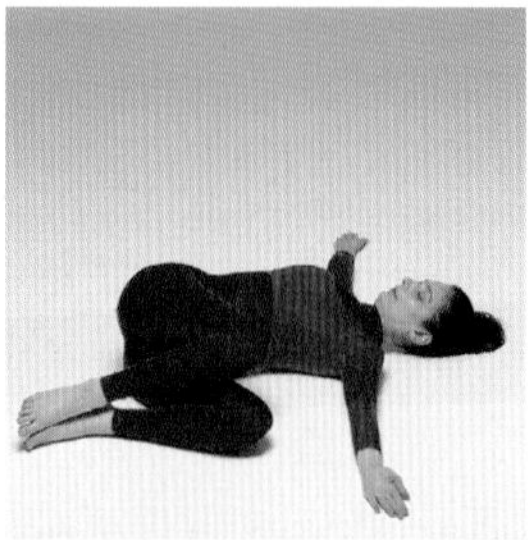

Exhale and take the legs down to the right, toward the arm; at the same time revolve the abdomen to the left and press the left shoulder down.

Place the right arm across the left knee. Press it down to intensify the rotation. Breathe evenly.

Stay in the pose for 20 to 30 seconds. Come to the center. Repeat on the other side.

To Progress

Keep the upper trunk flat on the floor, pressing both shoulder blades in and lifting the chest. Do not tilt the trunk.

शवासन *Śavāsana*

Corpse Pose

After much rotation the spine decompresses and relaxes well; this soothes the nerves.

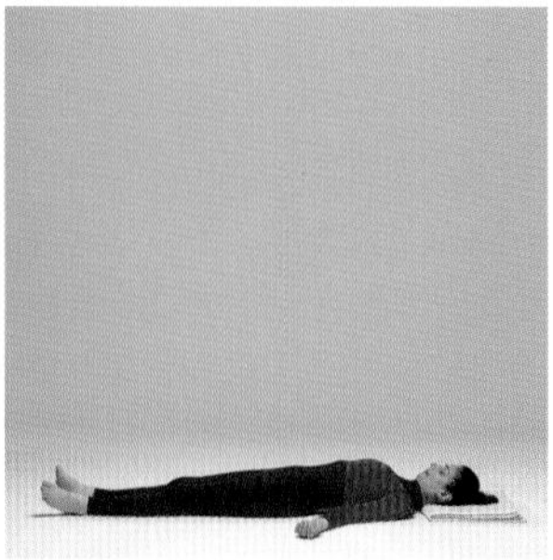

Follow the method given in Unit 1 (page 26).

To Progress

After relaxing the senses, be aware of the back of the head. Extend the span of awareness along the back of the body from the head to the feet. Maintain this flow of awareness uninterruptedly for a few minutes.

Meditation

KEY CONCEPT

Meditation Meditation is the ultimate in Yoga practice. It is considered to have two stages: object-supported and objectless. We might wonder how there can be meditation without an object. In reply, we can turn our attention to the experience of deep sleep. This differs from dreaming in that dreaming is a reflection of the waking state, but containing abnormal as well as normal objects. There is no object for the mind in deep sleep; instead there is awareness of the self shorn of all worldly adjuncts. This universally experienced state supports the concept of objectless meditation.

We have seen how Yoga analyzes the mind, its target, into five modes, which include three types of cognition, deep sleep, and memory. The last one is a veritable storehouse of innumerable traces left by experiences in this life and past lives; they are awakened when conditions are appropriate. The proximity of the soul prompts the mind, which is material in nature, to engage in its activities. These are suspended in deep sleep, meditation, and liberation. On this background, we will now go into further details of meditation, the central concern of Yoga.

Yoga is Education

Meditation is a very difficult process: that of channeling the mind toward the spiritual goal by gradually freeing it from its normal operations, in which it is virtually uncontrollable. In fact, normal human relations run smoothly because mental operations are invisible. We do not know what another person is thinking; it may be quite the opposite of what he says. This inability to know someone else's mind can even endanger human life and property, as it keeps a wrongdoer unknown till the crucial moment strikes. This peculiar character of the mind can thus promote or act against human interests. The mind directs us to act physically. Considering the mind's character, man has created a tool for developing it in such a way that it advances individual and group interests without involving serious conflict. This tool is general education. Yoga is nothing but education geared to a specific goal—spiritual development. This explains the approach of Yoga, which progresses from simple to difficult means, in keeping with the nature of the educational process, which starts with simple lessons and gradually introduces difficult ones.

This exposition has its own limitations. It explains the progressive stages of meditation, as stated by Patañjali, the highest authority on Yoga. For those without a background of Yogic meditative practice, it is bound to appear as a verbal exercise. We cannot verify its details, as we can, for instance, those of anatomy. And yet it is presented here to make the outline of the Yoga of Patañjali as complete as possible. The reader is requested to bear this in mind while reading the following details.

Object-based Meditation

Through this prolonged educational process, we are led by Patañjali to the top step of the ladder, deep meditation or absorption (*samādhi*). Meditation is conceived in two progressive categories: object based (*saṃprajñāta* or *sabīja*), in which the mind contemplates an object, and objectless (*asaṃprajñāta* or *nirbīja*), in which the mind is transcended. Though both are called meditation, only the first is included among the eight aids of Yoga, which, in its defined sense, is objectless meditation in which all mental operations are suspended.

Meditation on Tangible Objects

Object-based meditation has four stages. The first two stages concern tangible objects; the last two, intangible ones. The first stage involving tangible objects (for example, a book, tree, or mountain) is accompanied by a tripartite linguistic process involving word, meaning, and cognition. The cognition of a book involves the word "book" (or an equivalent word in a different language), the meaning of "book," and the understanding of "book." All these are inseparably tied together in normal communication, even though we are not aware of them. Ultimately, to transcend the mind, it is necessary to go beyond the network of language and thought.

In the second stage of meditation, focusing is on tangible objects as before but unaccompanied by the linguistic process. The Yogin is aware only of the object in this stage. Here a Yogin crosses the limits of normal cognition; for him, everything is envisioned by a preternatural perception. This kind of perception—one may call it insight or intuition—forms the basis of his knowledge. A Yogin who has developed Yogic aptitude opens, as it were, an inner eye when the physical eyes are closed; through this eye, visualizing of the unseen is made possible. There is no reliance on inference or traditional sources of authority, which are the normal means of knowing objects that are beyond perception by the senses. For the Yogin everything is a matter of intuitive knowledge, rather than intuitive perception.

Meditation on Intangible Objects

When accomplished in the meditation on tangible objects, the Yogin turns to intangible objects, such as the subtle essences of the five elements—smell, form-and-color, and so on. Thus, Yoga meditation refines contemplation progressively away from concrete phenomena toward the subtle, underlying cause from which they spring. In the third stage, awareness of space, time, and cause accompanies the meditation. All events in our normal life are characterized by a context of space, time, and cause. When, for instance, we walk, we do so on some place (the street, a garden), at a certain time (morning, evening), and for some reason (going to the office, for pleasure). This awareness is implied in the two early stages of meditation also; but they differ from the third because their objects are tangible rather than intangible.

The fourth stage begins when this awareness ceases and the mind is absorbed in progressively subtler principles, as posited in the *Sāṃkhya-Yoga* philosophy: the cosmic sense of self, the cosmic principle of intelligence, and Primordial Matter.

This is the picture of meditation as far as the object of meditation is concerned. Two more factors of cognition are left: the means (eyes, ears, and so on) and the ego as observer or subject. When meditation focuses on the means of cognition, the mind is filled with a sense of bliss; when it focuses on the individual ego, it is filled with the sense of individual existence involving the union of the soul with the individual identity.

Yogic Powers

The Yogin is said to gain miraculous powers while pursuing the path of Yoga. These develop as a result of his practice of the last three aids of Yoga—concentration, object-based meditation and absorption, and the resulting preternatural vision. We can compare this deep vision to the device of X-ray photography, which reveals what is invisible to ordinary sight. Patañjali informs us that by visualizing the essential elements of language, a Yogin is empowered to understand the communication of all creatures. By focusing his vision on the memory imprints in his mind, he can view his past lives; by focusing on the process of cognition, he can understand another person's mind; and so on. He is also the master of eight traditionally cited powers: to become minute; to become enormous; to become heavy; to become light; to reach anywhere in the world; to get what he wills; to control the elements (earth, fire, water, etc.); to change a thing into something else. In brief, the world is at the beck and call of a

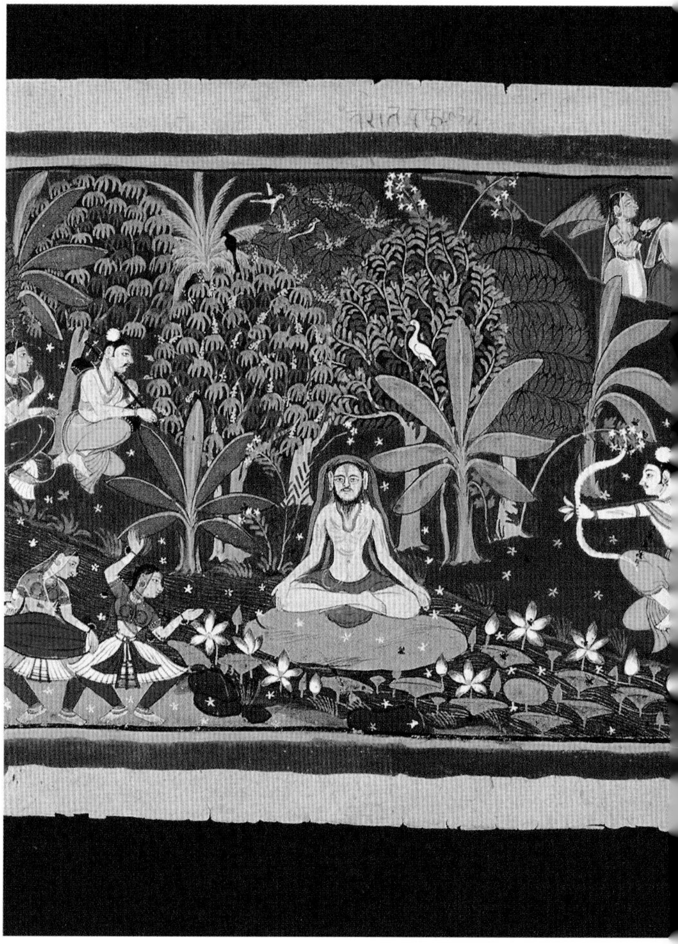

Indra attempts to disrupt Sage Mārkaṇḍeya's meditation.

Yogin at this stage. Patañjali gives a long list of such powers, but warns that, though seeming to be accomplishments, they are in fact obstacles to the ultimate goal of Yoga, liberation, as they may divert the Yogin from it.

Objectless Meditation

Having mastered object-based meditation, a Yogin can pass on to the higher stage of objectless meditation. On this plane all operations of the mind are suspended. What is left of the mind is only memory imprints and the Fates that guide and regulate our life. In other words, during this type of meditation, the mind is reduced practically to nil, albeit temporarily. It is the memory imprints that awaken the Yogin's memory at the end of the meditation and bring him back to normal functions—exactly as happens at the end of deep sleep.

In Brief

The mind is such a thing as cannot be grasped by another;
That is how deception can occur in respect of mind, speech, and deed.

Hence, to safeguard the interests of individuals and groups,
Men have introduced a means called education; Yoga is nothing but education of the mind.

Yoga masters have prescribed a long ladder of steps,
Easy to begin with but truly difficult; indeed, mind control is hard.

Thus meditation is of two types:
One, object based; the other, objectless.

The Yogin who is perfected in the meditation of subtle objects
Perceives everything; from this perception emerges authoritative knowledge.

Concentration, meditation, and absorption are together called deep vision.
Through deep vision of various objects, Yogins obtain miraculous powers.

Powers may be powers in ordinary life,
But in meditation all powers are only obstacles.

That meditation is called objectless in which all mind modes are checked,
In which the mind, remaining only as memory imprints, as if dissolves.

For a wider perspective...

Yoga in Fiction

Patañjali informs us that, at a certain stage in Yogic practices, the Yogin achieves miraculous powers. There are many stories about such powers in Sanskrit literature. One tale of great antiquity, dating from the third or fourth century B.C., is retold in an eleventh-century work called *The Ocean of Stories*; within this work is a series of stories narrated by a goblin to a king. Each ends in a riddle, which the king is called upon to solve or lose his life.

An old Yogin was living in a hut near a cemetery. His age would not permit him to continue his practices as vigorously as before. One day he discovered that the corpse of a young boy had been brought to the cemetery for cremation; a thought flashed in his mind. At that thought he first lamented and then danced in delight. Before the pyre was lit, the Yogin left his body and entered that of the boy. Seeing the dead boy restored to life, his relatives were overjoyed and hurriedly helped him down from the pyre. The Yogin, as the revived boy, told them that he had been sent back from death by god **Śiva** on the condition that he devote the rest of his life to Yogic practices. He asked them to leave him and go home. The boy's relatives did as asked, as the price for the very fact of his revival. When they left, the rejuvenated Yogin buried his old dead body.

The riddle the goblin put to the king was: Why did the Yogin first lament and then dance in delight? The king's reply was: The Yogin lamented as he was sorry to leave the body his parents had loved and brought up with care, and he was delighted at the thought of having a new lease on life in a young body, ensuring his Yogic practices for many years.

Unit 12

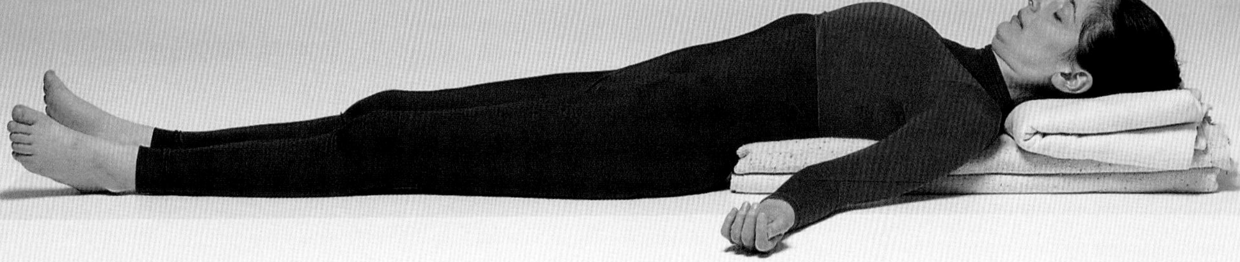

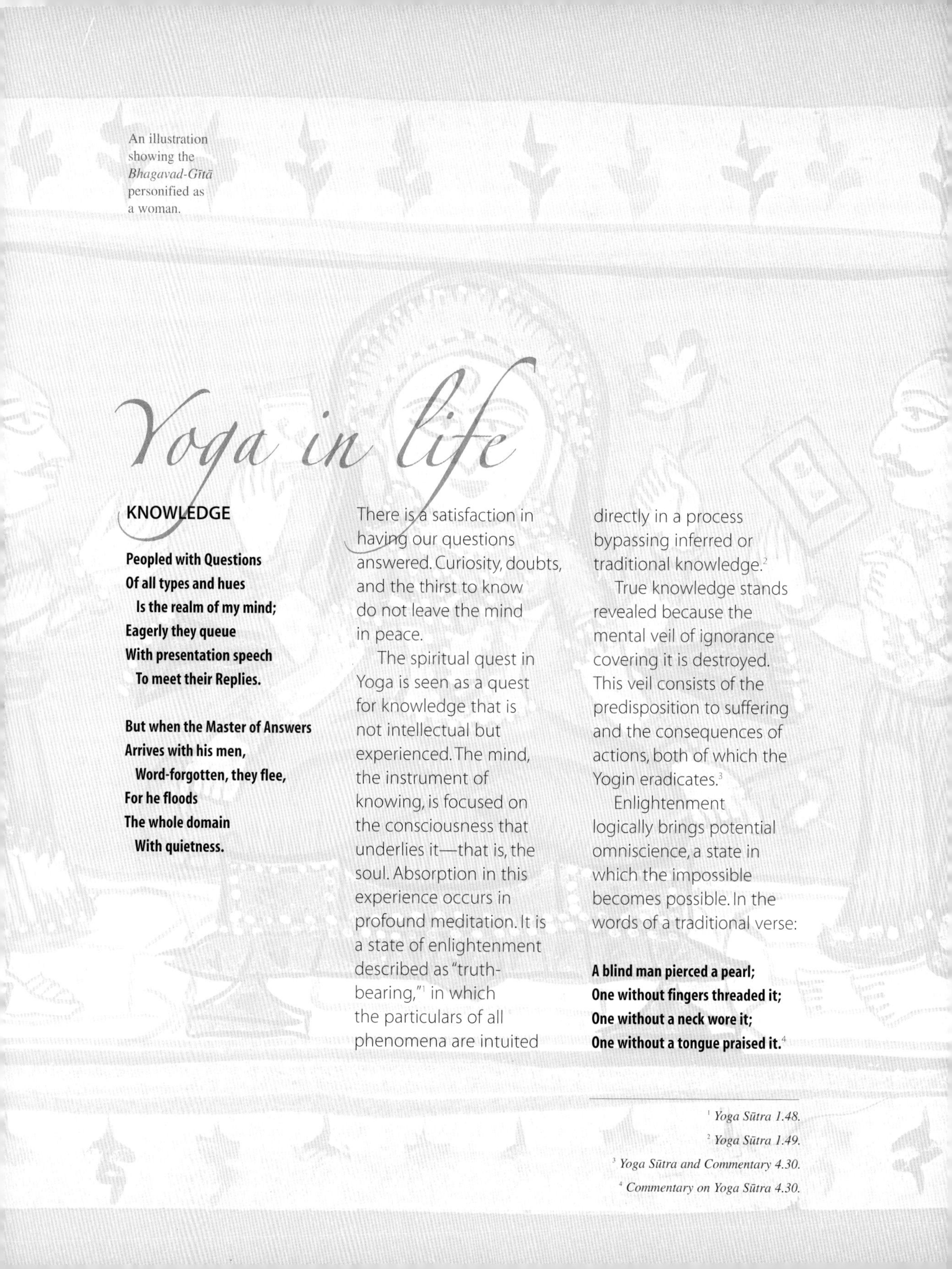

An illustration showing the *Bhagavad-Gītā* personified as a woman.

Yoga in life

KNOWLEDGE

Peopled with Questions
Of all types and hues
Is the realm of my mind;
Eagerly they queue
With presentation speech
To meet their Replies.

But when the Master of Answers
Arrives with his men,
Word-forgotten, they flee,
For he floods
The whole domain
With quietness.

There is a satisfaction in having our questions answered. Curiosity, doubts, and the thirst to know do not leave the mind in peace.

The spiritual quest in Yoga is seen as a quest for knowledge that is not intellectual but experienced. The mind, the instrument of knowing, is focused on the consciousness that underlies it—that is, the soul. Absorption in this experience occurs in profound meditation. It is a state of enlightenment described as "truth-bearing,"[1] in which the particulars of all phenomena are intuited directly in a process bypassing inferred or traditional knowledge.[2]

True knowledge stands revealed because the mental veil of ignorance covering it is destroyed. This veil consists of the predisposition to suffering and the consequences of actions, both of which the Yogin eradicates.[3]

Enlightenment logically brings potential omniscience, a state in which the impossible becomes possible. In the words of a traditional verse:

A blind man pierced a pearl;
One without fingers threaded it;
One without a neck wore it;
One without a tongue praised it.[4]

---

[1] *Yoga Sūtra 1.48.*

[2] *Yoga Sūtra 1.49.*

[3] *Yoga Sūtra and Commentary 4.30.*

[4] *Commentary on Yoga Sūtra 4.30.*

Mind and breath

When the breath moves, the mind moves;
When the breath is still, the mind is still.
The Yogin becomes still as a post;
Therefore one should restrain the breath.

So asserts a medieval manual on Yoga practice, the *Haṭha Yoga Pradīpikā*, voicing a widely accepted doctrine. Similarly, today it is well known that different breathing patterns accompany different mental states: for example, hyperventilation and anxiety, and deep breathing and composure.

Yoga postures can alter emotional states and induce calmness. When the mind is peaceful, another avenue opens, through which the mind can be controlled. This is the deliberate concentration on the breath.

As with all journeys with a set purpose, preparation is the key to success. There are two areas of need, corresponding to the two sides of the equation. Effective concentration requires the body and mind to be undisturbed by tensions. Effective concentration on the breath is not possible unless the lungs receive air in abundance.

Both needs are met by doing postures that expand the chest and promote relaxation. The process is started in supported supine poses. The release of mental tension continues in supported forward bends, in which the head rests: on the hairline in Dog Pose (*Adho-Mukha-Śvānāsana*), on the crown in Intense Stretch Pose (*Uttānāsana*) and on the forehead in the sitting poses. Inverted poses require concentration on the upper chest in order to keep it expanded. This trains the upper ribs and shoulder girdle to work more efficiently, sustaining an abundant intake of air.

All these poses are held for some length of time, ingraining their effects. The cumulative psychological effect of the whole series of poses is profoundly transformative, leading the mind from extroversion to introspection.

Finally, with physical ease and mental tranquillity well established, the mind is ready to focus on the breath.

The first step is to become aware of and observe the breath. As the eyes are closed this involves using an inner vision, the mind's eye. Rhythm, volume, duration, texture, passage through the nostrils, reception by each lung: noting all these things causes the breath to become familiar. Instead of a hidden, unmeasured force, it becomes an analyzable object. And by being known it becomes controllable.

Any and all of the characteristics of the breath are capable of being regulated. This is a separate area of Yoga practice, breath control (*prāṇāyāma*). It is developed on a foundation of a thorough and fruitful practice of postures. Even at an elementary level it brings an inexpressible experience of lucidity and quietude. And yet this is only a stepping stone toward the meditative heights offered by Yoga in its quest for the ultimate experience of the soul.

मत्स्यासन *Matsyāsana*

Fish Pose

The supported chest expands; the resulting freedom in breathing gives a sense of buoyancy.

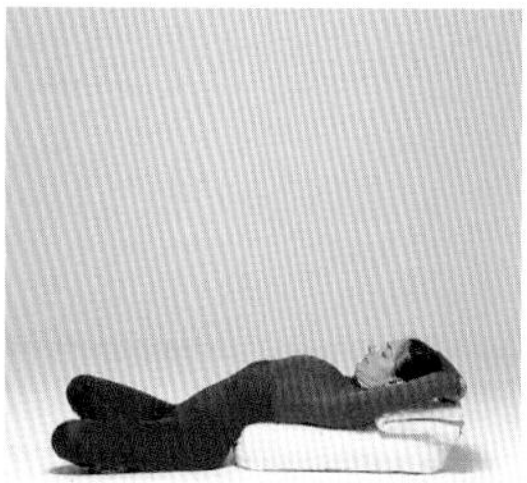

Follow the method given in Unit 4 (page 73). Fold the arms over the head.

To Progress

Lengthen the sides of the trunk when lying down.

सुप्त-बद्ध-कोणासन *Supta-Baddha-Koṇāsana*

Supine Bound-Angle Pose

When the breath settles down to be rhythmic and slow, thoughts become unhurried and the mind peaceful.

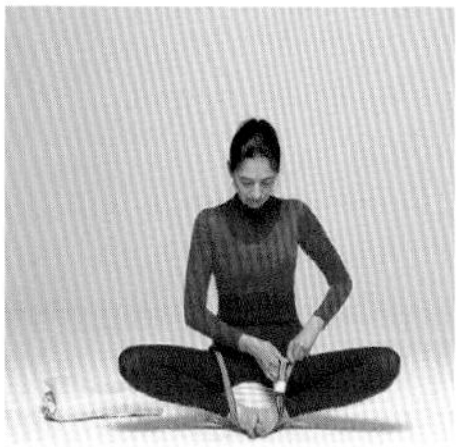

Sit on the end of a bolster. Bend the knees out to the sides and join the soles of the feet. Bring the heels toward the pubis. To maintain the legs close to the trunk without effort, tie the legs and trunk together. Pass a belt around the base of the lower back, over the tops of the thighs, and under the bottom shins. Pull it tight, with the buckle between the thigh and calf so that it does not press on the flesh of the leg.

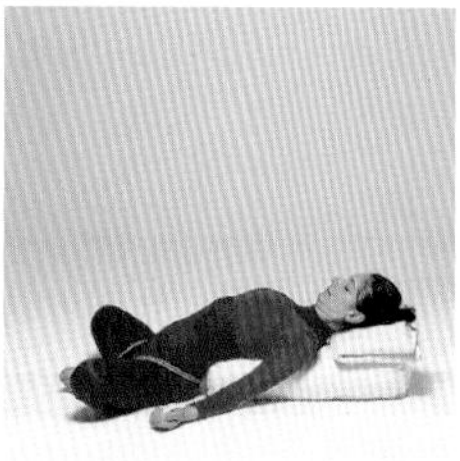

Slide down off the bolster and lie back on it. Place a folded blanket under the head and neck. Rest the arms on the floor beside the trunk. Breathe evenly and relax.

Stay for 3 to 5 minutes. Undo the belt, bring the knees together, turn to the side, and come up.

To Progress

Pull the belt tighter.

Help

- **If the hip joints or groin feel strained, place supports under the thighs.**

सुप्त-वीरासन *Supta-Vīrāsana*

Supine Hero Pose

The abdominal extension in this pose allays mental tension; the chest expansion enhances breathing and calmness, once the art of being comfortable is learned.

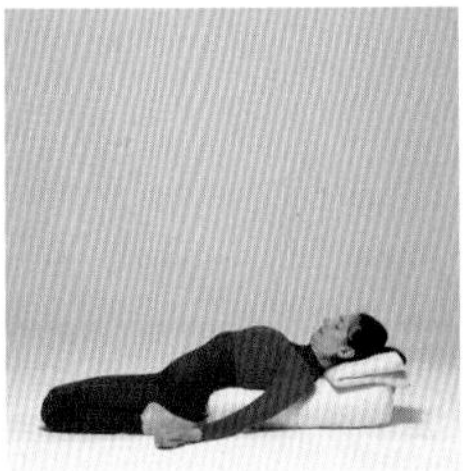

Sit in *Vīrāsana* (see Unit 6, page 107) with a bolster behind the back. Holding the bolster against the body, lie back on it. Place a folded blanket under the neck and head. Rest the arms beside the trunk. Breathe evenly and relax. Stay for 3 to 5 minutes. Come up. Bend forward in *Adho-Mukha-Vīrāsana* (see Unit 2, page 42).

To Progress

Bring the knees together (they tend to move apart initially).

Help

- **If the back and legs are stiff, sit on a support and raise the height of the support under the back.**
- **If the ankles are stiff, place a rolled blanket beneath them.**

अधोमुख-श्वानासन *Adho-Mukha-Śvānāsana*

Dog Pose, Head Down

When inverted, the spine and abdomen relax; this is soothing for the nerves and brain.

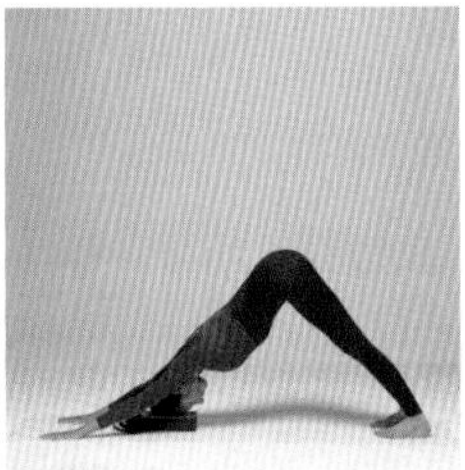

Follow the method given in Unit 4 (page 74).

To Progress

Lift the hips higher so that the abdomen moves back toward the spine. This increases the relaxing effect of the pose.

Help

- **Place the hands against the wall, with the thumbs and forefingers apart (see Unit 7, page 119).**

उत्तानासन *Uttānāsana*

Intense Stretch

When the abdomen relaxes, as in this pose, the chest feels ease and the lungs breathe more freely; all this contributes to mental calm.

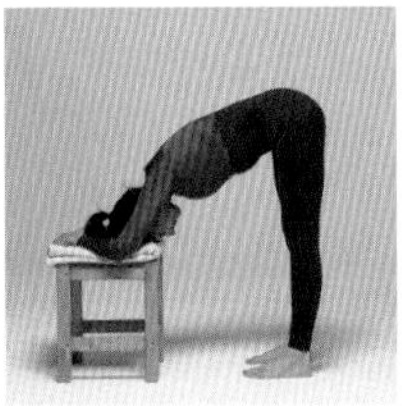

Follow the method given in Unit 4 (page 76).

To Progress

Reduce the height of the support under the head, to enable the trunk to lengthen downward.

अधोमुख-सुखासन *Adho-Mukha-Sukhāsana*

Comfortable Pose, Head Down

Abdominal softness increases when the legs are crossed.

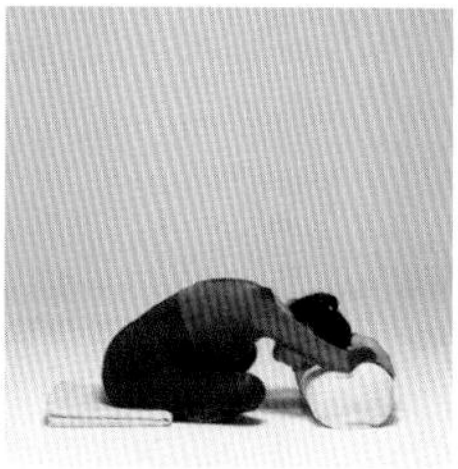

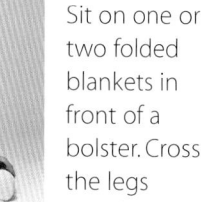

Sit on one or two folded blankets in front of a bolster. Cross the legs simply. Bend forward, and rest the head and arms on the bolster. Breathe evenly and relax. Stay for 1 to 2 minutes. Cross the legs the other way and repeat.

To Progress

Lengthen the front of the body and move the bolster a little farther away.

Help

- **If the pose is not comfortable, adjust the height of the support under the head or buttocks.**
- **If the hip joints or groins feel strain, support the thighs.**

जानुशीर्षासन *Jānuśīrṣāsana*

Head-to-Knee Pose

As the head is down, distractions from the outside world are minimized, and the mind can become introverted.

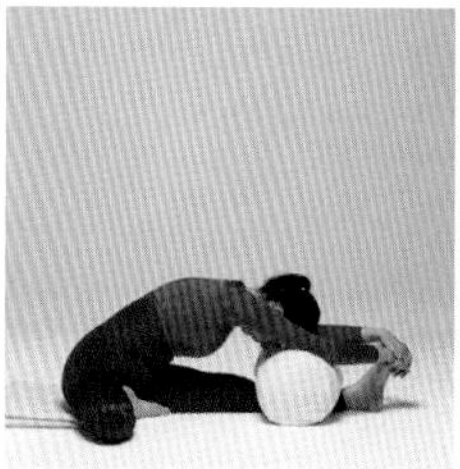

Sit on one or two folded blankets, and stretch the legs out in front. Bend the right leg to the side, bringing the heel to its own groin. Keep the left leg straight and the foot upright. Place a bolster on the shin. Exhale and bend forward, resting the forehead and arms on the bolster and catching the foot. Breathe evenly and relax.

Stay for 1 to 2 minutes. Inhale and come up. Repeat on the other side.

Help

- **If the back is stiff, sit higher or place a folded blanket on top of the bolster.**
- **If the hands do not reach the foot, use a belt to catch it.**

To Progress

As the back relaxes and the front of the body lengthens, move the bolster a little forward, without raising the head.

एकपादवीर-पश्चिमोत्तानासन *Ekapādavīra-Paścimottānāsana*

Posterior Intense Stretch with One Leg in Hero Pose

Each variation on a theme augments the effect; a different forward bend relaxes the body and mind in a slightly different way.

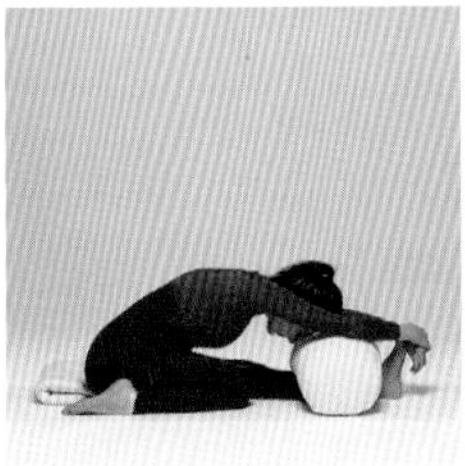

Sit on one or two folded blankets, and stretch the legs out in front. Move the blanket support so that it is under the left buttock. Bend the right leg back, taking the foot beside the buttock and keeping the knee facing forward. Keep the left leg straight and the foot upright. Place a bolster on the shin. Exhale and bend forward, resting the forehead and arms on the bolster. Breathe evenly and relax. Stay for 1 to 2 minutes. Inhale and come up. Repeat on the other side.

To Progress

As the back relaxes and the front of the body lengthens, move the bolster a little forward without raising the head.

Help

- **See *Jānuśirṣāsana*, page 211.**
- **If it is difficult to balance, sit higher.**
- **If the ankles are stiff, place a rolled blanket under the lower shin (see Unit 2, page 42).**
- **If the back aches after this series of forward bends, do *Parivṛtta-Sukhāsana* (see Unit 11, page 196).**

पश्चिमोत्तानासन *Paścimottānāsana*

Posterior Intense Stretch

With the head facing the legs and flanked by the arms, external stimuli do not excite the senses easily; this induces serenity.

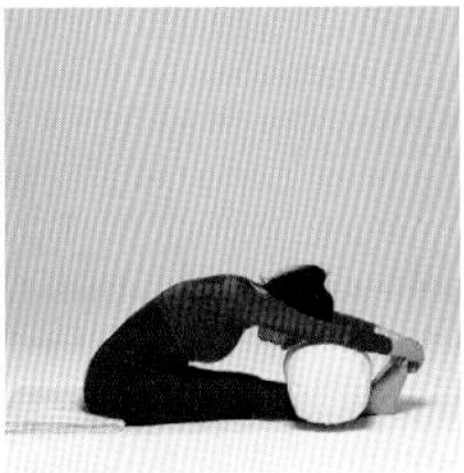

Sit on one or two folded blankets, with the legs stretched out in front. Straighten the knees and keep the feet upright. Place a bolster on the shins. Exhale and bend forward, resting the forehead and arms on the bolster. Breathe evenly and relax. Stay for 2 to 3 minutes. Inhale and come up.

Help **See *Jānuśirṣāsana*, page 211.**

To Progress

As the back relaxes and the front of the body lengthens, move the bolster a little forward without raising the head. Make sure that the forehead skin moves gently from the hairline to the brow; do not let it rub upward.

विपरीत-दण्डासन *Viparīta-Daṇḍāsana*

Inverted Staff Pose

A supported back arch combines chest and lung expansion with inversion of the head to give a feeling of quiet positivity.

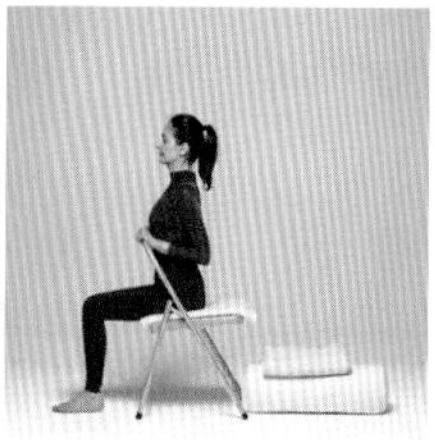

Place a nonslip mat and a folded blanket on a sturdy chair with a gap at the bottom of the back rest. Place a bolster and folded blanket lengthwise on the floor in front of the chair. Sit backward on the chair, taking the legs through the gap. It is helpful to tie the legs together at mid-thigh with a belt.

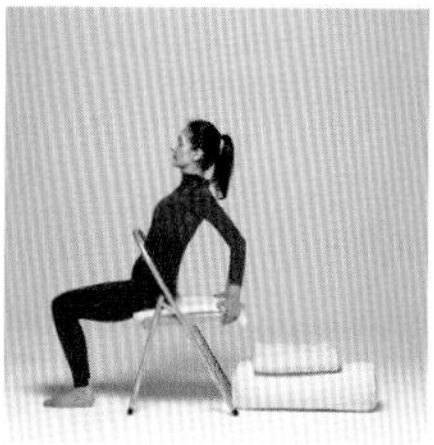

Move the buttocks forward and lean back, holding the seat of the chair.

Lie back on the seat so that the edge is below the shoulder blades. Rest the head on the support.

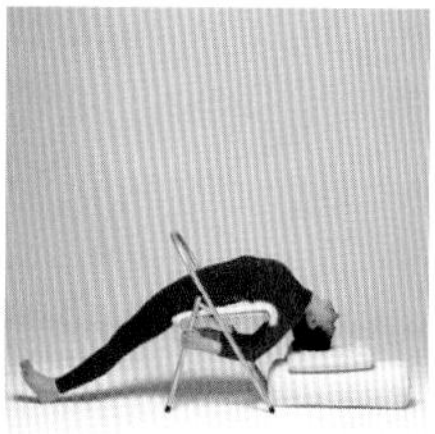

Straighten the legs. Take the arms under the seat of the chair, and hold the back legs of the chair. Breathe evenly and relax. Stay for 1 to 2 minutes. Breathe evenly and relax.

To come up, bend the legs and hold the top of the chair. Swing the trunk up, making the back concave and lifting the chest first and head last. Rest the front of the body against the back of the chair.

To Progress

Stay longer in the pose. Tighten the knees and stretch the legs. Roll the shoulders back, away from the head.

Help

- **If the back feels strained, raise the feet on a support.**
- **If the neck feels strained, raise the height of the support under the head.**
- **If nausea is felt, reduce the arch by raising the supports under both head and feet.**
- **If the shoulders feel constricted, hold the legs of the chair from outside.**

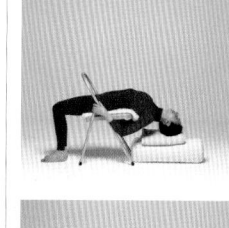

सर्वाङ्गासन *Sarvāṅgāsana*

Shoulder-Balance

Body and mind benefit from being able to stay in this supported inversion for a long time, enjoying its calming and rejuvenating effect.

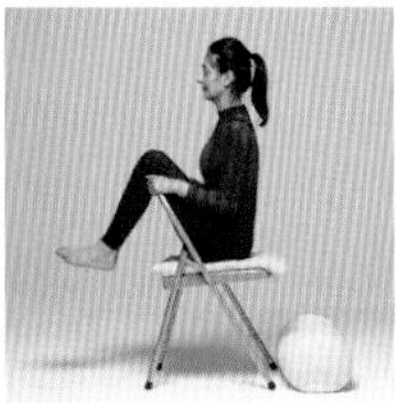

Place a folded blanket on a chair, preferably on top of a nonslip mat. Place a bolster horizontally on the floor in front of the seat. Sit backward on the chair, taking the legs over the back and holding onto it.

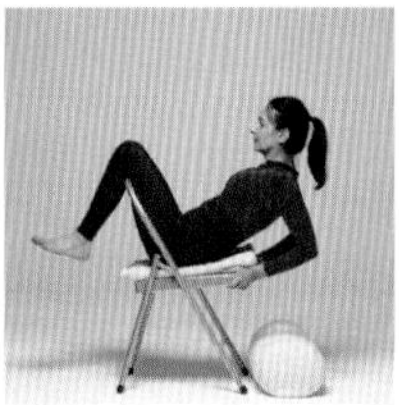

Lean back, moving the buttocks farther toward the back of the chair and holding the seat.

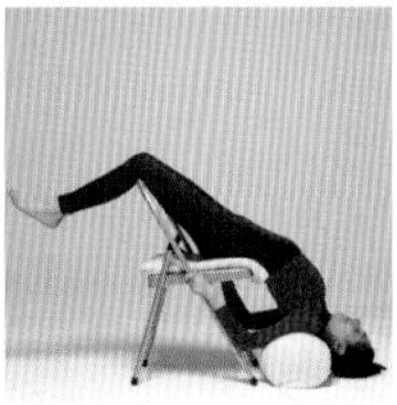

Curve the waist over the seat of the chair, and lower the shoulders onto the bolster and the head onto the floor. Adjust the position of the head and neck so that they are comfortable.

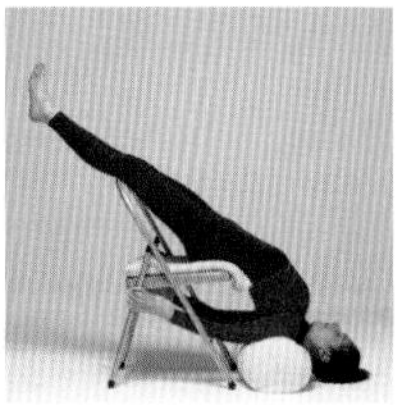

Straighten the legs up against the back of the chair. Take the arms under the seat of the chair, and hold the back legs of the chair. Stay for 3 to 5 minutes. Breathe evenly and relax.

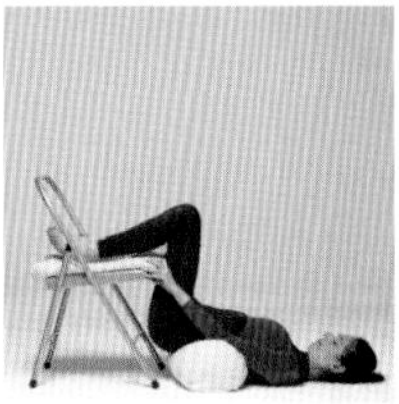

To come down, bend the legs and rest the feet on the back of the chair. Hold the back legs of the chair from outside. Holding the chair, slide backward and down off it until the lower back rests on the bolster.

To Progress

Press the shoulder blades in and lift the sternum (breastbone). Stay longer in the pose.

Help

- **If the back is stiff, place a second bolster or thickly rolled blankets lengthwise across the first one, so that the shoulders reach the support easily.**
- **If the knees bend over the chair back, place folded blankets on it to increase the height. For an even more relaxing pose, rest the feet against the wall. To do this, place the chair 1–1½ feet away from the wall.**

Cautions

See Unit 3 (page 62).

सेतुबन्ध-सर्वाङ्गासन

Setu-Bandha-Sarvāṅgāsana

Shoulder-Balance Bridge

Passive extensions and expansions such as this have powerful effects on the mind, releasing pent-up tension and replacing it with tranquillity.

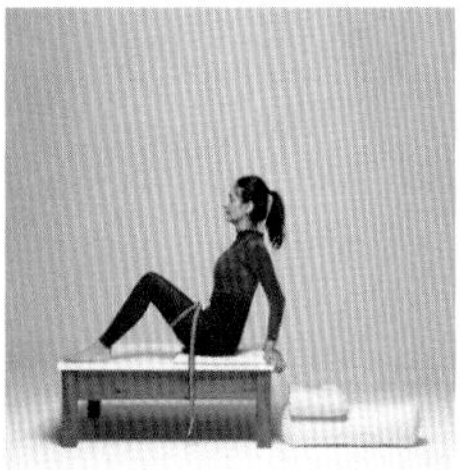

Place a nonslip mat and a folded blanket on one end of a sturdy bench or coffee table. Place a bolster and folded blanket lengthwise on the floor in front of the bench. Sit backward on it, with the feet up. Tie the legs together at mid-thigh with a belt.

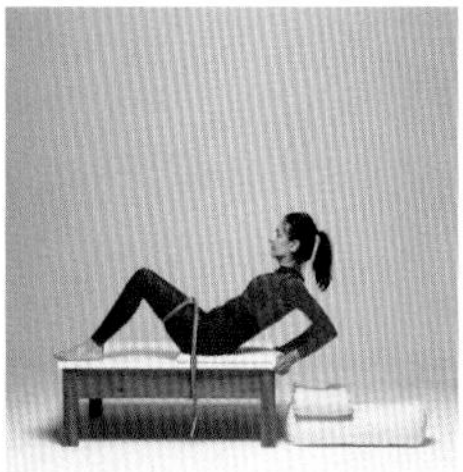

Holding the bench, move the buttocks a little forward and lean back.

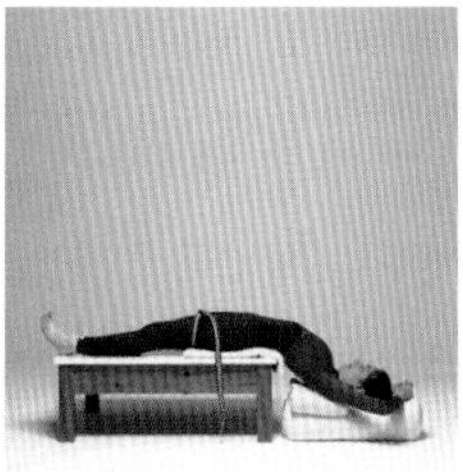

Curving the waist over the end of the bench, lower the trunk until the shoulders rest on the blanket and the head rests on the bolster. Straighten the legs. Take the arms over the head. Breathe evenly and relax. Stay for 3 to 5 minutes.

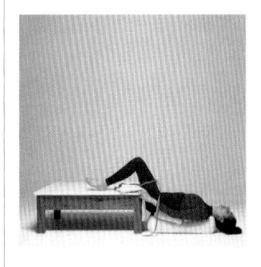

To come down, bend the legs, hold the bench, and slide backward off it until the lower back rests on the bolster.

Undo the belt. Sit on the bolster in simple cross-legs, and bend forward, resting the head on the bench.

To Progress

Before straightening the legs, lengthen the lower back away from the waist. From time to time tighten the knees and stretch the legs.

Help

- **If the back feels strained, bend the knees or raise the feet on a support.**

शवासन *Śavāsana*

Corpse Pose

With the chest lifted on a support, ease of breathing unites with profound relaxation, making this pose suitable for the initial practice of breath training, *prāṇāyāma*.

Follow the method given in Unit 4 (page 79).

After a few minutes proceed to:

To Progress

Lengthen the sides of the trunk when lying down.

उज्जायी प्राणायाम *Ujjāyī Prāṇāyāma*

Conquering Breath Control

The conquest referred to in the name is that of ailments; Yoga texts record breath control practices as curative of diseases.

Observe the breath as it flows into and out of the nose, throat, and lungs. Note its quality (soft or harsh) and rhythm, and whether it flows evenly on the right and left.

Gradually make the breath soft and steady. Fill and empty the two lungs equally. Let go of physical and mental tension during the exhalations. Relax the abdomen.

Observe how the abdomen deflates at the end of exhalation and how the chest inflates at the end of inhalation. This is the pattern of normal breathing.

Continue with normal breathing for a few minutes, then change to deep breathing. After exhalation, maintain the deflation of the abdomen and inhale. After inhalation, maintain the lift of the top chest and exhale.

Continue for a few minutes. Then lie quietly and breathe normally. Gently open the eyes, bend the knees and turn to the side, rolling down off the bolster. Keep the support for the head. Stay as long as the feeling of peaceful introversion lasts. Get up from the side.

To Progress

Do not strain. Keep the eyes relaxed and the mind focused on the breath. Breathe evenly on the right and left. Deliberately fill the sides of the lungs during inhalation. Control the speed of exhalation so that the rib cage does not collapse.

Help

- **If doing deep inhalation and exhalation continuously causes strain, take normal breaths between each cycle to recover. A cycle comprises one inhalation and one exhalation.**

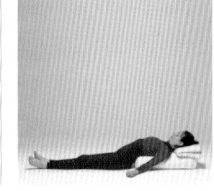

The eightfold scheme of Yoga

KEY CONCEPT

Aids of Yoga Patañjali's scheme of the aids of Yoga reveals that control of the mind starts from a disciplined and moral routine, a part of worldly life. At the same time, it should be remembered that, being a part of life, it is not relevant at the level of Ultimate Reality. It should be noted, too, that physical controls are also considered part of mind control. This shows how intimately the body and the mind are knit together. All these aids, including even the knowledge discriminating between mind and soul, are merely means, which a Yogin discards once he achieves his goal of liberation.

We now have a broad idea about meditation, the major concern of Yoga. Meditation, as conceived by Patañjali, consists of a progressive scheme that starts with the withdrawal of the senses from their stimuli, passes through an intermediate stage of fixing the mind on some object, and ends with meditation without a supporting object. For us, who are accustomed to normal thinking processes, meditation may sound as if it is the same thinking process more intensified. When, therefore, Patañjali talks about objectless meditation, it may sound absurd to us. All advanced knowledge is likely to sound absurd if subjected to commonsense methods. As we progress in it, the absurdity slowly turns into sense. We will now see the steps that progressively take the practitioner to the ultimate in meditation.

Primary Aids

The culmination of Yoga—the suspension of the mind in the absence of a supporting object—has eight aids; this explains its traditional description as eight-limbed or consisting of eight parts. These are: (1) moral discipline (*yama*), (2) personal discipline (*niyama*), (3) posture (*āsana*), (4) breath regulation (*prāṇāyāma*), (5) control of the sense organs (*pratyāhāra*), (6) fixation of mind on a selected object (*dhāraṇā*), (7) meditation (*dhyāna*), and (8) deep meditation or absorption (*samādhi*). It should be noted that this last, *samādhi*, is equivalent to Yoga and is employed in the sense of both means and goal. When deep meditation is object based, it is a means or aid; when it is objectless it is the goal.

The first five relate to general and physical discipline; the last three are part of mind discipline. The first five are treated as external or distant, and the remaining three

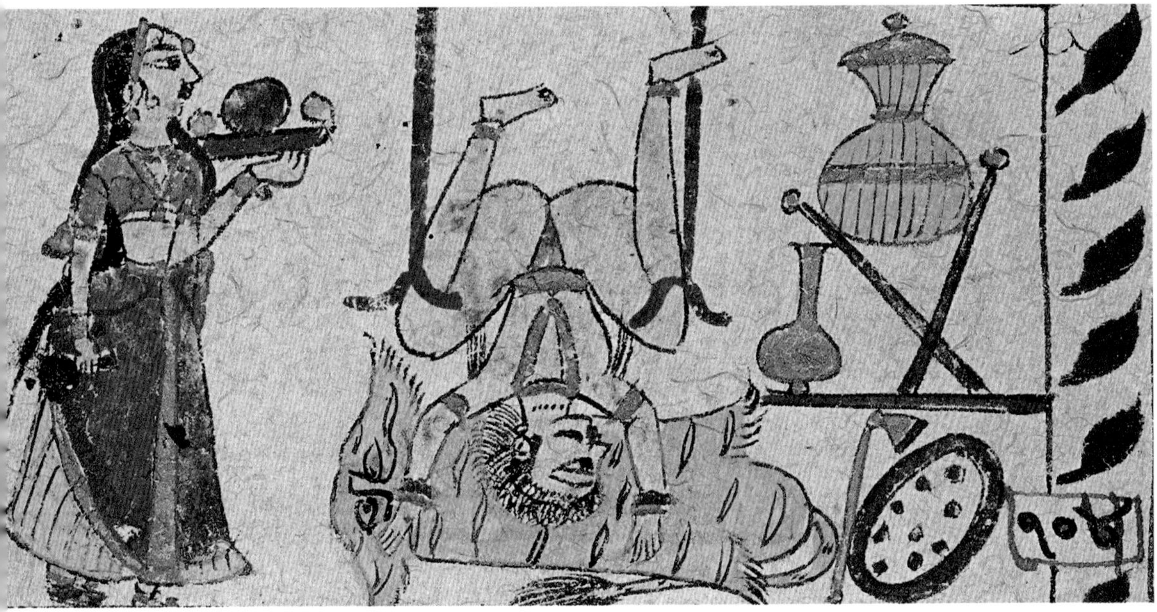

An illustration of a Yogi inverting himself—from the *Śiva Purāṇa* scripture, dated A.D. 1740.

as internal or close. This division is clear if we understand Yoga in its sense of absorption of the mind, which relates to the object-based type of meditation. In the context of objectless meditation, even the last three aids, being object based, are treated as external. Whether internal or external, these primary aids of Yoga call for total devotion to them by the practitioner. The first two aim at the purification of the mind, the rest are contributory to meditation, successively closer to it. The eight aids in their sequence are

1. Moral restraints or vows (*yamas*): nonviolence (*ahimsā*), truth (*satya*), refraining from theft (*asteya*), restraint of the sexual urge (*brahmacarya*), and rejection of possessions (*aparigraha*). Nonviolence is the basic moral restraint; the rest of the restraints and observances contribute to its perfection. Truth implies the fidelity of speech and thought to fact; it promotes the good of all creatures. Non-theft, in its ideal form, implies abstention even from the thoughts of theft. Mental abstention applies to other moral restraints also. To limit the restraints only to the physical aspect and let the mind run unbridled is to miss their purpose. This is comparable to the situation in which a man with double standards is called a hypocrite. This should make it clear that the ultimate aim of the moral restraints is the purification of the mind, and physical restraints are not a goal in themselves. When these moral restraints are observed without compromise, they are designated Great Vows. The development of moral attitudes includes the countering of thoughts of violence, and so on, by focusing on their opposites.

2. Daily observances (*niyamas*): purity of body and mind (*śauca*), contentment (*saṃtoṣa*), endurance of extremes like heat and cold (*tapas*), the study of philosophical texts or recitation of the sacred sound *Om* (*svādhyāya*), and the dedication of all actions to God (*īśvara-praṇidhāna*). Patañjali views God as the ultimate teacher and guide. Unlike ordinary souls, He is untouched by factors that involve the soul in worldly life, namely the fundamental predispositions to suffering, actions and their consequences, and fate. He may be compared to distilled water free from impurities causing diseases. It would be logical to think that Patañjali found the concept of God as the supreme teacher contributory to his main goal of cleansing the mind of worldly objects. Yoga is learning, and a teacher makes the process of learning easy.

3. Sitting postures (*āsanas*): the basic meaning of the term *āsana* is "sitting," and thus it logically refers to sitting postures. It is defined by Patañjali as a body position that is stable and comfortable. This precludes the popular concept of postures involving the maneuvering of the limbs, as developed by the *Haṭha* school of Yoga. Vyāsa refers to eleven postures, all of which relate to sitting. This reflects Patañjali's view on postures. Posture in Patañjali's scheme is said to be perfected when the practitioner ceases to make special efforts for it; the criterion for this perfection is the endurance of opposites like heat, cold, and so on.

4. Breath control (*prāṇāyāma*): this is defined as the holding or suspension of the movements of the air in relation to the body—that is, suspension of inhalation and exhalation. This can be done by holding the breath in or out after inhalation or exhalation, respectively. This act can be measured by (a) the distance the outgoing breath travels; (b) the duration of the suspension period; (c) the number of repetitions. A fourth variety of breath control is the suspension of breathing at any point, not necessarily after full inhalation or exhalation.

5. Withdrawal of the senses from their objects (*pratyāhāra*): the cessation of the operation of the senses as a result of that of the mind. This is compared to the movements of bees following those of the queen bee, an analogy as old as the *Upaniṣads*.

6. Fixation of the mind (*dhāraṇā*): the mind is focused on specific parts of the body such as the navel or heart, or on an external object such as a deity.

7. Meditation (*dhyāna*): this is defined as the flow of awareness of an object uninterrupted by the awareness of any other object, but accompanied by the awareness of the process of meditation.

8. Deep meditation or absorption (*samādhi*): this is called object-based meditation. It is characterized by the awareness of the object alone without the awareness of the process of meditation. Patañjali designates the last three aids together as deep vision (*saṃyama*), as this triad is needed for the acquisition of Yogic powers.

Secondary or Contributory Aids

The practice of Yoga is a complicated process. Following the eight aids of Yoga may be difficult for a beginner. Aware of this problem, Patañjali prescribes preliminary aids, which counter obstacles to meditation and/or prepare the ground for the primary aids. They are

1. Meditation on God;
2. A sympathetic or dispassionate attitude toward creatures of different tendencies—friendliness towards the happy; compassion for the distressed; delight at the pious; impartiality toward wrongdoers;
3. Control of the breath;
4. Perception of divine or subtle smells, tastes, and so on, which are said to be experienced by a Yoga practitioner during the process of meditation;
5. Focusing the mind on the heart or the sense of existence; focusing the mind on past Yogins;
6. Focusing the mind on a spiritually sublime object perceived in a dream, or on the peaceful state of sleep;
7. Meditation on a deity of one's choice;
8. The trio of daily observances—endurance of opposites, study of sacred texts and dedication of actions to God—which are the first three observances (*niyamas*).

This list seems to be a mix of the regular aids to Yoga with practical devices conducive to concentration of the mind. All are intended for removing the various difficulties encountered by the newcomer in the practice of the discipline. Controlling the mind by means of these aids, a Yogin gains self-realization and, ultimately, liberation.

In Brief

Yoga has eight limbs—morals, observances, posture,
Breath control and sense control; these are external.

Three are said to be internal—concentration, meditation,
And object-based meditation; these are known as deep vision.

The first two are for purifying the mind; the rest make it narrowly focused.
God is placed in the observances; He is thought of as the supreme teacher.

In Yoga, posture is an adjunct to meditation; it is defined as stable and comfortable.
For those who are not capable of these aids, there are easier means.

By these aids gradually restraining the mind from its host of objects,
A Yogin realizes his self and then attains liberation.

For a wider perspective...

Posture and Postures

Patañjali's concept of posture (*āsana*) is a body position that is conducive to meditation. He defines it as what is stable and comfortable. This obviously refers to a simple sitting posture, endorsed also by the *Bhagavad-Gītā* in the context of meditation, which uses the same Sanskrit word for "stable" as is used by **Patañjali**, and adds some more details, like keeping head, neck, and trunk in a straight line. **Vyāsa**, the commentator, gives a list of about a dozen postures by way of explanation. This should make it clear that posture was considered initially as a position of the body contributing to meditation.

The *Haṭha* Yoga tradition, on the other hand, views postures as a means to ensure the health and strength of the body, in tune with its aim to make it immortal. Under the rule of exaggeration, the possible number of postures soars to that of life species in the world—that is, 8.4 million. For practical considerations, however, it is brought down to 84, and finally, by some texts, to two: the Adept's Pose (*Siddhāsana*) and the Lotus Pose (*Padmāsana*).

Modern society appreciates Yoga mainly in the sense of postures and breath training as a means to maintain health. This is not incompatible with the major concerns of classical Yoga, which states that mastery of posture brings endurance and describes the miraculous body of a Yogin as excelling in beauty of form, strength, and diamondlike hardness.

Afterword

Dr. Patañjali, the Psychiatrist

A man once stepped into the clinic of Dr Patañjali, the renowned psychiatrist.

"What brings you here?" asked the doctor.

"Mental torture, of course," the patient replied.

"What is your name?" asked the doctor, taking out a registration form.

"You may call me Purusha for the time being," said the patient. "You must be aware of the problems of your patients."

"All right. Give me some details of your problem," the doctor responded.

"Sir, I am in love with a woman—we may call her Prakriti. She has stopped responding to my overtures and insists that I must fit myself in her formula. This is my problem."

"Then the simplest answer is that you fit yourself in *her* formula," observed the doctor.

"But, Sir, I am unable to do this because of the early ties deep-rooted in my mind." The patient continued, after a pause. "Don't you think that she should understand my difficulties and be agreeable to a compromise?"

"This means that you wish her to fit herself in *your* formula," the doctor remarked. "That is the way the human mind is molded: everyone has one's own set of formulas for others to fit in. This is the root cause of all suffering."

"Do you see a way one should take to get rid of this suffering?"

"Yes: isolation. Sever all ties with Prakriti – without and within," the doctor recommended.

"What do you mean? The Prakriti I love is only one, the one which is without, as you say," replied the perplexed patient.

"You are right, as far as normal understanding is concerned. But I am specialized in an area in which the starting point is: what is taken as normal is really abnormal," said the doctor.

"You confuse me," the patient complained.

"I am logical, as all scientists are. Let me explain. Your expectation that Prakriti should fit in your formula is rooted in your ego. Prakriti's expectation that you should fit in her formula is rooted in her ego. In other words, you have *your* ego, she has *hers*, which are in conflict with each other. In the absence of egos, different formulas have no chance to emerge, and there would be no scope for conflicts."

"How can you talk of an absence of ego which is born with us?" asked the patient, more confused.

"Again, try to understand the logic. Ego limited to an urge to live is natural—it is the manifestation of self-love; ego beyond that is a cultivated thing. Group ego certainly is—even that is ultimately rooted in self-love. Groups can be as small as a family, and as large as the world. In between, we have the group of humans, humanity. "Love thy neighbor," say the great. This privilege is restricted only to human beings; it is not comprehensive enough to include animals, which are slaughtered to feed humans. This shows the limitations of all so-called cultural values."

"This means, you accept individual ego as natural," retorted the patient.

"Natural, yes, insofar as one is born with it, but it is not real."

"What do you mean? What is universal must be real," asserted the patient.

"Now you come to the point: universality is not a proof of reality," said the doctor calmly.

"What proof can you adduce to support *your* thesis?" the patient asked.

"The proof lies in such of your states as is free from worldly influences. The only such state is deep sleep, in which one is aware of nothing but one's own existence. In this state, one has no nationality, no religion, no caste, no party, no sex distinction, no love, no hatred, no pleasure, no pain, not even an awareness of one's body and mind, much less the element of ego, indicating that the identification of the soul with ego is rooted in mistake, nay, an enormous basic blunder. We call it ignorance—ignorance of the pure nature of one's own self. In deep sleep, shorn of ego but not of ignorance, one experiences an indescribable bliss. It is absolute, and not relative in the slightest measure, as are all worldly pleasures and pains. One would get upset, even mad, if one were to have no sleep. The experience in deep sleep is what the philosopher considers a glimpse into the highest goal of human existence."

"This, again, means that the highest goal of philosophy is also as natural as ego. Everyone is born with an inherent ability to have this experience," the patient argued. "In other words, experience of pleasure and pain, as well as a release from it, are parts of life."

"True; the only problem is: this release is temporary as long as it is part of life. The recurrence of bond and release spells suffering in the final analysis. The philosopher's dream is that it could be made permanent," continued the doctor.

"How can one have such an unrealistic dream when all life is impermanent? From a practical point, all ends with death," the patient objected. "All talk of life-after-death in heaven or hell is a matter of belief—a carrot to drag the common man on."

"My theory is not in the least affected if heaven or hell are proved to be a figment of the imagination. My purpose is served if you accept the rebirth of a creature in the world we are aware of. I am talking of release or liberation from this *life* itself. Life, basically meaning breathing, is what imprisons the soul in the body-mind complex, gross or subtle; and its actions in one life shape its next life. This cycle of birth and death goes on unless and until the soul attains liberation," the doctor explained.

"Is not this theory of the cycle of births and deaths a matter of belief?" asked the patient.

"It is a hypothesis, not a belief. Hypotheses are offered to explain a matter of actual universal experience, and hence a part of rational thinking. Is not the scientist's explanation of the origin and expansion of the universe a hypothesis? When you accept such explanations, there is no reason why a philosopher's hypothesis be looked at with disapproval."

"It makes sense," the patient agreed, still dissatisfied. "Please go ahead."

"The cause-and-effect relation between the soul's actions and its rebirth is, on the one hand, a sequence of the universal law of cause and effect; and on the other, it is conceived to explain the born inequality of creatures on the levels or the order of life, as well as the upper and lower layers in the same order, and so on."

"How is all this related to my problem?" the patient asked impatiently.

"Take it easy. I have not lost sight of your problem; only that, instead of a temporary solution to it—I mean pills—I am trying to show you the way of a permanent one. Would you like me to recapitulate the ground we have covered?"

"Yes, please," the patient said, relieved.

The doctor summed up: "We have seen that:

(a) It is the ego, born with the body and mind, that is the cause of all suffering involving pleasure and pain.

(b) This ego, as our identity, is rooted in our ignorance of our self—the root cause all suffering.

(c) The intermediate links—between ignorance and suffering—are ego, attachment, and hatred, good and evil actions, and the chain of rebirths and re-deaths.

(d) To put an end to this chain, the root cause must be uprooted.

(e) With ignorance, the root cause, uprooted, the soul attains a state free from suffering, which is equivalent to the restoration of the soul to its own nature as experienced in deep sleep.

Have I made myself clear?"

"Absolutely," said the patient.

"That much is enough for today." The doctor gave him the next appointment.

Index of postures